中药 方剂 手册

HANDBOOK OF CHINESE HERBAL FORMULAS

楊謙志著

Him-che Yeung, L.Ac., O.M.D., Ph.D.
Los Angeles County, California, U.S.A.
June, 1995

Published by the Institute of Chinese Medicine,
602 San Gabriel Blvd., Rosemead, CA 91770, U.S.A.

Library of Congress Catalogue Card Number: TXu 151-173
International Standard Book Number: 0-9639715-1-4

First Edition: 1985, 1987, 1989, 1991
Second Edition: 1995

Printed in the United States of America

Table of Contents

Handbook of Chinese Herbal Formulas

Introduction

This book is originally the volume II of "The Handbook of Chinese Herbs and Formulas." These two books were first published in 1985. Since then, they have been reprinted numerous times to meet the need of the students that study Traditional Chinese Medicine over the United States and over the whole world. It has been assigned to be a required text book by the Acupuncture Committee of the California State Medical Board.

In this new version of the handbook, the pharmacological action of the Chinese herbs and formulas are added. The herbal formulas are arranged alphabetically according to the pin-yin system. The ingredients of each formula are arranged in groups and in the order of importance. The principal ingredient is generally the first one or two on the list. Most of these formulas are made into patent formulas, and are sold over the counter in the herb stores in China and all over the world. The generic name are given to facilitate the ordering or purchase of the products from the herbal stores, health food stores, and pharmaceutical companies.

Any person interested in both Western medicine and Traditional Chinese Medicine will find this book very helpful. The pharmacological action and indication are explained in TCM and modern medical terms. The herbal formulas have been used in China for thousands of years in the routine clinical setting. They are effective and predictable. They can be given to patients in the crude or pill form. Because of their low cost and effectiveness, they are getting more and more accepted by the general public. It is a pity that this precious method of herbal therapy is not treasured by the Chinese in the United States. I hope one of these days, we can get more Chinese students to study both the Chinese and Western medicine.

The process of compiling and revising this book has been a very long process. Explaining the TCM terms in English is difficult in the beginning. Learning to use the computer using the Dos and Windows, English and Chinese softwares are very frustrating experiences. It is like learning another foreign language. But thanks to the modern technology, I am able to make some corrections in the pin-yin and sisheng system. I have gone through two major computer break down in the last four years. However, with the technical support of many friends, technicians, and computer specialists, I am able to retrieve most of the documents back. With your advice, support, criticism and suggestions, I hope to bring you a finer copy of this textbook to all the students and health practitioners.

Writing these books have been the cross of my life. Teaching and taking care of patients have always been my joy. Painting is my second love. If I did not spend all these numerous hours on the computer, I would have painted many pictures with oil, ink or Chinese brushes. I hope that I can meet with everyone that use these books through the art show all over the world. Thanks to all your support. Without your letters and telephone calls requesting for the new edition, I would never have the endurance to finish this project. Enjoy this book, study it, and share your knowledge with your friends and patients.

Him-che Yeung, LAc., OMD, PhD.
Los Angeles County, U.S.A.
April, 1995.

ACKNOWLEDGMENT

The author would like to thank the following:

Homer Cheng, O.M.D.
Sung-you Cheng, O.M.D.
Hong-yen Hsu, Ph.D.
Martin S. Mok, M.D.
Steven Rosenblatt, L.Ac., Ph.D.
Cynthia Tantraphol, Pharm.D.
Franklin Wong, L.Ac., O.M.D.
Horatio Yeung, M.D.
Eugene Young, D.M.D.
Sophie C. Young, M.D.

for their invaluable guidance, suggestion, assistance and encouragement. And finally I would like to thank my belated parents for their love and patience.

The author would like to thank the following for their technical support:

Ardele Hui-yu Cao, George Chou, Peter Leimbigler, Kexing Li, Maxwell Li, Wil McKee, Edward Tantraphol, and Xiao-wen Zhang.

They are living in different parts of the world right now. But once in their life-time, they have helped me to accomplish a job that is meaningful to many people. Without anyone of them, I would not have learned the computer technology. My special thanks to Maxwell Li, for without the enduring support from him, this revised edition of the handbook will never be completed.

An ALPHABETICAL LIST of CHINESE HERBAL FORMULAS

A6

CLASSIFICATION OF CHINESE HERBAL FORMULAS

中藥方劑學之分類

I.   The Diaphoretics (解表劑)

II.   The Antipyretics or Febrifugal Formulas (清熱劑)

III.   The Mediating or Regulating Formulas (和解劑)

IV.   The Phlegm Expelling (Expectorant) Formulas (祛氮劑)

V.   The Antitussive and Anti-asthmatics (止咳，平喘劑)

VI.   The Warming Formulas (溫裡劑)

VII.   The Resolving or Discutient Formulas (消導劑)

VIII. The Tonifying Formulas (補益劑)

IX.   The Carminative Formulas (理氣劑)

X.   The Blood Regulating Formulas (理血劑)

XI.   The Purgative Formulas (瀉下劑)

XII.   The Diuretic Formulas (祛濕劑)

XIII. The Anticonvulsant Formulas (治風劑)

XIV.   The Moisturizing Formulas (治燥劑)

XV.   The Sedative or Tranquilizing Formulas (安神劑)

XVI.   The Resuscitating Formulas (開竅劑)

XVII. The Astringent Formulas (固澀劑)

XVIII. The Anthelmintic and Anti-parasitic Formulas (驅蟲劑)

XIV.   The Emetic Formulas (涌吐劑)

I. The Diaphoretics: (解表劑)

A. Diaphoretics with pungent and warm nature: (辛溫解表)
- Ma Huang Tang (麻黃湯)
- Gui Zhi Tang (桂枝湯)
- Xiao Qin Long Tang (小青龍湯)
- Xing Su San (杏蘇散)
- Xiang Ru San (香薷散)
- Cong Chi Tang (葱豉湯)
- Xiang Su San (香蘇散)
- Cang Er San (蒼耳散)
- Jing Fang Bai Du San (荊防敗毒散)
- Xin Yi San (辛夷散)

B. Diaphoretics with pungent and cool nature: (辛涼解表)
- Sang Ju Yin (桑菊飲)
- Yin Qiao San (銀翹散)
- Ma Xing Shi Gan Tang (麻杏石甘湯)
- Yue Bi Tang (越婢湯)
- Chai Ge Jie Ji Tang (柴葛解肌湯)
- Sheng Ma Ge Gen Tang (升麻葛根湯)
- Qiang Lan Tang (羌籃湯)

C. Diaphoretics with replenishing effect: (扶正解表)
- Ren Shen Bai Du San (人參敗毒散)
- Shen Su Yin (參蘇飲)
- Ma Huang Fu Zi Xi Xin Tang (麻黄附子細辛湯)
- Jia Jian Wei Rui Tang (加減葳蕤湯)

II. The Antipyretics or Febrifugal Formulas: (清熱劑)

A. Eliminating the heat in the Qi (inner defensive) system: (清氣分熱)
- Bai Hu Tang (白虎湯)
- Zhu Ye Shi Gao Tang (竹葉石膏湯)

B. Eliminating the heat in the Ying (Nutrient) system: (清營涼血)
- Qing Ying Tang (清營湯)
- Xi Jiao Di Huang Tang (犀角地黄湯)

C. Eliminating heat and toxin: (清熱解毒)
- Huang Lian Jie Du Tang (黃連解毒湯)
- Pu Ji Xiao Du Yin (普濟消毒飲)
- Wu Wei Xiao Du Yin (五味消毒飲)
- Si Miao Yong An Tang (四妙勇安湯)

D. Eliminating heat in the organs and visceras: (清臟腑熱)
　　　Dao Chi San （導赤散）
　　　Long Dan Xie Gan Tang （龍膽瀉肝湯）
　　　Yu Nu Jian （玉女煎）
　　　Wei Jing Tang （葦莖湯）
　　　Xie Bai San （瀉白散）
　　　Bai Tou Weng Tang （白頭翁湯）
　　　Ge Gen Huang Qin Huang Lian Tang （葛根黃芩黃連湯）
　　　Xie Xin Tang （瀉心湯）
　　　Yin Chen Hao Tang （茵陳蒿湯）

E. Eliminating the summer heat: (清熱袪暑)
　　　Liu Yi San （六一散）
　　　Qing Shu Yi Qi Tang （清暑益氣湯）

F. Eliminating the heat due to deficiency: (清虛熱)
　　　Qin Hao Bie Jia Tang （青蒿鱉甲湯）
　　　Qing Gu San （清骨散）
　　　Dan Gui Liu Huang Tang （當歸六黃湯）

III.　The Mediating or Regulating Formulas: (和解劑)

A. Regulating the Shao-yang channel: (和解少陽)
　　　Xiao Chai Hu Tang （小柴胡湯）
　　　Da Chai Hu Tang （大柴胡湯）
　　　Hao Qin Qing Dan Tang （蒿芩清膽湯）

B. Regulating the liver and spleen formulas: (調和肝脾)
　　　Si Ni San （四逆散）
　　　Xiao Yao San （消遙散）
　　　Chai Hu Shu Gan San （柴胡舒肝散）
　　　Tong Xie Yao Fang （痛瀉要方）

C. Regulating the stomach and intestines formulas: (調和腸胃)
　　　Ban Xia Xie Xin Tang （半夏瀉心湯）
　　　Huang Lian Tang （黃連湯）

D. Anti-malaria: (治瘧)
　　　Da Yuan Yin （達原飲）

IV. The Phlegm Expelling (Expectorant) Formulas: （祛氮劑）

A. Resolving phlegm and dampness: （燥濕化痰）
    Er Chen Tang （二陳湯）
    Wen Dan Tang （溫胆湯）

B. Eliminating heat and phlegm: （清化熱痰）
    Qing Qi Hua Tan Wan （清氣化痰丸）
    Xiao Luo Wan （消瘰丸）
    Xiao Xian Xiong Tang （小陷胸湯）

C. Expectorants with moistening effect: （潤燥化痰）
    Bei Mu Gua Lou San （貝母瓜蔞散）

D. Resolving phlegm caused by cold: （溫化寒痰）
    Ling Gan Wu Wei Jiang Xin Tang （苓甘五味薑辛湯）
    San Zi Yang Qing Tang （三子養親湯）
    Ling Gui Zhu Gan Tang （苓桂术甘湯）

E. Eliminating wind and phlegm: （治風化痰）
    Zhi Sou San （止嗽散）
    Ban Xia Bai Zhu Tian Ma Tang （半夏白术天麻湯）

V. The Antitussive and Anti-asthmatics: （止咳，平喘劑）

A. The Anti-tussives: （止咳）
    Zhi Sou San （止嗽散）
    Qing Zao Jiu Fei Tang （清燥救肺湯）
    Sang Xing Tang （桑杏湯）
    Bu Fei Tang （補肺湯）

B. The Anti-asthmatics: （平喘）
    Ding Chuan Tang （定喘湯）
    Su Zi Jiang Qi Tang （蘇子降氣湯）
    Ting Li Da Zao Xie Fei Tang （葶藶大棗瀉肺湯）

VI. The Warming Formulas: （溫裡劑）

A. Warming the Spleen and Stomach formulas: （溫中祛寒）
    Li Zhong Tang （理中湯）
    Wu Zhu Yu Tang （吳茱萸湯）
    Xiao Jian Zhong Tang （小建中湯）
    Da Jian Zhong Tang （大建中湯）
    Hou Po Wen Zhong Tang （厚朴溫中湯）

B. Formulas for Reinforcing the Yang (vital function) for the treatment of Prostration: (回陽救逆)
　　Si Ni Tang (四逆湯)
　　Shen Fu Tang (參附湯)
　　Zhen Wu Tang (真武湯)
　　Fu Zi Tang (附子湯)

C. Warming the Channels and Collaterals: (溫經散寒)
　　Dang Gui Si Ni Tang (當歸四逆湯)
　　Huang Qi Gui Zhi Wu Wu Tang (黃芪桂枝五物湯)
　　Yang He Tang (陽和湯)

VII. The Resolving or Discutient Formulas: (消導劑)

A. The Digestives: (消食導滯)
　　Bao He Wan (保和丸)
　　Zhi Zhu Wan (枳朮丸)
　　Mu Xiang Bing Lang Wan (木香檳榔丸)

B. Resolving Lumps: (消痞化積)
　　Shi Xiao Wan (失笑丸)

VIII. The Tonifying Formulas: (補益劑)

A. Replenishing the Qi (vital energy) (補氣)
　　Si Jun Zi Tang (四君子湯)
　　Shen Ling Bai Zhu San (參苓白朮散)
　　Bu Zhong Yi Qi Tang (補中益氣湯)
　　Sheng Mai San (生脈散)
　　Bai Zhu San (白朮散)

B. Replenishing Blood: (補血)
　　Si Wu Tang (四物湯)
　　Dang Gui Bu Xue Tang (當歸補血湯)
　　Gui Pi Tang (歸脾湯)

C. Replenishing both Qi (vital energy) and blood: (氣血雙補)
　　Ba Zhen Tang (八珍湯)
　　Zhi Gan Cao Tang (炙甘草湯)
　　Jia Jian Fu Mai Tang (加減復脈湯)
　　Tai Shan Pan Shi San (泰山盤石散)

D. Reinforcing the Yin (vital essence): （補陰）
    Liu Wei Di Huang Wan （六味地黃丸）
    Zuo Gui Yin （左歸飲）
    Zuo Gui Wan （左歸丸）
    Yi Guan Jian （一貫煎）
    Da Bu Yin Wan （大補陰丸）
    Hu Qian Wan （虎潛丸）

E. Reinforcing the Yang (vital function): （補陽）
    Jin Kui Shen Qi Wan （金匱腎氣丸）
    You Gui Yin （右歸飲）
    You Gui Wan （右歸丸）

IX. The Carminative Formulas: （理氣劑）

A. The Carminatives that regulate the flow of Qi (vital energy): （行氣劑）
    Yue Ju Wan （越鞠丸）
    Ban Xia Hou Po Tang （半夏厚朴湯）
    Gua Lou Xie Bai Bai Jiu Tang （瓜蔞薤白白酒湯）
    Tian Tai Wu Yao San （天台烏藥散）
    Liang Fu Wan （良附丸）
    Dao Qi Tang （導氣湯）
    Jin Ling Zi San （金鈴子散）
    Ju He Wan （橘核丸）

B. The Carminatives that oppress the ascending flow of Qi (vital energy): （降氣劑）
    Su Zi Jiang Qi Tang （蘇子降氣湯）
    Xuan Fu Dai Zhe Tang （旋覆代赭湯）
    Ding Xiang Shi Di Tang （丁香柿蒂湯）
    Xiao Ban Xia Tang （小半夏湯）
    Ju Pi Zhu Ru Tang （橘皮竹茹湯）
    Ding Chuan Tang （定喘湯）

X. The Blood Regulating Formulas: （理血劑）

A. Invigorating the blood ciruculation and remoing blood stasis: （活血祛瘀）
    Fu Yuan Huo Xue Tang （復元活血湯）
    Xue Fu Zhu Yu Tang （血府逐瘀湯）
    Tong Qiao Huo Xue Tang （通竅活血湯）
    Ge Xia Zhu Yu Tang （膈下逐瘀湯）
    Shao Fu Zhu Yu Tang （少腹逐瘀湯）
    Shen Tong Zhu Yu Tang （身痛逐瘀湯）
    Tao He Cheng Qi Tang （核桃承氣湯）

A. Invigorating the blood circulation and removing blood stasis:
  Bu Yang Huan Wu Tang （補陽還五湯）
  Wen Jing Tang （溫經湯）
  Sheng Hua Tang （生化湯）
  Shi Xiao San （失笑散）
  Dan Shen Yin （丹參飲）
  Gui Zhi Fu Ling Wan （桂枝茯苓丸）
  Tou Nong San （透膿散）

B. The Hemostatics: （止血劑）
  Shi Hui San （十灰散）
  Si Sheng Wan （四生丸）
  Huai Hua San （槐花散）
  Gu Jing Wan （固經丸）
  Huang Tu Tang （黃土湯）
  Jiao Ai Tang （膠艾湯）

XI. The Purgative Formulas: （瀉下劑）

A. Laxatives with cold nature: （寒下）
  Da Cheng Qi Tang （大承气湯）
  Da Huang Mu Dan Pi Tang （大黃牡丹皮湯）
  Da Xian Xiong Tang （大陷胸湯）
  Gan Sui Tong Jie Tang （甘遂通結湯）
  Liang Ge San （良膈散）
  Xiao Cheng Qi Tang （小承氣湯）

B. Laxatives with warm nature: （溫下）
  Da Huang Fu Zi Tang （大黃附子湯）

C. Emollients: （潤下）
  Ma Zi Ren Wan （麻子仁丸）
  Ji Chuan Jian （濟川煎）

D. Water-dispelling laxatives: （逐水）
  Shi Zao Tang （十棗湯）
  Ji Jiao Li Huang Wan （己椒藶黃丸）
  Zhou Che Wan （舟車丸）

E. Tonifying laxatives: （扶正攻下）
  Huang Long Tang （黃龍湯）
  Wen Pi Tang （溫脾湯）
  Zeng Ye Cheng Qi Tang （增液承氣湯）

XII. The Diuretic Formulas: (祛濕劑)

A. Eliminating dampness with fragrant aromatics: (芳香化濕)
      Ping Wei San (平胃散)
      Huo Xiang Zheng Qi San (藿香正氣散)

B. Eliminating heat and dampness: (清熱祛濕)
      Yin Chen Hao Tang (茵陳蒿湯)
      San Ren Tang (三仁湯)
      Gan Lu Xiao Du Dan (甘露消毒丹)
      Er Miao San (二妙散)
      Ba Zhen San (八正散)
      Xuan Bi Tang (宣痺湯)

C. The Diuretics: (利水滲濕)
      Wu Ling San (五苓散)
      Wu Pi Yin (五皮飲)
      Wei Ling San (胃苓散)
      Yin Chen Wu Ling San (茵陳五苓散)
      Fang Ji Huang Qi Tang (防己黃芪湯)
      Fang Ji Fu Ling Tang (防己茯苓湯)

D. Eliminating dampness by warming action: (溫化水濕)
      Ling Gui Zhu Gan Tang (苓桂术甘湯)
      Bei Xie Fen Qing Yin (卑薢分清飲)
      Ji Ming San (雞鳴散)
      Shi Pi San (實脾散)

E. Eliminating wind and dampness: (祛風勝濕)
      Qiang Huo Sheng Shi Tang (羌活勝濕湯)
      Du Huo Ji Sheng Tang (獨活寄生湯)
      Juan Bi Tang (蠲痺湯)

XIII. The Anticonvulsant Formulas: (治風劑)

A. Dispelling the endogenous wind formulas: (平熄內風)
      Ling Yang Gou Teng Tang (羚羊鉤藤湯)
      Tian Ma Gou Ten Yin (天麻鉤藤飲)
      Zhen Gan Xi Feng Tang (鎮肝熄風湯)
      Di Huang Yin Zi (地黃飲子)
      Da Ding Feng Zhu (大定風珠)
      San Jia Fu Mai Tang (三甲復脈湯)

B. Dispelling the exogenous wind formulas: (疏散外風)
    Chuan Xiong Cha Tiao San（川芎茶調散）
    Qian Zheng San（牽正散）
    Yu Zhen San（玉真散）
    Xiao Huo Luo Dan（小活絡丹）

XIV. The Moisturizing Formulas: (治燥劑)

A. Eliminating the external dryness: (清宣外燥)
    Sang Xing Tang（桑杏湯）
    Xing Su San（杏蘇散）
    Qing Zao Jiu Fei Tang（清燥救肺湯）

B. Eliminating the internal dryness: (滋潤內燥)
    Yang Yin Qing Fei Tang（養陰清肺湯）
    Bai He Gu Jin Tang（百合固金湯）
    Zeng Ye Tang（增液湯）
    Sha Shen Mai Men Dong Tang（沙參麥門冬湯）

XV. The Sedative or Tranquilizing Formulas: (安神劑)

A. Sedatives with heavy metals: (重鎮安神)
    Zhu Sha An Shen Wan（硃砂安神丸）
    Ci Zhu Wan（磁硃丸）

B. Sedatives with nourishing effect: (滋養安神)
    Suan Zao Ren Tang（酸棗仁湯）
    Tian Wang Bu Xin Dan（天王補心丹）
    Gan Mai Da Zao Tang（甘麥大棗湯）
    Huang Lian E Jiao Tang（黃連阿膠湯）

XVI. The Resuscitating Formulas: (開竅劑)

A. The resuscitating formulas of cold nature: (涼開)
    An Gong Niu Huang Wan（安宮牛黃丸）
    Zi Xue Dan（紫雪丹）
    Zhi Bao Dan（至寶丹）

B. The resuscitating formulas of warm nature: (溫開)
    Su He Xiang Wan（蘇合香丸）

XVII. The Astringent Formulas: (固澀劑)

A. The Anhidrotics: (固表止汗)
      Yu Ping Feng San (玉屏風散)
      Mu Li San (牡蠣散)
      Dang Gui Liu Huang Tang (當歸六黃湯)

B. Formulas for seminal emission: (澀精止遺)
      Sang Piao Xiao San (桑螵蛸散)
      Jin Suo Gu Jing Wan (金鎖固經丸)

C. The Anti-diarrhetics: (澀腸固脫)
      Zhen Ren Yang Zang Tang (真人養臟湯)
      Si Shen Wan (四神丸)
      Tao Hua Tang (桃花湯)

D. Formulas for leukorrhea: (固崩止帶法)
      Gu Chong Tang (固冲湯)
      Wan Dai Tang (完帶湯)

XVIII. The Anthelmintic and Anti-parasitic Formulas: (驅蟲劑)

      Wu Mei Wan (烏梅丸)
      She Chuang Zi Chong Xi Ji (蛇床子沖洗劑)
      Bu Dai Wan (布袋丸)

XIV. The Emetic Formulas: (涌吐劑)

      Gua Di San (瓜蒂散)

INTRODUCTION

Therapeutic Methods in the Chinese Herbal Formulas

There are eight methods of therapy in Traditional Chinese Medicine. These eight methods are related to the eight principal syndrome in diagnosis: *Yin* and *Yang*, exterior and interior, cold and heat, deficient and excessive syndromes. These eight therapeutic methods are as follows:

1. **Perspiration:** Inducing the body to perspire can eliminate the pathogenic factors to the surface and exterior of the body. It can improve the circulation of *Qi* (vital energy) and blood, and regulate the essential nutrients and defensive energy inside and outside of the blood vessels. It can relieve the swelling in edema and promote the eruption of measles. This method is divided into 2 kinds relating to the nature of the diseases: by herbs of pungent and cold, or pungent and warm nature. If a person is too weak and low in the immune system, the tonic herbs are also used in combination.

2. **Emetic method:** This method is used to remove the stagnation of phlegm, undigested food or toxic substances from the throat, chest and abdomen. It is also used to remove the stagnant *Qi* and blood in the chest. This method is a little painful, so it is usually used in the acute situations.

3. **Purgation:** This method is using purgatives to eliminate the undigested food, dry stools, constant heat, cold masses, blood stasis, phlegm and water retention. Because the nature of the diseases have heat/cold, or deficient/excessive, so it is divided into strong purgatives, warm purgatives, emollients, and water dispelling laxatives.

4. **Mediation:** This is a regulatory method to relieve symptoms in the Shaoyang channel and regulate *Qi* and blood of the related internal organs, such as the liver and the spleen, the liver and the stomach, the stomach and the intestines.

5. **Warming method:** This method is used to treat the interior cold syndromes in the abdomen, channels. It can be also used in resuscitation. Because interior cold is always related to weak constitution, so this method is usually combined with tonification.

6. **Cleansing method:** It is used to treat heat syndromes with herbs of cool or cold nature. Because the invasion of pathogenic heat, toxin, virus, bacteria usually produce fever in the body, so this method has anti-viral or anti-bacterial in nature. In the chronic stage, the person has low graded fever due to the depletion of *Yin* fluid. So the *Yin* tonics are generally added in the later stages of ailment.

7. **Elimination:** Elimination is used in the stagnation of *Qi*, blood, phlegm, food and water.

8. **Tonification:** This method is used to replenish *Qi* and blood, and regulate the balance of *Yin* and *Yang*. It is divided into *Yin* tonics, *Yang* tonics, *Qi* tonics and blood tonics. They are used singly or in conjunction with each other.

Classification of Herbal Formulas

In the Chinese classics "Nei Jing" (The Yellow Emperor's Canon of Internal Medicine), the formulas are divided into 7 kinds: heavy dosage, small dosage, drastic or acute dosage, mild or chronic dosage, and combination formulas.

Later on in the classic "Yao Tui", the formulas are divided into ten kinds: dispersing, penetrating, tonifying, purging, light, heavy, slippery, astringent, drying and wetting. In Song dynasty, cold and heat formulas are added. In Ming dynasty, ascending and descending formulas are added. Total are 14 kinds.

In Qing dynasty, the classic "Yi Fong Ji Jie" (Collections of Prescriptions with Exposition), Dr. Wang Ang divided the formulas into 22 kinds:

1. Tonifying
2. Dispersing
3. Emetic
4. Warming the interior
5. Superficial and Interior
6. Mediating or Regulating
7. Regulating the Qi
8. Regulating the Blood
9. Wind dispelling (Anti-convulsant)
10. Cold dispelling
11. Antipyretic or febrifugal
12. Diuretic
13. Purging the fire
14. Phlegm expelling
15. Resolving or Discutient
16. Astringent
17. Moisturizing
18. Anti-parasitic
19. Formulas for the eyes
20. Formulas for abscesses
21. Formulas for Obstetrics
22. Emergency formulas

In general, the classification of herbal formulas are generally divided according to different kind of diseases, symptoms, causes, interior organs, or method of therapies. In this textbook, 18 methods are listed. It is easy for the students to study and manipulate the formulas.

Composition of the Herbal Formulas

A. Principles of the therapies:

In writing an herbal prescription, one must not just keep on adding the number of herbs, or increasing the effects of the herbs. One must decide the method of therapy, and then select the herbs that are suitable for that specific condition.

In general, each formula consists of 4 groups of herbs:

1. Principal/Monarch herb: 君藥

Relieves the principal symptoms of the disease ailment.

2. Minister herb: 臣藥

Assists the principal herbs to increase the effect of therapy.

3. Assistant/Adjuvant herb: 左藥

Relieves the minor or secondary symptoms. If the principal herb is too toxic, the assistant herb is used to control the toxicity. Sometimes, the body is repelling the action of the herbs, then the adjuvant herb is added to treat from a different angle. For example, few cooling herbs are added in a formula that is warm in nature.

2

4. Conductant/Guiding herb: 使藥

Conducts the action of the herbs to the therapeutic channel; or tempers the action of other herbs.

Usually in an herbal formula, the dosage of the principal herbs are more than the others. The dosage of the minister herbs cannot exceed that of the principal's. The number of the principal herbs are few in number. There are usually more numbers of the minister or assistant herbs in a formula. The formulation is very flexible. There is no fixed amount or number of each group.

B. Variations in the herbal formulas:

1. **Variation in the dosage according to the symptoms:** Usually the minister or adjuvant herbs are varied in the dosage or number according to the difference in the minor or secondary symptoms. Also when the composition of the herbs in the formula are changed, the action of that formula are changed accordingly.

2. **Variation in the dosage of the herbs:** When the ingredients in the herbal formula are the same, but one of the ingredients is increased in the dosage, then the therapeutic effect is enhanced, and the action is also changed.

3. **Variation in the form of herbal formulas:** Usually if the formula comes in decoction form, the action is faster and more drastic. So decoction are usually in acute situations. Pills are slower and milder in action, but they are convenient to take and easy for storage.

Forms of the Herbal Formulas

1. **Decoction:** Water is added to the package of herbs in a clay or ceramic pot. Soak first before boiling. This method of preparation is used for general ailments and acute diseases. It can be used for internal intake or external wash. The effective ingredients in the herbs are easily absorbed by the body. It is easy for the doctor to modify the prescription by changes according to the individual patient or for specific conditions.

2. **Powder:** The herbs are crushed into powder. They can be taken internally or externally. For internal intake, the powder is finer and less in amount. For external uses, the powder is mixed and sprinkled over the abscess area. The powder herbs are simple to make, easy to carry and are easily absorbed into the body.

3. **Pills or bolus:** The herbs are crushed into powder, mix with water, honey, rice/flour paste, wine, vinegar or extracts from the decoction. Pills are absorbed slowly by the body, but the therapeutic action is more persistent. The pills are smaller in size, easy to swallow, carry, and storage. It is generally made for the patients that are weak and chronically ill.

The pills mixed with honey is softer and tastier. The therapeutic action is milder and is also tonifying. They are usually used for chronic patients.

The **water pills** are pills that are mixed with cold water, wine, vinegar or decoction. The water pills are easily dissolved and absorbed by the body. The size of the pills are small, and can be easily swallowed.

The **paste pills** are made by mixing the fine herb powder with rice or flour paste. They are more sticky and harder to dissolve. It take a long time to be absorbed in the body, so they are more long reacting therapeutically. The herbs that are more toxic or stimulatory are usually made into paste pills. Because of the complication in making these kind of pills, they are less applied in the industry.

The **concentrated pills** are made by mixing some fine herb powder with the concentrated extract of the decoction, then they are crushed and mixed with water or alcohol into fine pills. These pills are highly concentrated, small in size and dosage. They are easily absorbed and are used for treating different kinds of diseases.

4. **Extracts:** Extracts are made by decocting the herbs with water or vegetable oil and then concentrated. They can be taken internally or externally.

The **liquid extract** is made by extracting the effective ingredients with suitable solvent. Then part of the solvent is eliminated using steaming method. The thickness or the percentage of ethyl alcohol need to be adjusted to the desired concentration. In the liquid extract, 1 c.c. of the effective ingredient is equal 1 gm. of the crude herb. Both tincture and liquid extract contains alcohol, but the effective ingredient in the liquid extract is higher than tincture. The dosage is small and the side-effect from the alcohol or other solvent is also reduced.

The **semi-solid/dry extract** is made by extracting the soluble effective ingredients from the herbs into semi-solid or dry form using suitable kinds of solvent. After the extraction is done, the solvent is evaporated. The concentration is adjusted to the regulation. Usually 1 gm. of the dry extract is equal to 2-5 gm. of the crude herb. These extracts are highly concentrated, and they do not contain solvent, so there is no side-effect of the alcohol. The size and dosage are small. The semi-solid extract can be made into pills or tablets. The dry extract can be directly swallowed or placed in capsules.

The **soft extract** can also be called syrup. The herbs are boiled in water and then decanted. Honey or rock sugar are added and then concentrated by slow cooking. Because all the fibers and undesirable ingredients are removed, the volume is reduced. They are very tasty and nourishing. Because they are easily absorbed by the body, they are given to the weak or chronic patients.

The **medicated ointment** are made by mixing the herbs with suitable material, then applied over the skin or mucous membranes. The ointment is semi-solid in room temperature, and has a certain mucosity. It is slowly melted, and the effective ingredient absorbed by the body. Ointment is applied locally, suitable for abscesses or carbuncles.

The **adhesive plaster** are herbs mixed with lead or saponin based material, spread on paper or cloth, then applied on the skin. At room temperature, the plaster is in solid form. At 36-37 degree centigrade, it is softened and the effective ingredients are released to the skin or body. It is easy to use, carry, and storage. It is generally used for arthritis, bruises and trauma cases.

5. **Dan:** Dan are pills mixed with mercury, sulfur or other minerals and heated. It can be used internally or externally. In the clinical setting, usually the special or expensive herbal formulas are also called Dan. Some of the Dan are in powder, pill, liquid or tincture form.

6. **Tincture:** Tincture are herb extracts using rice or white wine as solvent to release the effective ingredient. It can be used internally or externally. It is usually for weak or chronic patients, or one with arthritis or soft tissue injuries.

7. **Medicinal Tea:** This kind of tea is made by mixing the crude herb powder with adhesive substances into solid form. It is shaped in small rectangular form and wrapped with paper. It is placed into a cup or a container with lid in time of use. Hot boiling water is poured into the cup and mixed before drinking. It is usually for flu or indigestion. Because the tea form is simple to use and therapeutic, so it is very popular.

8. **Distilled medicinal water:** The herbs that are fresh and have volatile substances are extracted by distillation with heat. The vapor is collected for medicinal use. It is fresh and aromatic, and is usually consumed in the hot summer time.

9. **Troche and medicated cake:** It is rectangular or cone-shaped preparation made with herbs in fine powder form and mixed with appropriate excipient. It can be taken internally or externally.

10. **Slender roll of medicated paper:** It is slender roll of paper made from mulberry bark. Herb powder can be applied over the slender roll and then inserted into the body for surgery use.

11. **Medicated thread:** Silk or cotton thread is soaked in herb liquid, boiled and then dried. It is usually used for patients with fistula.

12. **Moxa preparation:** The mugwort leaves are crushed into moxa wool. They are made into cone or stick form. It is heated to produce heat to warm up the body and some acupuncture points. It is used for therapy or prevention.

13. **Syrup:** Syrup are made of saturated sugar solution that may or may not contain herbs. The herbs are decocted and concentrated. Sucrose or cane sugar is added to make it into syrup. Average syrup contain 60-65% (gm./gm.) or 82-85% (gm./ml) of sucrose. Because the concentration of sugar and osmotic pressure are very high, the syrup do not need much preservatives. Because the syrup is sweet, they are suitable for children to take.

14. **Tablet:** Tablet is a processed or extracted form of herbs by pressing into small round tablet. It can be sugar coated or enteric coated. It is produced by machine. Its cost is low and efficiency is high, therefore it is a very popular form of herbal preparation.

15. **Infusion or medicinal granules:** Infusion is a mixture of concentrated liquid herbal extract and cornstarch, paste or sugar powder. The granules are being sieved, dried at 40-60 degree centigrade. Infusion can absorb moisture easily, therefore it is usually wrapped in plastic bags. It is fast reacting, light-weighed, and easy to carry.

16. **Injection:** Sterile solution for injection is extracted from herbs. It can be given subcutaneously, intramuscular or intravenous. The dosage is accurate, fast-acting and easily penetrated into the body tissues.

Method of Making a Decoction

The utensils used in making a decoction are silver, porcelain, clay, glass. Other pots made of metals such as iron, zinc, copper are not recommended, because they may have chemical reaction with the herbs and reduce the therapeutic results.

The water used are clear tap water, distilled water or water from the well. Usually 1 cup or bowl (200-300 c.c.) of water is added to 30 gm. of herbs.

Strong or high fire is used for decoction such as diaphoretics and carminatives for which only a short period of boiling is necessary. Slow or small fire is used for making tonic decoction which need a longer period of boiling. Generally, high fire is used first, then slow flame later.

Before decoction, place the herbs into the container. Add cold water and soak the herbs for a short while. After boiling, turn the flame lower. Opening the lid all the time will cause the loss of the effective ingredients. It is better to use high fire for the diaphoretics and antipyretics, so that the loss of the volatile substances. For the tonic herbs, it is better to use small flame and decoct longer to extract all the effective ingredients.

1. **Decocting first:** Certain shells and minerals are crushed first before decoction. Boil for 10 minutes first, then add the other ingredients such as tortoise shell and hematite.

2. **Decocting last:** The aromatic herbs with volatile and diffusible ingredients need to be added to the decoction last. It only need 4-5 minutes of boiling. Examples are the peppermint and saussurea.

3. **Decocting with the herbs wrapped:** Downy or powdered herbs or herbs containing much mucilage are usually wrapped with a piece of gauze or cheesecloth first before decoction. This can reduce the irritation to the throat and the digestive tract. Examples are red halloysite and inula flower.

4. **Decocting separately:** Some of the expensive herbs such as ginseng can be decocted separately in a double boiler for 2-3 hours. Others such as antelope horn and rhinoceros horn are cut into thin slices, and boil for 2 hours separately, or grounded into fine powder. This method of separate decoction can preserve the effective ingredient from mixing or being absorbed by other ingredients.

5. **Melting separately:** Maltose and donkey-hide gelatin are very sticky and can be melted easily. If they are boiled with other ingredients, they will stick to the pot and other herbs. It is better to decant the other herbs after boiling, then mix with the gelatin to dissolve it or cook for a short period of time.

6. **Steeping:** Some of the herbs contain volatile oils even if the dosage is small. These herbs are placed in the cup first and pouring water or herb concentrates are poured in. The cup is covered immediately, and the herb steeped for a few minutes. Examples are cinnamon and safflower.

7. **Taking medicine after pouring liquid on it:** Some of the Dan, pills, powder, fresh juice, and other herbs need to be prepared by pouring hot water or hot decoction over it with stirring. Examples are the powder of pseudoginseng, fresh lotus juice, and Liu Shen Wan.

8. **Taking medicinal powder after mixing it with liquid** such as a portion of hot decoction, water or wine.

Method of Taking the Herbal Medication

1. **Timing:** Generally, most herbs can be taken before the meal. The ones for the eyes or that may cause irritation in the GI-tract are taken after the meal. The greasy tonic herbs are taken empty-stomach. Anti-malaria herbs are taken 2 hours before the eruption. Sedatives are taken before sleep at night time. No specific time for acute conditions. For chronic conditions, the pills, powder, decoction, soft extract and tincture are taken at regular intervals of time. Most of the herbs are taken 3 times per day, Some of the herbs are taken like tea, no specification in time.

2. **Method:** Generally each pack of herbs are decocted once, and divide into 2-3 cups (first portion). The second day, it can be decocted again (second portion). Each time the patient can drink one cup. Generally, one pack can be used for 1 or 2 days. In acute situations, the herb tea is taken all at once, and 2 packages are needed on one day.

Decoction is generally taken warm. Sometimes it is better to take some porridge to enhance the effect of perspiration. For febrile disease, it is better to take the herb tea cold. For cold disease, it is taken hot. For situation that is true cold and false heat, the herb tea is taken cold. For true heat and false cold condition, it is taken hot. If the person vomits after the intake of herb tea, it is better to drink a little bit of ginger juice, or chew a small piece of citrus peel first.

In taking the strong, drastic, or toxic herbs, it is better to take a small dosage first, and slowly increase the dosage until the therapeutic result is reached. Overdosage may be life threatening.

Conversion of Units in Measurement of Weight

1 Jin = 16 Liang = 0.5 Kg. = 500 gm.

1 Liang = 31.25 gm.

1 Qian = 3.125 gm.

1 Fen = 0.3125 gm.

1 Li = 0.03125 gm.

Generally, we adopt the simple method of conversion in the handbook:

1 Liang = 30 gm.

1 Qian = 3 gm.

1斤 = 16兩 = 0.5公斤 = 500克

1市兩 = 31.25克

1市錢 = 3.125克

1市分 = 0.3125克

1市釐 = 0.03125克

簡單的來算:

1兩 = 30克

1錢 = 3克

PHARMACEUTICAL ACTIONS OF THE HERBS

1. The Diaphoretics

The diaphoretic formulas are used for relieving the infections in the upper respiratory tract and acute infectious diseases. There is damage to the center that control the body temperature by the endogenous pyrogens. There are changes in the contraction and dilation of the blood vessels in the brain and mucous membrane of the skin and respiratory tract. Other symptoms are such as fever, headache, aversion to cold, and with floating pulse.

Most of the diaphoretics are febrifugal, anti-viral, and anti-bacterial. Some herbs can induce perspiration and adjust the body temperature. Some herbs can adjust the blood flow to the brain and mucosa of the respiratory tract. Ephedra can assist and enhance the process of perspiration. Cinnamon can dilate the peripheral capillaries, increase the blood circulation in the skin. Fresh ginger is warm and pungent, thus it can induce perspiration and alleviate cold.

In exterior cold syndrome, there is reflex contraction in the blood vessels of the mucosa of the upper respiratory tract. The local resistance is reduced, thus the pathogens have the opportunity to invade the body and cause local inflammation. The herbs can relieve the contraction in the blood vessels of the mucosa caused by the cold, increase the immunity and blood circulation in the body.

In exterior heat syndrome, there is high fever at its peak temperature, contraction of the blood vessels, tight muscles, and increase in the pathogens. The fever is higher than the degree of aversion to cold. Most of the herbs of this group are anti-bacterial in nature.

A. Diaphoretics with pungent and warm nature:

麻 黄 Ma Huang (Ephedra) contains ephedrine, which is similar to epinephrine, but is milder and longer acting. It can induce heat sensation and perspiration. It has stimulatory action on the heart and the central nervous system. It can constrict the peripheral blood vessels and increase the heart beat and blood pressure. It can relax the bronchial smooth muscles and relieve asthma. δ-pseudo-ephedrine is a diuretic, and can increase the output of urine.

細 辛 Xin Xin (Asarum) can reduce the temperature of the body. It is antipyretic, analgesic and anti-inflammatory. It is diuretic, antitussive, and anti-histamine. dl-Demethyloclaurine is suspected to be the effective ingredient in eliminating the cold factor. Only small dosage of asarum is enough, high dosage can cause toxicity.

B. Diaphoretics with pungent and cool nature:

柴 胡 Chai Hu (Bupleurum) contains saikosaponin which is the effective ingredient that is antipyretic, antitussive, analgesic, anti-inflammatory, anti-viral, and anti-bacterial. Bupleurum can inhibit the increase in permeability caused by histamine. It can lower the blood cholesterol by increasing the secretion of bile and stool output. It can protect the liver cells from denaturalization and necrosis.

葛 根 Ge Gen (Pueraria) is antipyretic and anti-spasmodic, especially effective for patients with fever and stiff-neck. It can increase the blood flow to the coronary artery by relaxing the smooth muscles. It can lower the blood pressure, reduce heart beat and the resistance from the peripheral blood vessels.

菊 花 Ju Hua (Chrysanthemum flower) is anti-bacterial, anti-viral and anti-fungal. It is antipyretic, and has inhibitory action on the central nervous system. It is anti-hypertensive, anti-histamine. It is generally for the patients with fever, headache and blood-shot eyes.

薄　荷　Bo He (Mentha/peppermint) is antipyretic by dilating the capillaries of the skin and thus lowers the body temperature. Menthol can cause the reflex of cold sensation in the peripheral endings of the skin and mucosa. Menthone and menthol are anti-spasmodic, anti-inflammatory, and can increase the secretion of bile and bile salt.

蟬　蛻　Chan Tui (Ciccada slough) is antipyretic, anti-spasmodic and tranquillizing.

2. The Purgatives

Any herbal formulas that has purgative or emollient action are called purgatives. It is divided into 3 groups:

A. The Purgatives:

1. **Carthatics:** stimulate the bowel, induce increasing peristalsis and a subsequent bowel movement. Some herbs contains anthracene glycosides and other polyhydroxyanthroquinones from bacterial action in the large bowel. These substances are irritating and give delayed catharsis. They may also stimulate the nerve plexus in the bowel wall. Examples are: rhubarb, aloe, senna.

2. Anti-viral, antibacterial, and anti-fungal

大　黄　Da Huang (Rhubarb) has stimulatory action on the transverse and descending colon. It inhibits the reabsorption of water. The retention of water can cause the evaluation of the colon. The effective ingredient that cause carthatic action is sennoside, anthraquinone glycoside. In the process of prolonged boiling or processing, the effective ingredients may be hydrolyzed or oxidized. Therefore it is better to use the raw rhubarb for purging effect. Rhubarb also contain tannin which may cause secondary constipation after discontinued therapy. Rhubarb also contains rhein, emodin, aloe-emodin. These are ionized anthraquinone derivatives. They can inhibit the growth of staphycoccus, hemolytic streptococcus, bacillus, shigella, etc.

番瀉葉　Fan Xie Ye (Senna) contains sennoside A and B. It is absorbed in the stomach and small intestine, and decomposed in the liver. It can cause contraction in the large intestine and diarrhea. The action is so strong that it may cause abdominal cramps. It is more suitable for acute constipation.

芒　硝　Mang Xiao (Mirabilitum) contains sodium sulfate (96-98%) and magnesium sulfate. It is considered to be saline cathartics. The salts are not absorbable, and water is retained in the water through osmotic effect. The retained water distends the intestine, and thus stimulate peristalsis. This results in a brisk liquid bowel movement within a few hours. Because mirabilitum contains sodium, it is not advisable for patients with edema.

B. Emollient/Lubricants:

The emollients are simple oil and emulsion which soften and lubricate the bowel content. They are more suitable for weak and chronic patients, pre- and post-partum females, and elderly constipation.

火麻仁　Huo Ma Ren (Cannabis seed) contain fatty oil (oleic, linoleic, linolenic acid) and protein. The fatty oil lubricates the intestines. And on contact with the alkaline intestinal fluid, the fatty oil produce fatty acid which can stimulate the mucosa and increase peristalsis. It can also lower the blood pressure.

C. Drastic purgatives:

1. **Carthatics:** usually contain irritant oils or fatty acids which act on the small intestines and cause excessive purgation. For example, castor oil, croton oil. They

can increase the peristalsis action of the intestines, and the reabsorption of the small intestine.

2. Diuretics: There is an increase in the glomerular filtration or decrease in tubular reabsorption. The increased output of urine can alleviate the edema condition in glomerular nephritis or congestive heart failure.

車前子 Qian Niu Zi (Pharbitis seed) contains pharbitin which is decomposed in the intestines on contact with bile and intestinal fluid. It stimulates the intestinal mucosa, increases the secretion, and thus causes peristalsis. It also diuretic effect. So it is usually used for patients with edema and constipation.

甘 遂 Gan Sui (Kansui root) can stimulate the peristalsis the intestines, but has no diuretic action. The raw root is more purgative and toxic than the one processed with vinegar.

巴 豆 Ba Dou (Croton) contains croton oil. The croton oil contains "croton resin" which is reputed to be the most potent carthatic. It can increase the peristalsis action of the intestines, and the reabsorption of the small intestine. Its action is very drastic in 3 hours, with diarrhea, tenesmus, and abdominal cramp. Its action can last for 10-15 hours.

3. The Antipyretics or Febrifugals

The herbal formulas in this category are usually cold or cool in nature. They are used to alleviate the heat symptoms such as red face, blood shot eyes, bleeding, constipation, amber urine, delirium, mania, abscess, inflammation, tongue red with yellow coating, pulse rapid.

The pharmaceutical action of this group of formulas are as follows:

1. Anti-viral, anti-fugal and anti-bacterial: Herbs such as coptis, phellodendron, scutellaria, lonicera, isatis can inhibit the growth of gram positive cocci and gram negatives bacilli. Coptis, pulsatilla, brucea can inhibit the growth of amoeba. Pulsatilla can also inhibit trichomonas.

2. Increase the immunity of the body: Herbs such as oldenlandia, houttuynia, green chiretta can stimulate the reticulo-endothelial system, increase the phagocytosis of the white blood cells and the macrophages. Some herbs can increase the specific or non-specific immunity function of the body. Some herbs can also control the growth of the cancer cells.

3. Antipyretic: Herbs such as anemarrhena, wolfberry bark, moutan bark, gallstone can lower the body temperature.

4. Anti-hypertensive: Herbs such as gentiana, prunella, cassia seed can lower the blood pressure.

5. Sedative: Herbs such as gypsum, gardenia, lotus plumule, scutellaria, moutan bark has sedative action.

The antipyretics are divided into 5 major groups:

A. Herbs that can eliminate heat and fire:

These group of herbal formulas can inhibit the central nervous system, sympathetic nervous system, decrease the basal metabolic rate and heat production. They are diuretic and can low the blood pressure, and decrease the blood volume. They are used for high fever, inflammation, hypertension, delirium. The "fire" in Chinese medicine is related to lung, liver, heart and stomach fire. It is usually related to high fever and the excitory activity of the central nervous system.

石　膏 Shi Gao (Gypsum) contains calcium sulfate. It can lower the body temperature and reduce thirsty sensation. It can increase the phagocytosis of the macrophages. It can lower the blood sugar in the diabetic person. Bile can increase the absorption of calcium. The permeability of calcium in the intestines is higher than the other kind of calcium salt.

知　母 Zhu Mu (Anemarrhena) is antipyretic and antibacterial. It can reduce the side effects of the hydrocortisone if it is taken together, and can prevent the atrophy of the adrenal gland.

夏枯草 Xia Ku Cao (Prunella) is anti-bacterial and anti-hypertensive and is a diuretic. It can inhibit the growth of pseudomonas, E. coli, and mycobacteria.

B. Herbs that can eliminate heat by cooling the blood:

This group of herbs and formulas are antipyretic, cardiotonic, and cholagogue. They can inhibit the sympathetic nervous system, decrease the basal metabolic rate and heat production, and lower the blood pressure.

牛　黃 Niu Huang (Gallstone) contains bile acid and bilirubin. It can produce sedative, antipyretic and anti-inflammatory effect, but no analgesic or hypnotic effect. It is a cardiotonic by constricting the blood vessels and dilating the capillaries. The effective ingredient that lowers the blood pressure is the bilirubin. It can relax the sphincter and increase the secretion of bile.

牡丹皮 Mu Dan Pi (Moutan bark) contains paeonol which is anti-inflammatory. Its anti-inflammatory action is related to the inhibitory action against the agglutination of platelets, the plasminogen, and the activity of plasmin. It is also a sedative, an analgesic, antipyretic and anti-spasmodic.

C. Herbs that can eliminate heat and toxin:

This group of herbs and formulas have strong antibiotic effect. Some of them can inhibit the growth of virus, fungus, bacteria and even cancer cells. Some can also increase the immunity function of the body. They can destroy the endotoxin produced by the pyrogens. They can enhance the function of the adrenal cortex.

白花蛇舌草 Bai Hua She She Cao (Oldenlandia) is anti-bacterial and anti-inflammatory. It can increase the function of the reticulo-endothelial system, the production of white blood cells and antibodies, and enhance phagocytosis.

白頭翁 Bai Tou Weng (Pulsatilla) is an anti-bacterial, anti-amoebic. It inhibits the growth of staphylococci, pseudomonas, Bacillus subtilis and B. dysenteriae. It can inhibit the growth of amoebic trophozoite and trichomonas. It is also a cardiotonic. A constituent similar to digitalis can be extracted from the whole herb with the roots removed.

穿心蓮 Chuan Xin Lian (Green chiretta/kariyat) is more effective in the control of infectious diseases such as dysentery, intestinal and upper respiratory infections. Its anti-viral and anti-bacterial function is done by enhancing the phagocytic ability of the white blood cells. It is also an antipyretic and anti-inflammatory.

Other herbs such as houttuynia (Yu Xing Cao 魚腥草), lithospermum root (Ma Chi Xian 馬齒莧), and sophora root (Guang Dou Gen 廣豆根) all have similar actions.

D. Herbs that eliminate heat and dampness:

Heat and moisture are the required factors for the growth of yeast, bacteria, fungus, amoebiae, and trichomonas. So the herbs and formulas that belongs to this group can inhibit the growth of bacteria, and are used for dysentery, enteritis, leukorrhea, and vaginitis (caused by trichomonas). They are diuretic, cholalogue, and anti-inflammatory.

黄 連 Huang Lian (Coptis), 黄 芩 Huang Qin (Scutellaria)and 黄 柏 Huang Bai (Phellodendron) all have antipyretic and anti-bacterial actions. They are referred to as the "three Huangs". Generally speaking, scute is used for the upper part, scutellaria for the middle part, and phellodendron for the lower part of the body.

The effective ingredient in coptis and phellodendron is berberine. The anti-bacterial action of berberine is related to the inhibition in the oxidation of pyruvic acid, synthesis of DNA, RNA and protein. It increases the immunity and phagocytosis of the white blood cells. It lowers the blood pressure by dilating the peripheral blood vessels and increasing the production of acetylcholine. It is also a cholagogue.

Coptis is a sedative by prolonging the action of barbiturates, and interfering the transmission of impulses to the cortex.

Scutellaria is sedative, anti-spasmodic and anti-allergenic. Its anti-hypertensive action is related to the diuretic property. It is a cholagogue by increasing the secretion of bile, and decreasing the SGPT concentration in hepatitis patients.

Phellodendron contains berberine and phellodendrine. It can increase the contraction of the muscles of the uterus, bronchi, stomach, intestine and urinary bladder.

苦 参 Ku Shen (Sophora root) contains matrine and cystsine. It can inhibit the growth of bacteria, mycobacteria and trichomonas. It can prevent the loss of white blood cells during chemotherapy. It can reduce the heart rate, and the contraction of the heart muscles. It increases the output of salt and volume of urine. It is also antitussive and anti-asthmatic.

秦 皮 Qin Pi (Fraxinus bark) can inhibit the growth of staphylococci and Bacillus dysenteriae. It is analgesic and anti-inflammatory. It can increase the volume of urine and uric acid output from the normal people and arthritic patients.

E. Herbs that eliminate summer heat or low graded fever:

The symptoms of low graded fever are: chronic fever especially in the afternoon, annoying heat sensation in the heart, hands and feet, and even night perspiration.

青 蒿 Qing Hao (Artemisia/sweet wormwood) contains artemisinin. It can inhibit the maturation of malaria parasite. It is also anti-fungal and anti-bacterial. It is a pyretic, analgesic, antitussive, expectorant, and anti-asthmatic.

地骨皮 Di Gu Pi (Wolfberry bark) is very cold in nature, so it can lower the body temperature. It can inhibit the growth of typhoid, paratyphoid bacillus, and Flenxer's bacillus (shigella). It can also lower blood sugar and cholesterol. It lowers the blood pressure by dilation of the blood vessels and blockage of the peripheral sympathetic nerve.

4. The Antitussive

Cough may be nonproductive or productive of sputum. Suppression of the cough or periodic drainage of the sputum is necessary. Expectorants are agents which facilitate coughing in productive cough by thinning the sputum.

Inhalation of steam facilitates the movement of sputum by moistening and lubricating. Inhalation of carbon dioxide stimulates bronchial peristalsis and liquefies sputum. Some of the Chinese herbs and formulas have expectorant property. Some can increase the secretion in the respiratory tract. Some can dilate the bronchial smooth muscles, and relieve the tracheal spasms caused by pilocarpine, acetylcholine and histamine.

"Phlegm" in Chinese medicine includes sputum, goiter, scrofula and cholesterol deposit. If it is found in the lung, it will produce cough, asthma, emphysema, tracheitis, and bronchiectasis. If the phlegm is stagnant in the channels/meridians, it will produce goiter, scrofula, chronic lymphadenitis, convulsions, CVA and epilepsy.

The antitussives are divided into 4 major groups:

A. Eliminating cold phlegm with herbs of warm nature:

This group of herbs and formulas can increase the blood flow to the lung, bronchi and bronchioles. They can increase the cellular energy metabolic rate, reduce the edema in the respiratory tract.

天南星 Tian Nan Xing (Arisaema tuber) is an expectorant by increasing the secretion of mucous in the respiratory tract. It contains saponin, which can stimulate the gastric mucus membrane and augment gastric reflex. It has sedative, analgesic and tranquilizing effect. It is also an anti-convulsive. It is usually prepared with ginger to be used as an expectorant. It is prepared with bile to reduce its dryness and is used for epilepsy and convulsion.

B. Eliminating heat phlegm with cleansing herbs:

This group of herbs and formulas are antibacterial, antipyretic. They can lower the blood pressure, and decrease the blood flow to the lung, bronchi and bronchioles. They can increase the immunity of the body, and the energy metabolic rate of the tissues.

川貝母 Chuan Bei Mu (Tendrilled fritillary bulb) is an expectorant and antitussive by nourishing and moistening the lung. It can lower blood pressure with higher dosage. It is usually for tuberculosis, chronic cough with dryness or depletion of *Yin* fluid.

浙貝母 Zhe Bei Mu (Thunberg fritillary bulb) can dilate the smooth muscle of the bronchi and decrease the bronchial secretion. It is usually used in acute conditions of flu with cough, asthma, abscess, and scrofula.

C. Antitussive and anti-asthmatic:

This group of herbs and formulas can inhibit the excitatory state of the respiratory center, and the cough reflex. They can dilate the bronchi and the respiratory tract.

款冬花 Kuan Dong Hua (Tussilago flower) is an antitussive, expectorant and anti-asthmatic. Small dosage of it can dilate the bronchi, but large dosage can cause constriction. It is generally mixed with honey to relieve cough. Its action is not as strong as aminophylline when counteracting the tracheal spasm caused by histamine.

百 部 Bai Bu (Stemona) alkaloid can reduce the excitatory action on the respiratory center, inhibit the cough reflex. It can relax the tracheal spasm caused by histamine. It is antibacterial and anti-fungal, and anthelmintic. It is effective for lice, pinworm, head louse, trichomonas, schistosoma, etc.

紫 苑 Zi Wan (Aster root) can suppress cough and increase the tracheal secretions. It can inhibit the growth of gram negative bacilli and cancer cells. It is used for acute and chronic cough with asthma, and even whopping cough.

D. Herbs that relieve cough by moistening effect:

Drought is divided into external and internal dryness. External drought is caused by the dry weather and affection of flu. Internal drought is due to depletion of *Yin* fluid in the lung with symptoms of dry throat and dry cough, with no mucous, thin or bloody sputum.

If the kidney *Yin* fluid is depleted, there is heat sensation in the hand and feet, steaming sensation in the bone, and night perspiration. This group of herbs and formulas have moistening effect and can regulate the electrolyte balance.

百 合 Bai He (Lily bulb) is antitussive and anti-asthmatic. It can relieve cough and tracheal spasm caused by histamine. It can moisten the lung due to depletion of *Yin* fluid. It is a sedative and can alleviate insomnia and fidgetiness.

北沙参 Bei Sha Shen (Glehnia root) is an expectorant. It stimulates the bronchial mucosa to produce more secretions. It is good for dry throat, dry cough with no or thin sputum, constipation caused by dehydration of stomach fluids.

5. The Digestive

The digestive formulas can increase the digestion of fat, protein and carbohydrates. Some of them contain lipase and protease. Some can enhance the appetite by increasing the secretion of gastric acid, digestion, and evacuation. Some herbs contain vitamin B and C.

山 楂 Shan Zha (Hawthorn fruit) is also called crataegus fruit. It contains crataegolic acid, citric acid, lipase. It is used raw to remove blood stasis and lower blood pressure; stir-baked to remove stagnated food, and carbonized to treat dysentery. It dilates the blood vessels, and increase the blood flow to the coronary artery. It lowers blood pressure slowly but persistently. It lowers blood cholesterol, and increases the lecithin/cholesterol ratio, decreases the deposit of cholesterol in internal organs. It is a digestive because of its lipase and other enzymes in the stomach. It helps the contraction of uterus, thus leading to the passage of blood clots. This action can relieve menstrual pain and the recovery of the uterus after childbirth.

麥 芽 Mai Ya (Malt) is germinated barley. It contains diastases, peptidase, protease, lipase and choline. It is used raw as a carminative; stir-baked as digestive and lactifuge; and stir-baked to brown to remove food stagnation.

穀 芽 Gu Ya (Germinated rice) contains protease, peptidase and vitamin B. It can improve digestion and appetite, and remove food stagnation. It is generally used together with germinated barley to enhance the therapeutic action.

6. The Warming Herbal Formulas

This group of herbs and formulas are used for interior cold syndromes. One condition is caused by pathogenic cold acting on the spleen and stomach, leading to vomiting and diarrhea. The second kind of condition is the interior depletion of *Yang* energy, leading to lowered body temperature, cold extremities, and very weak pulse.

In general, the pharmacology of the warming herbs and formulas are as follows:

1. **Action on the digestive tract:** They are usually stomachic with pungent and spicy essential oils. They can increase the microcirculation and the excretion of gastric acid and protease. Thus they can evacuate gas and relax the intestinal muscles.

2. **Action on the cardiovascular system:** The depletion of *Yang* (vital energy) condition is the same as shock. Some cardiotonic herbal formulas can increase the blood pressure. They can also increase the tolerance of oxygen depletion in ischemic condition. Some can increase the renal blood flow, and some can increase the dilation of the peripheral skin blood vessels, and cause the body to feel warmer.

3. **Action on the Nervous system**: They have excitatory action on the central nervous system, and the sympathetic nervous system. They can increase the basal metabolic rate and calorie production.

附子/烏頭　　Fu Zi and Wu Tou (Aconite) contains aconitine which is a cardiotonic and can stimulate the central vagus nerve. The toxicity may be reduced by boiling in water or processing. It is analgesic, anesthetic, anti-hypertensive and anti-inflammatory. It can extend the sleeping time of cyclo-barbiturates. It can reduce the lowering of body temperature, and prolong the life of living creatures in fatal cold condition.

肉　桂　Rou Gui (Cinnamon bark) is a stomachic. Cinnamon oil is a mild stimulant on the stomach and the intestines. It can increase the secretion of saliva and gastric juice, improve digestion, relieve GI-spasms and evacuate gas. It lowers blood pressure by dilating the blood vessels centrally and peripherally. It can also cause the congestion of blood in the uterus, leading to menstruation.

丁　香　Ding Xiang (Cloves) is a carminative and stomachic by relieving flatulence and increasing the digestive functions. It is an analgesic, anti-emetic, and anti-inflammatory. It can inhibit the growth of bacteria, parasites and tapeworm.

吳茱萸　Wu Zhu Yu (Evodia) is an antibacterial and anti-parasitic. It is an analgesic, stomachic, and anti-emetic. It can cause the peristalsis of the intestines, evacuation of gas and prevent any extraordinary fermentation process.

花　椒　Hua Jiao (Zanthoxylum) is pungent and warm in nature. It can warm up the abdomen, increase appetite, induce perspiration and urine output, and increase peristalsis of the intestines. It is a sedative, analgesic (can increase the effect of morphine in the body). It is an anticonvulsant, and is effective for epilepsy.

7. The Tonics

The chronic patients are usually very weak and depleted. Usually it is caused by depletion or asthenia of *Qi* (vial energy), blood, *Yin* (vital essence) and *Yang* (vital function). Depletion of these four essence in different organs will reflect different symptoms. It is possible to have depletion of one or more factors.

The pharmacology of the tonic herbal formulas are as follows:

A. **Action on the immunity of the body:**

1. On non-specific cellular immunity:

a. Increase the production of T-lymphocytes, prevent the loss of white blood cells caused by cyclophosphamide which is an anti-tumor agent.

b. Increase the phagocytic ability of white blood cells, the reticulo-endothelial system and the production of interferon.

2. On specific humoral immunity:

a. Increase rate of formation of the E-rosette, and increase the B-lymphocytes.

b. Increase the concentration of the immunoglobulins IgG and IgM.

B. **Increase the adaptability of the body:** The tonics can control the activity of the adrenalin, the sudden decrease of blood pressure, and excessive gastric bleeding.

C. **Action of the endocrine and the nervous system:** The tonics can enhance the action of the adrenal cortex, and prevent the degeneration of the thyroid, pituitary, adrenal cortex, testis and uterus.

D. **Action on metabolism:** The tonics can regulate the metabolism of glucose, protein, cholesterol, white blood cells and red blood cells.

E. **Increase the productivity of the body at work:** The tonics can reduce stress and fatigue, improve memory and mentality.

The tonic herbal formulas are divided into 4 major groups:

A. The Qi Tonics:

This group of herbs and formulas can:

1. Act on the CNS and sympathetic nervous system. It can increase the cAMP, and energy metabolic rate. It can also stimulate cellular bioelectricity.

1. Increase the specific and non-specific immunity of the body by increasing the phagocytosis of the cells.

2. Increase the adaptability and increase the resistance to the invasion of foreign bodies

3. Increase the physical ability and the thinking capability of the brain

4. Regulate the function of the endocrine, and increase the function of the sex hormones and the adrenal cortical hormones.

人 参 Ren Shen (Ginseng) can increase the function of the adrenal cortex, immunity and resistance to diseases by stimulating the production of immunoglobulins. It stimulates the pituitary gland to produce more sex hormones. It increases the ability of analysis and reduce fatigue. It has similar action as the adaptogen. It shortens the period of healing in injury. It increases the body metabolism, and reduces the blood sugar and cholesterol.

党 参 Dang Shen (Codonopsis) increases the production of white blood cells, and phagocytosis of reticulo-endothelial system and increase the ability to fight against diseases. It increase the production of hemoglobin and red blood cells in anemia or bleeding conditions. It lowers blood pressure by dilating the peripheral blood vessels. It can decrease protein in urine in chronic nephritis.

黄 芪 Huang Qi (Astragalus) is a cardiotonic by increasing the contraction of the heart. It increases phagocytosis and the production of antibodies. It lowers blood pressure by dilating the blood vessels. It is a diuretic by increasing the secretion of sodium ions.

甘 草 Gan Cao (Licorice) contains glycyrrhizin. It has similar action as the mineral corticoid and glucocorticoid. It is anti-histamine and anti-inflammatory. It can relieve the spasms of the intestines caused by histamine or acetylcholine. It lowers the gastric acidity. It can reduce or neutralize the toxicity of other herbs in the formula. Licorice may cause edema and hypertension if it is taken for a long period of time. The mechanism is due to adrenocortical action resulting in the retention of water in the body and sodium ions, but the excretion of potassium ions.

白 术 Bai Zhu (White atractylodes) can increase body weight and muscle strength. It increases the secretion of stomach and intestinal juice. It lowers blood sugar, and also prevent the loss of glycogen in liver. It has the action as an anti-coagulant, increasing the prothrombin time and clotting time.

灵 芝 Ling Zhi (Ganoderma) is a dried fructification of the fungus Ganoderma lucidum. It contains ergosterol, fungal lysozyme and albumin. It inhibits the action of the central nervous system. It is a sedative and analgesic. It increases the circulation of blood to the coronary artery and the cardiac muscles. It increases the WBC and immunity of the body. It is anti-tussive, expectorant and anti-hypertensive.

16

B. The Blood Tonics:

This group of herbs anf formulas can increase the production of peripheral white blood cells and red blood cells. There is regeneration of the blood cells, and the maturation of the reticulocyte. It is believed in Chinese medicine that the production of *Qi* can influence the production of blood.

當 歸 Dang Gui (Chinese angelica root) contains folic acid, vitamin B_{12}, and vitamin A. It is good for anemia and pernicious anemia. It is a sedative, analgesic, and anti-inflammatory. It increases the flow of blood to the coronary artery and prevent myocardial ischemia. It has action similar to quinidine and has therapeutic effect on auricular fibrillation. It can relax the spasmodic muscles of the uterus. The whole root is used to regulate menstruation and blood disorders. The head of the root is hemostatic, body is nourishing, and tail is used to invigorate the circulation of blood. It is processed with wine to invigorate blood circulation, with honey as an emollient, and carbonized as a hemostatic.

地 黄 Di Huang (Rehmannia root) can increase the contraction of cardiac muscles and increase blood pressure. It also has diuretic action. It can lower the blood sugar that is caused by adrenaline or ammonium chloride. It is antibacterial, antifungal, and anti-inflammatory. It is hemostatic, and can promote the coagulation of blood and shorten the bleeding time. The fresh root is used for the treatment of thirst, and bleeding due to existence of heat. The dried root is used for bleeding due to blood deficiency and to nourish the vital essence.

白 芍 Bai Shao Yao (White peony) is anti-spasmodic and has inhibitory action on the smooth muscle of the stomach and uterus. It is sedative, analgesic, anti-ulcer, anti-convulsive, anti-inflammatory. It can lower the body temperature and dilate the blood vessels. It inhibits the agglutination of platelets. It can inhibit the growth of gram positive and negative bacteria.

何首烏 He Shou Wu (Polygonum/fleeceflower root) contains lecithin which is the essential ingredient in the formation of nerve tissues, blood cells and other cell membranes. It can lower blood cholesterol, and prevent the deposit of cholesterol in liver and the formation of atherosclerosis. It is a laxative because of the anthraquinone (rhein and emodin). It has action similar to adrenal-corticoid hormone.

C. The *Yang* (vital function) Tonics:

This group of herbs and formulas have similar actions as the *Qi* tonics. They can increase the action on the hormones and the endocrines: the pituitary gland, adrenalin, norepinephrine, glucocorticoid, erythropoietin, vasopressin and renin. They have strong action on metabolism and increase of the metabolic rate.

鹿 茸 Lu Rong (Pilose antler) is the hairy, young horn of male deer or stag. It contains oestrone, oestradiol, gelatin, protein and amino acids. It increases the regeneration of hemoglobin, red blood cells, and reticulocytes. It can increase the consumption of oxygen in the brain tissues. It reduces fatigue, and increases appetite and capability to work. It increases the healing of fractured bones and ulceration. There is no experimental proof that it has male or female sex hormonal action.

淫羊藿 Yin Yang Huo (Epimedium) can increase the secretion of semens and copulation. Its action is similar to male sex hormone. It is antitussive, expectorant, anti-asthmatic, anti-bacterial, and anti-hypertensive.

冬蟲夏草 Dong Chong Xia Cao (Cordyceps) is a fungus growing on the larvae of caterpillar. It increases the phagocytosis of the macrophages, and the action of the adrenal gland. It is hypnotic and tranquilizing. It is anti-bacterial and anti-cancer cells.

補骨脂 Bu Gu Zhi (Psoralea) can dilate the coronary artery and increase the heart rate. It has similar action as meladinine in causing the skin to produce new color pigment locally. It can shorten the bleeding time and volume, and is used for uterine bleeding.

D. The *Yin* (vital essence) Tonics:

It is believed in Chinese medicine that blood anemia will generally lead to depletion of fluid and electrolyte. This group of herbs and formulas can enhance the function of the parasympathetic nervous system, increase cGMP, increase the cellular and hormular immunity. They are diuretic, can lower the blood pressure. They can decrease the energy metabolic rate. They can increase the production of peripheral blood cells, and prevent the loss of white blood cells caused by cyclophosphamide.

枸杞子 Gou Qi Zi (Lycium/wolfberry fruit) can enhance the nonspecific immunity, phagocytosis of the macrophages, and the production of T-lymphocytes. It can inhibit the deposit of fat in liver cells and promote regeneration. It can lower blood cholesterol and prevent the formation of atherosclerosis. It can lower the concentration of blood sugar in diabetes.

麥門冬 Mai Men Dong (Ophiopogon root) can increase the tolerance in oxygen deficit. It can lower the blood sugar and regenerate the beta cells of the islets of Langerhans of the pancreas.

石 斛 Shi Hu (Dendrobium) is analgesic, antipyretic, and anti-inflammatory. It increases the peristalsis of the stomach and intestines, and the secretion of gastric juice.

玉 竹 Yu Zhu (Polygonatum rhizome) is a cardiotonic. Small dosage of it can increase the heart beat rapidly, but large dosage will slow down the process. It can increase the blood sugar first after oral intake and then decrease slowly.

8. The Carminatives

The stagnation of *Qi* flow means the abnormal function of the smooth muscles of the blood vessels, the intestines and the skeletal muscles. Any stagnation of flow in the body/organs/channels will lead to local pain, distention or oppression. The pharmacology of the carminatives are as follows:

A. **Regulatory action on the digestive tract:** both excitatory and inhibitory on the smooth muscles of the intestines.

1. Inhibitory action on the alimentary tract: Herbs such as citrus peel, green tangerine peel can reduce the tension of the intestinal tubules. They are used for regurgitation, hiccough, diarrhea, abdominal pain and other hyperactive symptoms.

2. Excitatory action on the alimentary tract: Herbs such as immature bitter orange, saussurea, lindera can enhance the contraction of the GI-tubules. They are used for indigestion, abdominal distention, constipation, and other hypo-active symptoms.

3. Increase the secretion of gastric juice: The carminatives all have certain kinds of essential oils which can stimulate the local sites, increase the peristalsis of the intestines and the bowel movements, evacuate gas and relieve the distention caused by overeating.

B. **Relaxation of the smooth muscles:** relax the smooth muscles of the bronchi and blood vessels, and the tension of the respiratory skeletal muscles.

C. **Cholagogue:** increase the secretion of bile. They can regulate the smooth muscles of the liver, bile duct, breast, uterus and the digestive tract. They can increase the hepatic blood flow to the liver.

陳 皮 Chen Pi (Citrus peel) can increase the secretion of gastric juice and improve digestion. It is an expectorant and anti-asthmatic. It stimulates the mucosa of the respiratory tract and increase secretion and dilution of phlegm. It is anti-ulcer and anti-inflammatory. Its action is stronger if used in comminution with vitamin C and K. It maintains the regular osmotic pressure of the blood vessels, decreases the fragility of the vessels and the bleeding time.

青 皮 Qing Pi (Green tangerine peel) is an expectorant and anti-asthmatic. It can relax the bronchial spasms caused by histamine. It is a stomachic, and can speed up the evacuation of gas. It can increase the blood pressure.

枳 殼 Zhi Ke (Bitter orange) has milder action than immature bitter orange (Zhi Shi 枳 實), and is better used for removing stagnation of Qi and food in the spleen and stomach. Both of them can cause the muscles of the uterus and alimentary tract to contract with force and rhythm. Both can increase the contraction of heart muscles and the output volume of blood. Both can inhibit the release of histamine transmitter substances.

香 附 Xiang Fu (Cyperus) inhibits the contraction of the uterus and relieves spasms. It is an analgesic and can increase the pain threshold. It has anti-acetylcholine action with decrease of tension on the intestines. It is anti-bacterial and anti-inflammatory. Is has weak estrogenic action. It is generally prepared with vinegar to relieve pain; with wine to penetrate all the meridians; with salt to moisten the dryness; with ginger juice to resolve phlegm; and with charcoal to stop bleeding.

9. Herbs for Blood Regulation
by invigorating blood circulation and removing blood stasis

Blood stasis is generally caused by bleeding, stagnation of Qi flow, asthenia of Qi, pathogenic heat or cold factors, or external trauma. Any blockage in circulation (especially microcirculation) causing inflammation, abnormal growth, fibroid, metabolic or autoimmune disorders can be relieved by eliminating blood stasis.

The pharmacology of this groups of herbs and formulas are as follows:

A. In circulation:

1. Regulate the metabolism of the cardiac muscles, reduce the oxygen consumption, reduce heart beat, prevent ischemia condition.

2. Dilate the coronary artery, increase the blood flow in the artery and cardiac muscle. Some can even lower blood pressure by dilating the blood flow to the peripheral blood vessels in the brain and kidney.

3. Inhibit the agglutination of the platelets, increase the activity of plasmin (fibrinolysin), reduce fibrin stabilizing factors, prevent the formation of thrombus, and enhance thrombolysis.

4. Lower blood cholesterol, prevent the formation of atherosclerosis.

B. In inflammation:

1. Anti-viral and anti-bacterial

2. Improve local circulation and permeability of the capillaries.

3. Increase phagocytosis

C. For metastasis:

1. Inhibit the growth of the cancer cells by increasing the monocytes and phagocytes.

2. Inhibit the formation of collagen and regulate the metabolism of the connective tissues.

D. For soft tissue injury:

Increase the phagocytosis of the monocytes and macrophages, increase the regeneration of blood cells and the repair of the soft tissues.

E. Effects on the immune system:

Regulate the function of the humoral and cellular immune systems. Inhibit the abnormal growth of the tumor cells and tissues. Effective for conditions such as nephritis, scleroderma, newborn hemolytic anemia, nodular periarteritis, and systemic lupus erythematosus.

The herbs of this group are divided into 2 groups:

A. The Blood Regulating Herbs:

赤芍藥 Chi Shao Yao (Red peony) can dilate the coronary artery, and increase the blood flow. It is anti-spasmodic by inhibiting the action on the smooth muscles of the stomach and uterus. It has synergistic action together with the extract from licorice in alleviating spasms. It is sedative, analgesic, and anti-convulsive. It is anti-bacterial, antipyretic and anti-inflammatory. It inhibits the secretion of gastric juice and can prevent the formation of ulcer.

丹 參 Dan Shen (Salvia root) can improve the micro-circulation by increasing the peripheral circulation, increase anoxia tolerance under normal and low pressure, and increase capillary vascular net. It dilates the coronary artery, increase blood flow, improve myocardial contraction and adjust the heart rate. It promotes the repair and regeneration of tissues, and inhibits the growth of cancer cells. It inhibits the coagulation of blood and activates the fibrinolysis.

川 芎 Chuan Xiong (Ligusticum root) can increase the blood flow to the brain, coronary artery, and the extremities. It can decrease the consumption of oxygen in the cardiac muscles, and the resistance of the peripheral blood vessels. It reduces the agglutination and the peripheral activities of the platelets. It has very good effect in lowering the blood pressure if used in combination with reserpine. It can prevent nutritional cerebral disease caused by vitamin E deficiency.

紅 花 Hong Hua (Safflower) can produce rhythmic contraction on the uterus, and has excitatory action on the smooth muscles of the bronchi, intestines and blood vessels. It inhibits the aggregation of platelets, increase the activity of plasmin (plasmolysin), and inhibits the formation of thrombus. It lowers the content of blood cholesterol, total lipid and triglyceride.

桃 仁 Tao Ren (Persica seed) contains amygdalin which is antitussive and anti-asthmatic. Its emollient action is due to the content of 45% of fatty oil. It is anti-allergenic, can be used for urticaria and dermatitis. It can inhibit the formation of allergenic antibodies and hemolytic plague forming cells.

延胡索 Yan Hu Suo (Corydalis tuber) is a good analgesic, but not as strong as the effect of morphine. It is a sedative, hypnotic and anti-spasmodic. It suppresses the secretion of gastric juice, decreases gastric acidity and ulceration.

薑 黃 Jiang Huang (Tumeric rhizome) contains curcumin (tumeric yellow) which increases the secretion of bile and resolve sandy gallstone. It inhibits the agglutination of platelet and increases fibrinolysis. It is an analgesic and anti-inflammatory, It is used for angina, atherosclerosis and rheumatoid arthritis.

B. The Hemostatic:

The hemostatic herbs and formulas can:

1. Shorten the process of coagulation by increasing the number of platelets and thrombin. They can shorten the bleeding time.

2. They can constrict the local blood vessels

3. They can improve the function of the membranes of the blood vessels. They can increase the resistance of the capillaries, and decrease vascular permeability.

4. They can inhibit fibrinolysin.

仙鶴草 Xian He Cao (Agrimony) is used for all kinds of bleeding. It can increase the platelet count and shorten the bleeding time. It can increase blood pressure because of the cardiotonic action and constriction of peripheral blood vessels. It is anti-fungal and anti-bacterial. It can inhibit the growth of malaria, tapeworm and trichomonas.

三 七 San Qi (Pseudoginseng/Notoginseng) is a hemostatic by shortening the coagulation time and prothrombin time. It is anti-inflammatory for arthritis condition. It increases the blood flow to the coronary artery, but decreases the oxygen consumption in the cardiac muscle. It can lower blood sugar, and increase the accumulation of glycogen. It is a diuretic and can increase the output of urine by 5 folds.

10. Diuretic Herbal Formulass that can resolve Dampness

The diuretics are agents which increase the rate of urine flow. There are increased glomerular filtration or decreased tubular reabsorption. The most effective diuretics influence the excretion of sodium ion rather than the water itself.

This group of herbs and formulas have the following properties:

1. **Diuretics:** Most of the herbs contain increased potassium ion, and can increase the excretion of sodium ion or the output of urine. Examples are: poria, polyporus, alisma, plantago seed.

2. **Antibacterial:** This group of herbs can also inhibit the growth of bacilli in the urinary tract infections. Examples are: akebia, lysimachia, pyrossia leaf, alisma, polygonum, dianthus, talc, lygodium spores.

3. **For hepatitis:** Hepatitis in Chinese medicine is considered to be related to "dampness". The icteric color of the skin reveals 2 kinds of conditions: bright yellow is related to heat and dampness, dull yellow is related to cold and dampness. They are all cholagogue, protecting the damage of liver and gallbladder. Examples are: oriental wormwood (capillaris), lysimachia, lobelia, corn stigma, alisma.

4. **The aromatic:** Accumulation of dampness in the spleen and stomach is related to hypofunction of the digestive tract with symptoms of indigestion, loss of appetite, abdominal distention, thick and greasy tongue. The aromatic all contain essential oils which can stimulate the movement of the bowels, evacuation of the food content and elimination of the cellular edema in the GI-tract. Examples are agastache, and magnolia bark.

The diuretic formulas are divided into 3 major groups:

A. The diuretics:

They can increase the output of sodium ion and urine output, and are used to relieve edema or oliguria.

茯　苓 Fu Ling (Poria) is the sclerotium of the fungus. It contains pachyman polysaccharide. Its diuretic effect is not quite understood, but its effect is slow and prolonged. It can increase the excretion of sodium, potassium and chloride ions. It is a sedative. It can also reduce the concentration of blood sugar.

豬　苓 Zhu Ling (Polyporus) can increase the output of sodium, potassium and chloride ions, and the volume of urine. Its diuretic action is stronger than caffeine, akebia or poria. The mechanism is due to the inhibition of reabsorption of water and electrolytes in the renal tubules. It inhibits the growth of gram positive and negative bacteria, and tumor cells.

澤　瀉 Ze Xie (Alisma) can increase the output of urine, excretion of urea, potassium and chloride ions. It can lower blood sugar and cholesterol, and has similar action to choline and lecithin.

防　己 Fang Ji (Stephania) contains tetrandrine, and trilobine. Small dosage can stimulate the kidney and increase the urine output, but large dosage can inhibit the action. It is an analgesic, antipyretic, anti-bacterial, anti-histamine, anti-inflammatory, and anti-hypertensive. It is also a muscle relaxant.

半邊蓮 Ban Bian Lian (Lobelia) is a diuretic and anti-hypertensive. It has excitatory action on the vagus nerve, but inhibitory action on the vasomotor center, cardiac muscles. It can shorten the bleeding time and increase the production of bile.

B. The herbs for eliminating heat and dampness:

木　通 Mu Tong (Akebia) is a diuretic and cardiotonic. Its action is similar to digitalis. It can increase the contraction of the heart muscles. Its cardiotonic action may be related to the content of calcium ion and tannin.

萹　蓄 Bian Xu (Polygonum) contains avicularin and potassium, which can increase the output of urine, sodium and potassium ions. It can also lower blood pressure.

金錢草 Jin Qian Cao (Lysimachia) is a diuretic, possibly because of its potassium content. It is a cholagogue and lithagogue. It can increase the production of bile by the liver cells, and the break down of stones in the gallbladder.

茵陳蒿 Yin Chen Hao (Capillaris) contains capillarisin which is a very strong cholagogue. It increases the secretion of bile, bile salt and bilirubin. It can lower blood cholesterol and lipoprotein. It can lower blood pressure by its diuretic action and by dilation of the blood vessels in the internal visceras.

車前子 Che Qian Zi (Plantago seed) can increase the output of water, urea, sodium chloride, uric acid. It is an antitussive and expectorant. It can increase the secretion in the trachea and bronchi.

滑　石 Hua Shi (Talcum) is hydrous magnesium silicate. It forms a protective layer on the skin by adsorbing toxin or chemical substances. Internally it can protect the inflamed GI-tract. It is an anti-diarrhetic, antiemetic, and anti-inflammatory.

C. The aromatic herbs that can relieve dampness:

藿　香 Huo Xiang (Agastache or pogostemon herb) contain the essential oil patchouli alcohol. It can stimulate the gastric mucous membrane and increase the secretion of gastric juice to improve digestive function, and inhibit the excessive peristalsis of the GI-tract. It is antibacterial, anti-fungal, and inhibit the growth of spirochetes. It can be used together with ginger as antiemetic.

厚　朴 Hou Po (Magnolia bark) contain essential oils to reduce flatulence in the alimentary tract. It is antibacterial, anti-fungal, and anti-amoebic. It can relax the skeletal muscles. It is considered to be a non-depolarizer type of muscle-relaxant. It can also lower the blood pressure.

11. The Anti-rheumatic

In Chinese medicine, the "bi" syndrome includes rheumatic arthritis, rheumatoid arthritis, sciatica and all kinds of muscular pain. They are all caused by wind, cold and dampness factors. This group of herbs can alleviate pain, increase *Qi* and blood circulation and strengthen the tendons.

The pharmacology of this group of herbal formulas are as follows:

1. **Anti-inflammatory:** They have similar action as sodium salicylate. Some has excitatory action on the hypophysis-adrenal gland system.

2. **Analgesic:** They can increase the pain threshold in the body. They have sedative action and can loosen the skeletal muscles.

3. **Diuretic:** They can dilate the blood vessels and lower the blood pressure.

秦　艽 Qin Jiao (Gentiana) contains gentianine which has similar action as sodium salicylate. It is a sedative and analgesic. It is antipyretic, anti-bacterial, anti-histamine, anti-hypertensive. It can release adrenalin, thereby increase blood sugar and decrease glycogen.

威靈仙 Wei Ling Xian (Clematis) can increase the peristalsis of the digestive tract. For a person with a piece of fish bone stuck in the throat, the decoction of clematis can relax the muscles. It is a diuretic and an analgesic, and can relieve arthritic pain with spasm.

臭梧桐 Chou Wu Tong (Glorybower leaf) is analgesic and anti-inflammatory. It is good for arthritis with numbness in the extremities. It can lower blood pressure by dilating the blood vessels, and correct the other symptoms such as headache, insomnia, and dizziness.

桑寄生 Sang Ji Sheng (Mulberry mistletoe) is a sedative, diuretic and anti-hypertensive. The mechanism is by the inhibition of the excitatory activities of the sympathetic nervous system and the vasomotor centers. It can lower blood cholesterol. It has similar action as vitamin P to maintain the resistance ability of the capillaries.

12. The Sedatives

Sedatives are agents used to calm or induce sleeping status. Sleep is a state of rest and repair. It is a conditioned reflex. Tranquilizer implies mental calmness without depression of mental activity or alertness.

This group of herbs and formulas are divided into 2 kinds:

A. The heavy sedatives:

They are the heavy minerals or shells such as oyster shell, cinnabar, magnetite, and amber/succinum. They are found to have inhibitory action on the CNS. They can prolong the sleeping time caused by barbiturates, reduce activity, and reduce shock.

硃　砂 Zhu Sha (Cinnabar) is a mineral used internally as a sedative, tranquilizer, anti-spasmodic and anti-convulsive. Externally it is an antibacterial and anti-parasitic, and is used for boils and furuncle.

牡 蠣 Mu Li (Oyster shell) is rich in calcium carbonate, phosphate, sulfate, and magnesium. It is a sedative, astringent and tranquilizer. It is calcined to be used as an astringent and anti-acid agent for seminal emission, leukorrhagia, and gastric hyperacidity.

琥 珀 Hu Po (Amber/succinum) is a diuretic, sedative, tranquilizer, and anti-convulsant. It contains succinic acid which is related to the metabolism of r-aminobutyric acid in the central nervous system.

B. The herbal nourishing sedatives:

They contain protein, vitamins, and glucosides. They are nourishing to the heart and replenish more *Yin* fluid. They can improve the integrity, mental spirit, and thinking process of the brain. They can lower the blood pressure. They can be hypnotic and anti-convulsive.

酸棗仁 Suan Zao Ren (Zizyphus; wild jujube) is a sedative and tranquilizer. It has synergistic action with the barbiturates. It can lower the body temperature, blood pressure and reduce pain. It is generally made into sleeping pills and is taken before retiring to bed.

遠 志 Yuan Zhi (Polygala root) is an expectorant by stimulating the gastric mucosa and inducing mild degree of nausea and thus increasing the bronchial secretion by reflex action. It is a sedative, tranquilizer and anti-convulsant.

茯 神 Fu Shen (Poria) is the central part of the sclerotium of the fungus adhering to the pine tree. It is a sedative, but not hypnotic. It can induce the animals into the sleeping status, but not the sleeping phenomenon.

13. The Anti-convulsant

Epilepsy occurs as major convulsive seizures (grand mal), or momentary pauses of consciousness (petit mal). In Chinese medicine, it is related to the imbalance of liver *Yang*, endogenous wind and phlegm, with symptoms of spasms, dizziness, and convulsions.

The pharmacology of this group of herbs and formulas are:

1. **Anti-hypertensive**

2. **Anti-convulsant and anti-epileptic**

3. **Sedative and hypnotic**

天 麻 Tian Ma (Gastrodia) contains gastrodin. It is an analgesic, sedative and anti-convulsant. It can prolong the sleeping period caused by barbiturates. It can increase the secretion of bile. It can lower the blood pressure and slow down the heart beat. It can increase the tolerance of oxygen depletion, and protect the heart from anoxic condition. It can also dilate the blood flow to the cerebral and peripheral blood vessels, and reduce the pressure in the brain.

鉤 藤 Gou Teng (Uncaria/Gambir stem with hooks) is sedative, but not hypnotic. It lower the excitation of the cerebral cortex, destroy some positive conditioned reflex, and prolong the time of the conditioned reflex. It is anti-hypertensive and anti-epileptic. It has significant effect on renal hypertension. It can counteract the action of histamine, and relax the spasm of the smooth muscles.

珍珠母 Zhen Zhu Mu (Mother of pearl) contains 80-90% of calcium carbonate. It is used for cataract, blood-shot eyes and night-blindness. It can protect the liver damage in the hepatitis patients. It can inhibit the contraction of intestines caused by histamine. It can also neutralize the gastric ulcer caused by hyperacidity.

14. The Astringents

The astringents contains tannin, organic acids or inorganic salts. They usually have sour and astringent taste. Tannin can combine with the protein in the tissues after contact with the mucosa, and form a protective layer from the foreign toxin. The protein can coagulate with blood and block the injured capillaries, thus tannin can help to stop bleeding.

This group of herbs and formulas can regulate the smooth muscles of the urinary-genital tract, digestive tract, respiratory tract and blood vessels. They can inhibit the secretion of mucous and sweat glands. They can inhibit the exuation and effusion in wounds and inflammations. They are used for cough, diarrhea, bleeding, leukorrhea, spermatorrhea, excessive urination, night or spontaneous perspiration.

五味子 Wu Wei Zi (Schisandra) can regulate the excitatory and inhibitory action of the central nervous system. It increases one's working capacity and reduces fatigue. It has excitatory action on the respiratory center and the smooth muscle of the uterus. It is also a cardiotonic by increasing the blood circulation and contraction of the heart muscles. Its acid constituent is a very strong expectorant.

烏 梅 Wu Mei (Mume) can increase the secretion of bile. It inhibits the growth of tinea and ascariasis. It is anti-bacterial, anti-fungal, and anti-parasitic. Externally it is used for callus, corn and psoriasis.

赤石脂 Chi Shi Zhi (Kaolin) has adhesive action on the toxin and bacteria. It can reduce the stimulation to the intestinal membrane and stop diarrhea.

15. The Anthelmintic

The anthelmintic are agents against tapeworm, roundworm, flukeworm, and many other parasites.

A. Agents against roundworm (ascaris):

使君子 Shi Jun Zi (Quisqualis fruit) is effective against pork ascaris (Ascaris suis), earthworm, pinworm and hookworm. The potassium salt of quisqualic acid is the effective ingredient against ascaris and tapeworm. It can paralyze the head of pork ascaris, but cannot kill it. This herb can also improve digestion, and is good for malnutrition and indigestion of children. It can be taken together with aloe vera juice. To achieve the best effect, take sodium sulfate or magnesium sulfate 3 hours after the intake of the quisqualis fruit.

苦楝皮 Ku Lian Pi (Melia bark) has excitatory action on the head and middle segment of pork ascaris. It results in increase of spontaneous movement, and severe contraction intermittently. This destructive rhythmic movement can last for about 10-24 hours. This direct excitatory action on the muscles of the worm causes contractible fatigue and spasms. Finally the worm loses adherence to the intestinal membrane and is passed out of the body.

B. Agents against tapeworm:

南瓜子 Nan Gua Zi (Pumpkin seed): 30% extract of the pumpkin seed can paralyze the middle and end part of the tapeworm. It causes the segments to become thinner and broader.

檳 榔 Bing Lang (Areca seed): 30% of the areca seed can paralyze the head part of the tapeworm. Since these 2 herbs can complement each other, they are usually used in conjunction. Clinically it is better to take 80-120 gm. of pumpkin seed powder or extract in the early morning before breakfast. 1/2 to 2 hours later, take 60-100 gm. of areca seed. Then take 30 gm. (or 60 c.c. of the 50% extract) of magnesium sulfate half hour later. Usually the worm will be excreted 3 hours later. Most of the patients will pass out the worm in the afternoon or the next day.

16. Herbs and Formulas for Cancer

The pharmacology of this group of herbs and formulas have the following actions:

A. Eliminate toxin and abscess:

This group of herbs can directly or indirectly kill or inhibit the growth of the cancer cells. Some are anti-viral or anti-bacterial, and can eliminate toxin and abscesses. Some can increase the immunity of the person by increasing the number and functions of the white blood cells, lymphocytes and macrophages. Some can increase the function of the adrenal cortex and ACH (adreno-cortical hormone), and enhance the therapeutical effect of the chemical or radiological radiation.

白花蛇舌草　Bai Hua She She Cao (Oldenlandia) can inhibit the mitosis process of the tumor cells, and can cause degeneration and necrosis of the tumor tissues. There are changes in the density of the argentaffin in liver, spleen and lymph nodes. This argentaffin can enwrap the cancer nests, making the infiltration and metastasis more difficult.

半枝蓮　Ban Zhi Lian (Barbat skullcap) is a detoxicant. It is also used for hepatitis, snake and insect-bite. It is generally used in combination with oldenlandia for tumors.

鴉膽子　Ya Dan Zi (Brucea fruit) can inhibit the growth of spermaocytes. It can cause the karyorrhexis of the nucleus and the nuclear membrane, karyopyknosis, vacuolation of the nucleus, and mild nuclear hyperchromatism. Its chloroform extract can inhibit the growth of fibrocyte.

B. Increase blood circulation and resolve blood stasis:

Patients with fixed or chronic pain are caused by stagnation of blood (either with heat or cold nature). The tongue is usually dark red with purplish spots. Herbs of this group can invigorate the circulation of *Qi* and blood, increase blood permeability, soften the connective tissues, reduce pain and inflammation. Some herbs can increase the proteolytic action of the fibrin, and decrease the stability of the fibrin surrounding the tumor cells. The herbs can destroy the agglutination of the fibrin, increase the volume of blood and improves the micro-circulation.

大薊　Da Ji (Cirsium) can increase the hemolytic plaque in the spleen, and the formation of E-rosette. It can increase both the cellular and humoral immunity of the body. It can shorten the bleeding time and clotting time similar to the action of prothrombin.

莪术　E Zhu (Zedoary) can destroy the tumor cells by degeneration, necrosis, shedding and diminution. It can increase the number of white blood cells, the phagocytosis and the immunity of the body. It can improve the micro-circulation, and prevent the formation of fibrin clots.

C. Eliminate phlegm and nodules:

The herbs can inhibit the growth of the tumor cells, disperse the mass or nodules of the benign tumors, and decrease the secretion around the malignant tumor cells. It is better to use in combination with the carminatives or digestive to reduce phlegm.

天花粉　Tian Hua Fen (Trichosanthis peel and the fruit (Gua Lou Ren 瓜蔞仁) can dilate the coronary artery and increase the flow of blood. It can also increase the tolerance of the body against environmental low blood pressure with decreased oxygen content. It is an expectorant, and can moisten the lung and resolve phlegm.

It is used to relieve chest pain, pulmonary infection and stuffiness sensation in the chest.

夏枯草 Xia Ku Cao (Prunella) can be used for cancer of the liver, throat, thyroid and the mammary gland.

D. Eliminate tumor and masses:

These herbs can kill or inhibit the growth of the tumor cells. Some have purgative action. They are usually used in combination with the herbs that can invigorate blood circulation.

大黄 Da Huang (Rhubarb) is a strong purgative. The purgative effect is observed 6-8 hours after oral intake. The action of evacuation is increased, leading to defecation. The effective ingredient rhein and emodin can inhibit the synthesis of DNA and the multiplication of cancer cells. It is boiled together with other herbs to achieve anti-tumor effect.

E. Tonification:

The cancer patients are usually weak and progressively losing weight. The tumor cells proliferate very fast. Deficiency of *Qi* and *Yang* usually indicate the deterioration of the organic functions of the body. Deficiency of *Yin* and blood usually indicate the depletion of blood and body fluid. The herbs can increase the phagocytosis of the tumor cells, and immunity of the body. They can enhance the function of the pituitary-adrenal glands. Some can increase the number of cAMP, or regulate the ratio of cAMP and cGMP, and inhibit the growth of the tumor cells.

人参 Ren Shen (Ginseng) can increase the production of white blood cells, lymphocytes, and immunoglobulins (IgG and IgM). It increases the synthesis of DNA, RNA, protein and lipid. It has similar action as the adaptogen, and can increase the defense mechanism of the body.

黄芪 Huang Qi (Astragalus) can increase the content of cAMP and inhibit the growth of the tumor cells. It increases the sensitivity to interferon which is similar to adenylate cyclase in action. It increases the production of macrophages, plasma cells and antibodies, and has effect against the immunosuppressants. It is effective for both cellular and humoral immunity.

靈芝 Ling Zhi (Ganoderma) can increase the number of white blood cells, the lymphocytes and the formation of E-rosette. It can improve the function of the adrenal cortex and prevent the radiological damage to the tissues. It is a cardiotonic, and can improve the blood circulation to the coronary artery and the cardiac muscles.

COMMONLY USED

CHINESE HERBAL FORMULAS

Ān Gōng Niú Huáng Wán　安宫牛黄丸
(An-Kung-Niu-Huang-Wan)
(Bezoar Resurrection Pills)

Constituents:

牛 黃	Niu Huang (Bos calculus)	.5-1 gm.	*Calculus Bovis*
犀 角	Xi Jiao (Rhinoceros horn)	.5-1 gm.	*Cornus Rhinoceri*
麝 香	She Xiang (Musk)	.25 gm.	*Moschus*
黃 連	Huang Lian (Coptis)	1-3 gm.	*Rhizoma Coptidis*
黃 芩	Huang Qin (Scutellaria)	1 gm.	*Radix Scutellariae*
栀 子	Zhi Zi (Gardenia)	1 gm.	*Fructus Gardeniae*
雄 黃	Xiong Huang (Realgar)	1 gm.	*Arsenic Disulfide*
郁 金	Yu Jin (Curcuma)	3-9 gm.	*Radix Curcumae*
冰 片	Bing Pian (Borneol)	.25 gm.	*Borneolum*
硃 砂	Zhu Sha (Cinnabar)	.5-1 gm.	*Cinnabaris*
珍 珠	Zhen Zhu (Pearl)	.5-1 gm.	*Concha Margaritifera Usta*
金箔衣	Jin Bo (Gold sheets)		

Action:

1. To eliminate heat and toxin
2. Resuscitating

Indication:

For a person with febrile disease and coma. The symptoms are: high fever, irritability, delirium, difficulty of speech, coma, convulsions.

Application:

Japanese encephalitis, epidemic cerebral-spinal meningitis, dysentery, uremia, cerebral vascular accident, hepatitis, hepatic coma, infantile convulsions.

Generic Name:

An Kung Niu Huang Wan;
Bos and Curcuma Formula

Bā Xiān Cháng Shòu Wán (Mài Wèi Dì Huáng Wán)
八仙長壽丸 (麥味地黃丸)
(Pa-Chian-Chang-Shou-Wan) (Mai-Wei-Ti-Huang-Wan)
(The Longevity Pill)
(Ophiopogon, Schisandra and Pills of Six Herbs with Rehmannia)

Constituents:

麥門冬	Mai Men Dong (Ophiopogon)	6-9 gm.	*Radix Ophiopogonis*
五味子	Wu Wei Zi (Schisandra)	6-9 gm.	*Fructus Schisandrae*
熟地黃	Shu Di Huang (Prep. rehmannia)	20-25 gm.	*Radix Rehmanniae Praeparatae*
山茱萸	Shan Zhu Yu (Cornus)	10-15 gm.	*Fructus Corni*
山 藥	Shao Yao (Dioscorea)	10-15 gm.	*Rhizoma Dioscoreae*
澤 瀉	Ze Xie (Alisma)	9-12 gm.	*Rhizoma Alismatis*
牡丹皮	Mu Dan Pi (Moutan bark)	6-9 gm.	*Cortex Moutan Radicis*
茯 苓	Fu Ling (Poria)	9-12 gm.	*Poria*

Action:

1. To replenish the *Yin* (vital essence) of kidney & lung
2. Anti-tussive and anti-asthma

Indication:

For a person with deficiency of *Yin* (vital essence) of the kidney and the lung. The symptoms are: cough with blood, asthma, tidal fever, night perspiration, nocturnal emission, spermatorrhea.

Tongue: red
Pulse: thready and rapid

Application:

Cough, asthma, hemoptysis, pulmonary tuberculosis, spermatorrhea, diabetes, mellitus, chronic nephritis.

Generic Name:

Ba Xian Chang Shou Wan

Bā Zhēn Tāng　八珍湯

(Pa-Chen-Tang)
(The Eight Precious Ingredients Decoction)

Constituents:

人　參	Ren Shen (Ginseng)	6-9 gm.	Radix Ginseng
熟地黄	Shu Di Huang (Prep. rehmannia)	9-12 gm.	Radix Rehmanniae Praepaparatae
白　术	Bai Zhu (White atractylodes)	9-12 gm.	Rhizoma Atractylodis Macrocephalae
當　歸	Dang Gui (Chinese angelica)	9-12 gm.	Radix Angelicae Sinensis
白　芍	Bai Shao Yao (White peony)	6-9 gm.	Radix Paeoniae Alba
川　芎	Chuan Xiong (Ligusticum)	6-9 gm.	Rhizoma Ligustici Chuan-xiong
茯　苓	Fu Ling (Poria)	9-12 gm.	Poria
炙甘草	Zhi Gan Cao (Baked licorice)	3-6 gm.	Radix Glycyrrhizae
生　薑	Sheng Jiang (Fresh ginger)	1-3 gm.	Rhizoma Zingiberis Recens
大　棗	Da Zao (Jujube)	3-5 pc.	Fructus Ziziphus Jujubae

Action:

To replenish *Qi* (vital energy) and blood

Indication:

For a person with deficiency of both *Qi* (vital energy) and blood. The symptoms are: face pale or sallow, dizziness, general fatigue, shortness of breath, palpitation, loss of appetite.

      Tongue: light with thin white coating
      Pulse: thready and weak, or gigantic and weak

Application:

Anemia, irregular menstruation, uterine bleeding, chronic abscess, chronic diseases of all kinds.

Modification:

1. For deficiency of *Qi*, blood and *Yang* with coldness, add:
黄芪　Huang Qi (Astragalus)　　　*Radix Astragali*
肉桂　Rou Gui (Cinnamon bark)　　*Cortex Cinnamomi*
This is called Shi Quan Da Bu Tang (Ginseng and Tang-kuei Ten Combination) (十全大補湯)

2. For irregular menstruation with abdominal pain during menstruation, leukorrhea, back pain, fatigue, decreased appetite, add:
益母草 Yi Mu Cao (Leonurus)　　　*Herba Leonuri*
This is called Ba Zhen Yi Mu Tang （八珍益母湯）

Generic Name:

Women's Precious Pills; Tang-kuei and Ginseng Eight Combination

Bā Zhèng Sàn   八正散
(Pa-Cheng-San)
(Powder of Eight Ingredients to Correct Urinary Disturbances)

Constituents:

木 通	Mu Tong (Akebia stem)	6-9 gm.	*Caulis Akebiae*
瞿 麥	Qu Mai (Dianthus; Pink)	6-9 gm.	*Herba Dianthi*
萹 蓄	Bian Xu (Polygonum)	6-9 gm.	*Herba Polygoni Avicularis*
滑 石	Hua Shi (Talc)	10-15 gm.	*Talcum*
燈心草	Deng Xin Cao (Juncus)	6-9 gm.	*Medulla Junci*
車前子	Che Qian Zi (Plantago seed)	6-9 gm.	*Semen Plantaginis*
梔 子	Zhi Zi (Gardenia fruit)	3-6 gm.	*Fructus Gardeniae*
大 黃	Da Huang (Rhubarb)	6-9 gm.	*Radix et Rhizoma Rhei*
炙甘草	Zhi Gan Cao (Baked licorice)	3-6 gm.	*Radix Glycyrrhizae Praeparatae*

Action:

1. To clear the true heat and dampness in the urinary bladder
2. Diuretic

Indication:

For a person with heat and dampness in the lower burner. The symptoms are: frequent and painful urination, scanty or obstructed flow of urine, abdominal distention, mouth and throat dry, urine with amber color.

Tongue: red, with yellow coating
Pulse: rapid and forceful

Application:

Acute urinary tract infection, urolithiasis, cystitis, urethritis, acute prostatitis, stones in the urinary tract, acute nephritis, acute pyonephritis.

Contraindication:

For a person of chronic disease with weak constitution; a pregnant woman.

Modification:

1. For acute urinary tract infection, add:

小 薊	Xiao Ji (Small thistle)	*Herba Cephalanoploris*
白茅根	Bai Mao Gen (Imperata rhizome)	*Rhizoma Imperatae*

2. For urolithiasis, add:

金錢草	Jin Qian Cao (Lysimachia)	*Herba Lysimachiae*
海金沙	Hai Jin Sha (Lygodium spores)	*Spora Lygodii*

Generic Name:

Dianthus Formula

Bǎi Hé Gù Jīn Tāng　　百合固金湯

(Pai-Ho-Ku-Chin-Tang)
(Decoction of Lily Bulb to Consolidate the Lung)

Constituents:

百　合	Bai He (Lily bulb)	6-9 gm.	*Bulbus Lilii*
熟地黃	Shu Di Huang (Prep. rehmannia)	9-12 gm.	*Radix Rehmanniae Praeparatae*
生地黃	Sheng Di Huang (Raw rehmannia)	6-9 gm.	*Radix Ophiopogonis*
麥門冬	Mai Men Dong (Ophiopogon)	6-9 gm.	*Radix Paeoniae Alba*
白芍藥	Bai Shao Yao (White peony)	6-9 gm.	*Radix Paeoniae Alba*
玄　參	Xuan Shen (Scrophularia)	6-9 gm.	*Radix Scrophulariae*
川貝母	Chuan Bei Mu (Tendrilled fritillary)	6-9 gm.	*Bulbus Fritillariae Cirrhosae*
當　歸	Dang Gui (Chinese angelica)	6-9 gm.	*Radix Angelicae Sinensis*
桔　梗	Jie Geng (Platycodon)	3-6 gm.	*Radix Platycodi*
甘　草	Gan Cao (Licorice)	3-6 gm.	*Radix Glycyrrhizae*

Action:

1. To eliminate heat and nourish the *Yin* (vital essence)
2. To moisten the lung and resolve sputum

Indication:

For a person with deficiency of *Yin* (vital essence) of both lung and kidney, thus with inflammation of the weak fire. The symptoms are: dry and painful throat, cough and asthma with bloody sputum, heat sensation in the palm of the hands and feet.

Tongue: red, with little coating
Pulse: thready and rapid

Application:

Tuberculosis, cough, asthma, hemoptysis.

Counteraction:

For a person with cough due to Shi (excessive) syndromes.

Modification:

For tuberculosis with cavity, add:

白　芨	Bai Ji (Bletilla tuber)	*Rhizoma Bletillae*
仙鶴草	Xian He Cao (Agrimony herb)	*Herba Agrimoniae*
紫珠草	Zi Zhu Cao (Purple pearl)	*Herba Callicarpae*

Generic Name:

Lily Combination

Bái Hú Jiā Guì Zhī Tāng　白虎加桂枝湯
(Pai-Hu-Chia-Kuei-Chi-Tang)
(White Tiger Decoction plus Cinnamon)

Constituents:

桂　枝	Gui Zhi (Cinnamon)	6-9 gm.	*Ramulus Cinnamomi*
石　膏	Shi Gao (Gypsum)	20-30 gm.	*Gypsum Fibrosum*
知　母	Zhi Mu (Anemarrhena)	9-12 gm.	*Rhizoma Anemarrhenae*
粳　米	Jing Mi (Oryza)	15-30 gm.	*Semen Oryzae*
炙甘草	Zhi Gan Cao (Baked licorice)	3-6 gm.	*Radix Glycyrrhizae Praeparatae*

Action:

To relieve arthritic pain caused by wind, heat and dampness.

Indication:

For a person with arthralgia due to wind, heat and dampness. The symptoms are: joints painful with swelling and burning sensation, pain is relieved by cold, difficulty of joint movements in one or more areas, fever, thirst, restlessness.

> Tongue: red with yellow coating
> Pulse: slippery and rapid

Application:

Arthralgia

Bái Hú Jiā Rén Shēn Tāng　白虎加人參湯

(Pai-Hu-Chia-Sheng-Tang)
(White Tiger Decoction plus Ginseng)

Constituents:

人　參	Ren Shen (Ginseng)	10-15 gm.	*Radix Ginseng*
石　膏	Shi Gao (Gypsum)	20-30 gm.	*Gypsum Fibrosum*
知　母	Zhi Mu (Anemarrhena)	9-12 gm.	*Rhizoma Anemarrhenae*
粳　米	Jing Mi (Oryza)	15-30 gm.	*Semen Oryzae*
炙甘草	Zhi Gan Cao (Baked licorice)	3-6 gm.	*Radix Glycyrrhizae Praeparatae*

Action:

1. To eliminate heat in the *Qi* (secondary defensive) system and the Yang-ming channel. (Febrifugal)
2. To promote the secretion of body fluids and to replenish vital energy.

Indication:

For a person with heat in the *Qi* (Secondary defensive) system and the Yang-ming channel. The symptoms are: high fever, headache, mouth dry, thirst with desire to drink water, increased urination, profuse perspiration.

> Tongue: red in the tip and sides
> Pulse: forceful and rapid

Application:

Diabetes mellitus, encephalitis B, epidemic meningitis.

Generic Name:

Ginseng and Gypsum Combination

Bái Hú Tāng   白虎湯
(Pai-Hu-Tang)
(White Tiger Decoction)

Constituents:

石 膏	Shi Gao (Gypsum)	20-30 gm.	*Gypsum Fibrosum*
知 母	Zhi Mu (Anemarrhena)	9-12 gm.	*Rhizoma Anemarrhenae*
粳 米	Jing Mi (Oryza)	15-30 gm.	*Semen Oryzae*
炙甘草	Zhi Gan Cao (Baked licorice)	3-6 gm.	*Radix Glycyrrhizae Praeparatae*

Action:

1. To eliminate the heat in the *Qi* (secondary defensive) system and the Yang-ming channel
2. To promote the secretion of body fluids

Indication:

For a person with heat in the *Qi* (secondary defensive) system and the Yang-ming channel. The symptoms are: high fever, headache, mouth dry, very thirsty, excessive perspiration, face red, aversion to heat.

Tongue: red with yellow and dry coating
Pulse: forceful and gigantic, or slippery and rapid.

Application:

Diabetes, gingivitis, encephalitis B, epidemic meningitis.

Modification:

1. With deficiency of vital energy and body fluids, add
人 參 Ren Shen (Ginseng)   *Radix ginseng*
This formula is called Bai Hu Jia Ren Shen Tang

2. With arthritic pain, add:
桂 枝 Gui Zhi (Cinnamon twig)   *Ramulus Cinnamomi*
This formula is called Bai Hu Jia Gui Zhi Tang

3. For encephalitis and meningitis, add:
金銀花 Jin Yin Hua (Lonicera flower)   *Flos Lonicerae*
連 翹 Lian Qiao (Forsythia)   *Fructus Forsythiae*
4. With convulsions, add:
鈴羊角 Ling Yang Jiao (Antelope horn)   *Cornus Antelopis*
鉤 藤 Gou Teng (Uncaria)   *Ramulus Uncariae*

Generic Name:

Gypsum Combination

Bái Tóu Wēng Tāng　白頭翁湯
(Pai-Tou-Weng-Tang)
(Decoction of Pulsatilla)

Constituents:

白頭翁	Bai Tou Weng (Pulsatilla)	10-15 gm.	*Radix Pulsatillae*
黃 連	Huang Lian (Coptis)	6-9 gm.	*Rhizoma Coptidis*
黃 柏	Huang Bai (Phellodendron)	9-12 gm.	*Cortex Phellodendri*
秦 皮	Qin Pi (Fraxinus)	10-15 gm.	*Cortex Fraxini*

Action:

To eliminate heat and toxin in the stomach and intestines (Febrifugal)

Indication:

For a person with dysentery (heat type). The symptoms are: abdominal pain with tenesmus, diarrhea with blood and pus, leukorrhea with bloody discharges, thirst with desire to drink water, burning sensation around the anus.

> Tongue: red with yellow coating
> Pulse: wiry/taut and rapid

Application:

Dysentery (both bacterial and amoebic)

Modification:

1. With exterior symptom-complex, with fever and aversion to cold, and interior heat, add:

葛 根	Ge Gen (Pueraria root)	*Radix Puerariae*
金銀花	Jin Yin Hua (Lonicera flower)	*Flos Lonicerae*

2. With tenesmus and insufficient flow of vital energy, add:

木 香	Mu Xiang (Saussurea root)	*Radix Saussureae*
檳 榔	Bing Lang (Areca seed)	*Semen Arecae*

3. With abdominal pain (refused to be pressed), thick and greasy tongue coating, indicating indigestion, add:

山 楂	Shan Zha (Crataegus fruit)	*Fructus Crataegi*
枳 實	Zhi Shi (Immature bitter orange)	*Fructus Aurantii Immaturus*

4. With epidemic dysentery, with purplish blood, add:

生地黃	Sheng Di Huang (Fresh rehmannia)	*Radix Rehmanniae*
牡丹皮	Mu Dan Pi (Moutan bark)	*Cortex Moutan Radicis*

Generic Name:

Anemone Combination

Bái Zhú Sàn (Qī Wèi Bái Zhú Sàn)　白术散 (七味白术散)
(Pai-Chu-Sam) (Chi-Wei-Pai-Chu-San)
(The White Atractylodes Powder)

Constituents:

人 參	Ren Shen (Ginseng)	6-9 gm.	Radix Ginseng
白 术	Bai Zhu (White atractylodes)	10-15 gm.	Rhizoma Atractylodis
茯 苓	Fu Ling (Poria)	10-15 gm.	Poria
葛 根	Ge Gen (Pueraria)	10-15 gm.	Radix Puerariae
藿 香	Huo Xiang (Agastache)	10-15 gm.	Herba Agastachis
木 香	Mu Xiang (Saussurea)	3-6 gm.	Radix Saussureae
炙甘草	Zhi Gan Cao (Baked licorice)	1-3 gm.	Radix Glycyrrhizae Praeparatae

Action:

1. To tonify the spleen and stomach
2. To resolve dampness
3. Antiemetic and anti-diarrhea

Indication:

For a person with weakness and deficiency of spleen and stomach. The symptoms are: decreased intake of food, abdominal pain, diarrhea, vomiting, thirst with desire to drink water, fatigue.

Tongue: with white and greasy coating
Pulse: slow and weak

Application:

Infantile diarrhea, infantile malnutrition, vomiting and diarrhea, diabetes.

Generic Name:

Atractylodes and Pueraria Formula

Bàn Xià Bái Zhú Tiān Má Tāng　半夏白术天麻湯

(Pan-Hsia-Pai-Chu-Ten-Ma-Tang)
(Decoction of Pinellia, White Atractylodes and Gastrodia)

Constituents:

半 夏	Ban Xia (Pinellia tuber)	6-9 gm.	*Rhizoma Pinelliae*
天 麻	Tian Ma (Gastrodia tuber)	3-6 gm.	*Rhizoma Gastrodiae*
白 术	Bai Zhu (White atractylodes)	6-9 gm.	*Rhizoma Atractylodis Macrocephalae*
茯 苓	Fu Ling (Poria; Hoelen)	6-9 gm.	*Poria*
陳 皮	Chen Pi (Citrus peel)	3-6 gm.	*Pericarpium Citris Reticulatae*
甘 草	Gan Cao (Licorice)	3-6 gm.	*Radix Glycyrrhizae*
生 薑	Sheng Jiang (Fresh ginger)	3-6 gm.	*Rhizoma Zingiberis Recens*
大 棗	Da Zao (Jujube)	3-5 pc.	*Fructus Ziziphus Jujubae*

Action:

1. To resolve phlegm caused by endogenous wind
2. To strengthen the spleen and dispel dampness

Indication:

For a person with wind phlegm. The symptoms are: vertigo, headache, profuse sputum, feeling of oppression and stuffiness in the chest.

Tongue: white with greasy coating
Pulse: soft and slippery

Contraindication:

For a person with vertigo that is not caused by wind and phlegm.

Application:

Auditory vertigo (Meniere's disease), neurotic vertigo.

Modification:

1. If vertigo is severe, add:

僵 蠶	Jiang Can (White-stiff silkworm)	*Bombyx Batryticatus*
胆南星	Dan Nan Xing (Arisaema with bile)	*Rhizoma Arisaematis*

2. For excessive accumulation of phlegm causing coma, headache, coldness of extremities, add:

黄 柏	Huang Bai (Phellodendron bark)	*Cortex Phellodendri*
蒼 术	Cang Zhu (Atractylodes)	*Rhizoma Atractlodis*
黄 芪	Huang Qi (Astragalus root)	*Radix Astragali*
人 參	Ren Shen (Ginseng)	*Radix ginseng*
澤 瀉	Ze Xie (Alisma tuber)	*Rhizoma Alismatis*
麥 芽	Mai Ya (Germinated barley)	*Fructus Hordei Germinatus*
神 曲	Shen Qu (Medicated leaven)	*Massa Fermentata Medicinalis*

Generic Name:

Pinellia and Gastrodia Combination

Bàn Xià Hòu Pò Tāng 半夏厚朴湯
(Pan-Hsia-Hou-Pu-Tang)
(Decoction of Pinellia and Magnolia Bark)

Constituents:

半　夏	Ban Xia (Pinellia tuber)	6-9 gm.	*Rhizoma Pinelliae*
厚　朴	Hou Po (Magnolia bark)	6-9 gm.	*Cortex Magnoliae Officinalis*
紫蘇葉	Zi Su Ye (Perilla leaf)	6-9 gm.	*Folium Perillae*
茯　苓	Fu Ling (Poria; Hoelen)	9-12 gm.	*Poria*
生　薑	Sheng Jiang (Fresh ginger)	10-15 gm.	*Rhizoma Zingiberis Recens*

Action:

1. To regulate the flow of *Qi* (vital energy) and disperse lumps
2. To resolve phlegm

Indication:

For a person with globus hystericus. The symptoms are: blockage in the throat, difficulty in swallowing or vomiting, cough with profuse sputum.

Tongue: white and moist, or slippery and greasy
Pulse: wiry/taut, or wiry and slippery

Application:

Globus hystericus, hysteria, gastro-intestinal neurosis, esophagiospasm, chronic laryngitis, tracheitis.

Modification:

1. For a person with deficiency of *Qi* (vital energy), add:

人　參	Ren Shen (Ginseng)	*Radix Ginseng*
檳　榔	Bing Lang (Areca seed)	*Semen Arecae*
沉　香	Chen Xiang (Aquilaria wood)	*Lignum Aquilariae Resinatum*
烏　藥	Wu Yao (Lindera root)	*Radix Linderae*

which is the formula called Si Mo Yin (四磨飲)

2. If the obstruction of flow of *Qi* (vital energy) is severe, add:

柴　胡	Chai Hu (Bupleurum)	*Radix Bupleuri*
郁　金	Yu Jin (Curcuma root)	*Radix Curcumae*
香　附	Xiang Fu (Cyperus tuber)	*Rhizoma Cyperi*
青　皮	Qing Pi (Green tangerine peel)	*Pericarpium Citri Reticulatae Viridae*

3. If vomiting with sputum, but no thirst, just use:

半　夏	Ban Xia (Pinellia tuber)	*Rhizoma Pinelliae*
生　薑	Sheng Jiang (Fresh ginger)	*Rhizoma Zingiberis*

This mini formula is called Xiao Ban Xia Tang (小半夏湯)

Generic Name:

Pinellia and Magnolia Combination

Bàn Xià Xiè Xīn Tāng 半夏瀉心湯

(Pan-Hsia-Hsieh-Hsin-Tang)
(The Stomach Purging Decoction with Pinellia)

Constituents:

半 夏	Ban Xia (Pinellia)	9-12 gm.	*Rhizoma Pinelliae*
黃 連	Huang Lian (Coptis)	3-6 gm.	*Rhizoma Coptidis*
黃 芩	Huang Qin (Sctellaria)	6-9 gm.	*Radix Scutellariae*
乾 薑	Gan Jing (Dry ginger)	9-12 gm.	*Rhizoma Zingiberis*
人 參	Ren Shen (Ginseng)	6-9 gm.	*Radix Ginseng*
炙甘草	Zhi Gan Cao (Baked licorice)	3-6 gm.	*Radix Glycyrrhizae Praeparatae*
大 棗	Da Zao (Jujube)	3-5 pc.	*Fructus Ziziphus*

Action:

1. To reverse the flow of vital energy of the stomach
2. To relieve the fullness sensation caused by cold and heat factors

Indication:

For a person with disharmony between the stomach and the intestines with interaction of cold and heat factors. The symptoms are: epigastric fullness but no pain, retch or vomiting, borborygmus, diarrhea.

Tongue: with thin yellow and greasy coating
Pulse: wiry/taut and rapid

Application:

Acute gastroenteritis

Modification:

1. For interaction of water and heat in the stomach, add:
生 薑 Sheng Jiang (Fresh ginger)　　　*Rhizoma Zingiberis*
and eliminate Gan Jiang (Dry ginger) (乾薑)

This formula is now called Sheng Jiang Xie Xin Tang (Pinellia and Ginger Combination) (生薑瀉心湯)

2. For deficiency of *Qi* (vital energy) of the stomach, increase the amount of baked licorice to 60 gm. This formula is called Gan Cao Xie Xin Tang (Pinellia and Licorice Combination) (甘草瀉心湯)

Generic Name:

Pinellia Combination

Bǎo Hé Wán   保和丸

(Pao-Ho-Wan)
(Pills for Indigestion)

Constituents:

山 楂	Shan Zha (Crataegus)	9-12 gm.	*Fructus Crataegi*
神 曲	Shen Qu (Medicated leaven)	6-9 gm.	*Massa Fermentata Medicinalis*
萊菔子	Lai Fu Zi (Raphanus seed)	9-12 gm.	*Semen Raphani*
半 夏	Ban Xia (Pinellia)	6-9 gm.	*Rhizoma Pinelliae*
陳 皮	Chen Pi (Citrus peel)	3-6 gm.	*Pericarpium Citri*
茯 苓	Fu Ling (Poria; Hoelen)	6-9 gm.	*Poria*
連 翹	Lian Qiao (Forsythia)	6-9 gm.	*Fructus Forsythiae*

Action:

To promote the digestion function of the stomach and remove stagnated food (Digestive)

Indication:

For a person with food stagnation. The symptoms are: fullness and distension in the gastric region, belching, acid regurgitation, loss of appetite, constipation or diarrhea.

Tongue: yellow with greasy coating
Pulse: slippery

Application:

Indigestion, diarrhea, abdominal pain, gastro-intestinal flu.

Contraindication:

For a person with gastric and abdominal distention due to deficiency syndromes.

Modification:

1. If abdominal distress is severe, add:

枳 實	Zhi Shi (Immature bitter orange)	*Fructus Aurantii Immaturus*
厚 朴	Hou Po (Magnolia bark)	*Cortex Magnoliae Officinalis*

2. With bad breath, add:

黃 芩	Huang Qin (Scutellaria)	*Radix Scutellariae*
黃 連	Huang Lian (Coptis)	*Rhizoma Coptidis*

3. With constipation, add:

大 黃	Da Huang (Rhubarb)	*Radix et Rz. Rhei*
檳 榔	Bing Lang (Areca seed)	*Semen Arecae*

4. With flu symptoms, add:

紫蘇根	Zi Su Gen (Perilla stem)	*Rhizoma Perillae*
藿 香	Huo Xiang (Agastache)	*Herba Agastachis*

Generic Name:

Po Chi Pills; Citrus and Crataegus Formula

Bèi Mǔ Guā Lóu Sàn　　貝母瓜蔞散

(Pei-Mu-Kua-Lou-San)
(Power of Fritillary and Trichosanthes Fruit)

Constituents:

川貝母	Chuan Bei Mu (Tendrilled fritillary)	6-9 gm.	*Bulbus Fritillariae Cirrhosae*
瓜蔞子	Gua Lou Zi (Trichosanthes fruit)	9-12 gm.	*Fructus Trichosanthis*
天花粉	Tian Hua Fen (Trichosanthes root)	9-12 gm.	*Radix Trichosanthis*
茯　苓	Fu Ling (Poria)	6-9 gm.	*Poria*
橘　紅	Ju Hong (Tangerine peel)	3-6 gm.	*Pericarpium Citri*
桔　梗	Jie Geng (Platycodon)	6-9 gm.	*Radix platycodi*

Action:

1. To resolve the dryness in the lung
2. Carminative and expectorant

Indication:

For a person with phlegm and dryness in the lung. The symptoms are: cough with sputum, but with difficulty to spit, throat dry and sore, dyspnea.

    Tongue: red and dry
    Pulse: rapid

Application:

Sore throat, bronchitis, tracheitis, aphonia, pulmonary emphysema.

Modification:

1. With severe dry and sore throat, add:

麥門冬	Mai Men Dong (Ophiopogon)	*Radix Ophiopogonis*
玄　參	Xuan Shen (Scrophularia)	*Radix Scrophlariae*

2. With cough and irritability of throat, add:

前　胡	Qian Hu (Peucedanum)	*Radix Peucedani*
牛蒡子	Niu Bang Zi (Arctium fruit)	*Fructus Arctii*

3. With blood in the sputum, add:

沙　參	Sha Shen (Glehnia)	*Radix Glehniae*
阿　膠	E Jiao (Donkey-hide gelatin)	*Colla Cortii Asini*

    and eliminate:

橘　紅	Ju Hong (Tangerine peel)	*Pericarpium Citri Reticulatae*

Bì Xiè Fēn Qīng Yǐn   萆薢分清飲
(Pi-Hsieh-Fen-Ching-Yin)
(Decoction of Hypoglauca Yam)

Constituents:

萆 薢	Bi Xie (Hypoglauca yam)	9-12 gm.	*Rhizoma Dioscoreae*
益智仁	Yi Zhi Ren (Black cardamon)	6-9 gm.	*Fructus Alpiniae*
烏 葯	Wu Yao (Lindera)	6-9 gm.	*Radix Linderae*
石菖蒲	Shi Chang Pu (Acorus)	3-6 gm.	*Rhizoma Acori Graminei*
	May add:		
茯 苓	Fu Ling (Poria)	6-9 gm.	*Poria*
甘 草	Gan Cao (Licorice)	3-6 gm.	*Radix Glycyrrhizae*

Action:

1. To resolve dampness by warming the kidney
2. To purify the turbidity

Indication:

For a person with cloudy urine or gonorrhea caused by deficiency of kidney *Qi* (vital energy) with coldness. The symptoms are: frequent urination, cloudy urine, white and mucoid.

> Tongue: pale with white coating
> Pulse: sinking, slow and weak

Application:

Milky or cloudy urination, chronic prostatitis, gonorrhea.

Contraindication:

For a person with deficiency of kidney *Yin* (vital essence).

Modification:

If the patient also has symptoms of spleen and stomach *Qi* deficiency, use in combination with the formula Si Jun Zi Tang (Four Major Herb Combination) 四君子湯

Generic Name:

Tokora Combination

Bù Dài Wán   布袋丸

(Pu-Tai-Wan)
(The Pills in a Bag)

Constituents:

使君子	Shi Jun Zi (Quisqualis)	10-15 gm.	*Fructus Quisqualis*
蕪 荑	Wu Yi (Stinking elm)	6-9 gm.	*Herba Ulmi*
夜明砂	Ye Ming Sha (Bat's dung)	6-9 gm.	*Faeces Vesperitilionis*
人 參	Ren Shen (Ginseng)	6-9 gm.	*Radix Ginseng*
白 术	Bai Zhu (White atractylodes)	6-9 gm.	*Rhizoma Atractylodis Macrocephalae*
茯 苓	Fu Ling (Poria)	6-9 gm.	*Poria*
蘆 薈	Lu Hui (Aloe)	6-9 gm.	*Aloe*
甘 草	Gan Cao (Licorice)	3-6 gm.	*Radix Glycyrrhizae*

Grind the above ingredients into powder and made into pills. Put the pills into a bag and decoct with pork.

Action:

1. Anthelmintic
2. To reinforce the spleen *Qi*

Indication:

For a person with infantile malnutrition due to helminth infestation. The symptoms are: sallow face, emaciation, high body temperature, skinny hands and feet, abdominal distention, eyes dull and very dry.

> Tongue: pale
> Pulse: weak

Application:

Infantile malnutrition, ascariasis, parasitic infestations.

Bǔ Fèi Tāng 補肺湯 （补肺汤）
(Pu-Fei-Tang)
(Tonifying the Lung Decoction)

Constituents:

人 参	Ren Shen (Ginseng)	6-9 gm.	Radix Ginseng
黄 芪	Huang Qi (Astragalus)	6-9 gm.	Radix Astragali
熟地黄	Shu Di Huang (Prep. rehmannia)	9-12 gm.	Radix Rehmanniae
五味子	Wu Wei Zi (Schisandra)	6-9 gm.	Fructus Schisandrae
紫 菀	Zi Wan (Aster root)	6-9 gm.	Radix Asteris
桑白皮	Sang Bai Pi (Mulberry bark)	6-9 gm.	Cortex Mori Radicis

Action:

1. To replenish the Qi (vital energy) of the lung
2. Antitussive, expectorant

Indication:

For a person with deficiency of Qi (vital energy) of the lung. The symptoms are: cough, asthma, with thin and scanty sputum, low in energy, voice low and weak, intolerance of cold, spontaneous perspiration, face pale, malaise.

Tongue: pale with thin white coating
Pulse: feeble and weak

Application:

Chronic cough and asthma, pulmonary tuberculosis.

Bǔ Gān Tāng 補肝湯 (补肝汤)

(Pu-Gan-Tang)
(Tonifying the Liver Formula)

Constituents:

熟地黃	Shu Di Huang (Prep. rehmannia)	10-15 gm.	*Radix Rehmanniae*
當 歸	Dang Gui (Chinese angelica)	9-12 gm.	*Radix Angelicae Sinensis*
川 芎	Chuan Xiong (Ligusticum)	6-9 gm.	*Rhizoma Ligustici Chuanxiong*
白芍藥	Bai Shao Yao (White peony)	9-12 gm.	*Radix Paeoniae Alba*
麥門冬	Mai Men Dong (Ophiopogon)	12-15 gm.	*Radix Ophiopogonis*
酸棗仁	Suan Zao Ren (Wild jujube)	6-9 gm.	*Semen Ziziphi Spinosae*
木 瓜	Mu Gua (Chaenomeles)	6-9 gm.	*Fructus Chaenomelis*
甘 草	Gan Cao (Licorice)	3-6 gm.	*Radix Glycyrrhizae*

Action:

To replenish the liver *Yin* fluid

Indication:

For a person with deficiency of liver *Yin* fluid. The symptoms are: headache, dizziness, eyes dry, photophobia, blurred or decreased vision, face red, numbness in the limbs, muscles with cramps or twitching, irritability.

Tongue: red
Pulse: rapid, thready or wiry

Application:

Anemia, malaise, headache, dry eyes, photophobia, muscle cramps, chronic fatigue syndrome.

Modification:

1. With severe headache, dizziness, muscle cramps, add:

石決明	Shi Jue Ming (Abalone shell)	*Concha Haliotidis*
菊 花	Ju Hua (Chrysanthemum flower)	*Flos Chrysanthemi*
鉤 藤	Gou Teng (Uncaria stem with hooks)	*Ramulus Uncariae cum Uncis*

2. With dry eyes, photophobia, decreased vision, add:

枸杞子	Gou Qi Zi (Lycium fruit)	*Fructus Lycii*
女貞子	Nu Zhen Zi (Ligustrum fruit)	*Fructus Ligustri Lucidi*

3. With numbness in the limbs, add:

雞血藤	Ji Xue Teng (Millettia stem)	*Caulis Milletti*
絲瓜絡	Si Gua Luo (Luffa)	*Fasciculus Vascularia Luffae*

4. With irritability and bad temperament, with dark urine or constipation, add:

龍膽草	Long Dan Cao (Gentiana)	*Radix Gentianae*
黃 芩	Huang Qin (Scutellaria root)	*Radix Scutellariae*
梔 子	Zhi Zi (Gardenia)	*Fructus Gardeniae*

Bŭ Yáng Huán Wŭ Tāng 補陽還五湯 (补阳还五汤)

(Pu-Yang-Huan-Wu-Tang)

(Decoction for Reinforcing Vital Function and Restoring Normal Function of the Five Visceras)

Constituents:

黄 芪	Huang Qi (Astragalus)	10-15 gm.	Radix Astragali
當 歸	Dang Gui (Chinese angelica)	6-9 gm.	Radix Angelicae Sinensis
川 芎	Chuan Xiong (Ligusticum)	6-9 gm.	Rhizoma Ligustici Chuanxiong
赤芍藥	Chi Shao Yao (Red peony)	6-9 gm.	Radix Paeoniae Rubra
地 龍	Di Long (Earthworm)	3-6 gm.	Lumbricus
桃 仁	Tao Ren (Persica seed)	6-9 gm.	Semen Persicae
紅 花	Hong Hua (Carthamus)	6-9 gm.	Flos Carthami

Action:

To replenish vital energy, invigorate the blood circulation in the collaterals.

Indication:

For a person with post-cerebral apoplexy syndromes with symptoms of hemiplegia, deviation of the mouth and eyes, difficulty of speech, salivation, frequent urination or incontinence of urination.

Tongue: with white coating
Pulse: moderate

Application:

Apoplexy, hemiplegia, cerebral vascular accident, infantile paralysis.

Modification:

1. With coldness of the limbs, add:

制附子 Fu Zi (Prepared aconite)   Radix Aconiti Praeparatae

2. With spleen and stomach asthenia, add:

人 參 Ren Shen (Ginseng)   Radix Ginseng
白 术 Bai Zhu (White atractylodes)   Rhizoma Atractylodis Macrocephalae

3. With profuse sputum, add:

半 夏 Ban Xia (Pinellia tuber)   Rhizoma Pinelliae

Bǔ Zhōng Yì Qì Tāng　補中益氣湯　(补中益气汤)

(Pu-Chung-I-Chi-Tang)
(Decoction for Reinforcing the Middle Burner and Replenishing the Vital Energy)

Constituents:

黄 芪	Huang Qi (Astragalus)	6-15 gm.	*Radix Astragali*
人 參	Ren Shen (Ginseng)	6-9 gm.	*Radix Ginseng*
白 术	Bai Zhu (White atractylodes)	9-12 gm.	*Rhizoma Atractylodis Macrocephalae*
炙甘草	Zhi Gan Cao (Baked licorice)	3-6 gm.	*Radix Glycyrrhizae Praeparatae*
當 歸	Dang Gui (Chinese angelica)	6-9 gm.	*Radix Angelicae Sinensis*
升 麻	Sheng Ma (Cimicifuga)	3-6 gm.	*Rhizoma Cimicifugae*
柴 胡	Chai Hu (Bupleurum)	6-9 gm.	*Radix Bupleuri*
陳 皮	Chen Pi (Citrus peel)	3-6 gm.	*Pericarpium Citri Recticulatae*

Action:

1. To replenish the vital energy and tonify the spleen and stomach
2. To uplift the *Yang* (functional activity)

Indication:

For a person with *Qi* (vital energy) deficiency with prolapse of the visceras. Other symptoms are: fever, headache, irritability, shortness of breath, fatigue, spontaneous perspiration, intolerant of cold, reduced food intake, loose bowels, thirst.

　　　　Tongue: light color with white coating
　　　　Pulse: feeble, large (gigantic), weak

Application:

Gastroptosis, prolapse of the rectum and uterus, uterine bleeding, myasthenia gravis

Modification:

To increase the effect in treatment of gastroptosis, hysteroptosis, prolapse of the rectum, add:

枳 殼 Zhi Ke (Bitter orange)　　　　　　*Fructus Aurantii*

Generic Name:

Bu Zhong Yi Qi Wan;
Ginseng and Astragalus Combination

Cāng Ěr Sàn 蒼耳散

(Chang-Er-San)
(Powder of Xanthium Fruit)

Constituents:

蒼耳子	Cang Er Zi (Xanthium fruit)	6-9 gm.	*Fructus Xanthii*
辛 夷	Xin Yi (Magnolia flower)	3-6 gm.	*Flos Magnoliae*
白 芷	Bai Zhi (Angelica)	3-6 gm.	*Radix Angelicae*
薄 荷	Bo He (Mentha)	3-6 gm.	*Herba Menthae*

Action:

1. To disperse wind
2. To open the orifices

Indication:

For a person with nasal sinusitis. The symptoms are: fever, purulent nasal discharges, frontal and temporal headache.

Tongue: with white coating
Pulse: floating

Application:

Nasal sinusitis, chronic rhinitis, allergic rhinitis, accessary nasal sinuses.

Modification:

1. With increased heat in lung, add:

地骨皮	Di Gu Pi (Lycium bark)	*Cortex Lycii Radicis*
桑白皮	Sang Bai Pi (Morus bark)	*Cortex Mori Radicis*

2. With profuse nasal discharges, add:

金銀花	Jin Yin Hua (Lonicera flower)	*Flos Lonicerae*
鵝不食草	E Bu Shi Cao (Centipeda)	*Herba Centipedae*
甘 草	Gan Cao (Licorice)	*Radix Glycyrrhizae*

Chái Gé Jiě Jì Tāng (Gé Gēn Tāng) 柴葛解肌湯 (葛根湯)
(Chai-Ko-Chieh-Chi-Tang)
(Decoction of Bupleurum and Pueraria)

Constituents:

柴 胡	Chai Hu (Bupleurum)	6-9 gm.	Radix Bupleuri
葛 根	Ge Gen (Pueraria root)	9-12 gm.	Radix Puerariae
羌 活	Qiang Huo (Notopterygium)	6-9 gm.	Rhizoma Seu Radix Notopterygii
白 芷	Bai Zhi (Angelica root)	6-9 gm.	Radix Angelicae
黃 芩	Huang Qin (Scutellariae)	6-9 gm.	Radix Scutellariae
石 膏	Shi Gao (Gypsum)	15-20 gm.	Gypsum Fibrosum
白芍藥	Bai Shao Yao (White peony)	6-9 gm.	Radix Paeoniae Alba
桔 梗	Jie Geng (Platycodon)	3-6 gm.	Radix Platycodi
甘 草	Gan Cao (Licorice)	3-6 gm.	Radix Glycyrrhizae
生 薑	Sheng Jiang (Fresh ginger)	3-6 gm.	Rhizoma Zingiberis Recens
大 棗	Da Zao (Jujube)	3-5 pc.	Fructus Ziziphus Jujubae

Action:

1. To dispel exterior wind and cold (Diaphoretic)
2. To eliminate internal heat

Indication:

For a person with common cold caused by wind and cold factors, but with inflammation (interior heat) in the muscles. The symptoms are: fever, intolerance of cold, headache, muscle-ache, blood-shot eyes, nose dry, insomnia, mouth bitter.

Tongue: red with thin yellow coating
Pulse: full, or slippery and rapid

Application:

Common cold, toothache, trigeminal neuralgia, influenza.

Contraindication:

For a person with common cold caused by wind and heat factors.

Modification:

1. With thirst and dry tongue, add:
知 母 Zhi Mu (Anemarrhena)　　　Rhizoma Anemarrhenae
天花粉 Tian Hua Fen (Trichosanthes root)　Radix Trichosanthis
2. With cough and sticky sputum, add:
瓜蔞皮 Gua Lou Pi (Trichosanthes peel)　Pericarpium Trichosanthis

Generic Name:

Bupleurum and Pueraria Combination

Chái Hú Shū Gān Sàn   柴胡舒肝散
(Chai-Hu-Shu-Kan-San)
(Powder to Disperse Vital Energy in Liver)

Constituents:

柴　胡	Chai Hu (Bupleurum)	9-12 gm.	*Radix Bupleuri*
白芍藥	Bai Shao Yao (White peony)	6-9 gm.	*Radix Paeoniae Alba*
枳　殼	Zhi Ke (Bitter orange)	6-9 gm.	*Fructus Aurantii*
川　芎	Chuan Xiong (Ligusticum)	3-6 gm.	*Rhizoma Ligustici Chuanxiong*
香　附	Xiang Fu (Cyperus tuber)	6-9 gm.	*Rhizoma Cyperi*
甘　草	Gan Cao (Licorice)	1-3 gm.	*Radix Glycyrrhizae*

Action:

To relieve pain by dispersing the circulation of vital energy and blood in the liver.

Indication:

For a person with stagnancy of *Qi* (vital energy) and blood in the liver. The symptoms are: mental depression, moodiness, hypochondriac distention and pain, chest fullness, belching, indigestion, abdominal distention, constipation.

> Tongue: with thin white coating
> Pulse: wiry/taut

Application:

Hypochondriac pain, hypertension, mania, dysmenorrhea, irregular menstruation, breast distention.

Modification:

1. With belching and acid regurgitation, add:

瓦楞子	Wa Leng Zi (Ark shell)	*Concha Arcae*
海螵蛸	Hai Piao Xiao (Cuttlefish bone)	*Os Sepiellae*

2. Severe abdominal pain, add:

延胡索	Yan Hu Suo (Corydalis tuber)	*Rhizoma Corydalis*
川楝子	Chuan Lian Zi (Sichuan chinaberry)	*Fructus Melia Toosendan*

3. With mouth bitter, add:

黄　連	Huang Lian (Coptis)	*Rhizoma Coptidis*
黄　芩	Huang Qin (Scutellaria)	*Radix Scutellariae*

Comment:

Similar product from China: Shu Gan Wan

Chuān Xiōng Chá Tiáo Sàn   川芎茶調散

(Chuan-Chiung-Cha-Tiao-San)
(Decoction or Tea with Ligusticum)

Constituents:

川 芎	Chuan Xiong (Ligusticum)	6-9 gm.	*Rhizoma Ligustici Chuanxiong*
羌 活	Qiang Huo (notopterygium)	6-9 gm.	*Rz. Seu Radix Notopterygii*
白 芷	Bai Zhi (Angelica)	6-9 gm.	*Radix Angelicae Dahuricae*
細 辛	Xi Xin (Asarum)	3-6 gm.	*Herba Asari*
荆 芥	Jing Jie (Schizonepeta)	6-9 gm.	*Herba Schizonepetae*
防 風	Fang Feng (Ledebourella)	6-9 gm.	*Radix Ledebourellae*
薄 荷	Bo He (Mentha)	3-6 gm.	*Herba menthae*
甘 草	Gan Cao (Licorice)	3-6 gm.	*Radix Glycyrrhizae*
茶 葉	Cha Ye (Green tea leaves)		

Grind the above ingredients into powder. Take 6 gm. of the powder with the green tea each time.

Action:

1. Analgesic 2. To dispel pathogenic wind

Indication:

For a person with headache caused by wind. The symptoms are: headache (frontal, occipital, bilateral, vertical or migraine), vertigo, stuffy nose, fever, intolerance of chill.

Tongue: white with thin coating
Pulse: floating and tight

Application:

Flu with headache, migraine, chronic rhinitis, nasal sinusitis, neuralgic headache.

Contraindication:. For a person with headache caused by wind and heat.

Modification:

1. With severe intolerance of chill, add:

生 薑 Sheng Jiang (Fresh ginger)   *Rhizoma Zingiberis Recens*
紫蘇葉 Zi Su Ye (Perilla leaf)   *Folium Perillae*

2. For chronic rhinitis and nasal sinusitis, add:

辛夷花 Xin Yi Hua (Magnolia flower)   *Flos Magnoliae*
蒼耳子 Cang Er Zi (Xanthium fruit)   *Fructus Xanthii*

3. For headache due to wind and heat, with dizziness and vertigo, add:

菊 花 Ju Hua (Chrysanthemum flower)   *Flos Chrysanthemi*
僵 蠶 Jiang Can (White-stiff silkworm)   *Batryticated Silkworm*
炙甘草 Zhi Gan Cao (Baked licorice)   *Radix Glycyrrhizae*

This formula is called Ju Hua Cha Tiao San (菊花茶調散)

Generic Name: Cnidium and Tea Formula

Cí Zhū Wán (Shén Qū Wán)　磁硃丸（神曲丸）
(Chi-Chu-Wan, Shen-Chu-Wan)
(Sedative Pills with Magnetite and Cinnabar)

Constituents:

磁　石	Ci Shi (Magnetite)	20-30 gm.	*Magnetitum*
硃　砂	Zhu Sha (Cinnabar)	3-6 gm.	*Cinnabaris*
神　曲	Shen Qu (Medicated Leaven)	9-12 gm.	*Massa Fermentata Medicinalis*

Action:

1. Sedative (Tranquilizing)
2. To subdue the excessive fire of the heart
3. To brighten the eyes

Indication:

For a person with up-flaring fire of the heart due to deficiency of vital essence in the kidney. The symptoms are: insomnia, palpitation, tinnitus, deafness, blurry vision, headache, dizziness.

Application:

Cataract, glaucoma, tinnitus, deafness, retinitis, epilepsy, schizophrenia.

Modification:

1. With profuse phlegm in epilepsy, add:

胆南星	Dan Nan Xing (Arisaema tuber)	*Rhizoma Arisaemae*
半　夏	Ban Xia (Pinellia)	*Rhizoma Pinelliae*
僵　蠶	Jiang Can (White-stiff silkworm)	*Batrytricated Silkworm*

2. For schizphrenia, add:

黄　連	Huang Lian (Coptis)	*Rhizoma Coptidis*
梔　子	Zhi Zi (Gardenia fruit)	*Fructus Gardeniae*
胆南星	Dan Nan Xing (Arisaema tuber)	*Rhizoma Arisaemae Praeparatae*

3. With severe deficiency of vital essence of kidney, add:

枸杞子	Gou Qi Zi (Wolfberry fruit)	*Fructus Lycii*
女貞子	Nu Zhen Zi (Ligustrum fruit)	*Fructus Ligustrii*
菟絲子	Tu Si Zi (Cuscuta seed)	*Semen Cuscutae*
熟地黄	Shu Di Huang (Prep. rehmannia)	*Radix Rehmanniae Praeparatae*

Generic Name:

Tze Zhu Pills

Cōng Chǐ Tāng　　葱豉湯

(Chong-Chi-Tang)
(Decoction of Allium Bulb and Soya)

Constituents:

葱　白	Cong Bai (Allium bulb)	9-12 gm.	*Bulbus Allii Fistulosumi*
淡豆豉	Dan Dou Chi (Prepared soybean)	9-15 gm.	*Semen Sojae Praeparatae*

Action:

To dispel exterior wind and cold (Diaphoretic)

Indication:

For the initial stage of common cold. The symptoms are: fever, no perspiration, headache, stuffy-nose, and intolerance of cold.

Tongue: with thin white coating
Pulse: floating and tight/tense

Application:

Common cold, influenza

Modification:

1. With muscle-ache, add:

羌　活	Qiang Huo (Notopterygium)	*Rz. seu Radix Notopterygii*
荆　芥	Jing Jie (Schizonepeta)	*Herba Schizonepetae*
防　風	Fang Feng (Ledebouriella)	*Radix Ledebouriellae*
紫蘇葉	Zi Su Ye (Perilla leaf)	*Fructus Perillae*

2. With sore-throat, add:

金銀花	Jin Yin Hua (Lonicera flower)	*Flos Lonicerae*
連　翹	Lian Qian (Forsythia fruit)	*Fructus Forsythiae*
蒲公英	Pu Gong Ying (Dandelion)	*Herba Taraxaci*
板藍根	Ban Lang Gen (Isatis root)	*Radix Isatidis*

3. With cough and sputum, difficult to spit, add:

桔　梗	Jie Geng (Platycodon)	*Radix Platycodi*
前　胡	Qian Hu (Peucedanum root)	*Radix Peucedani*
杏　仁	Xing Ren (Apricot seed)	*Semen Armeniacae Amarum*

4. With nausea, chest and abdominal distention, add:

陳　皮	Chen Pi (Citrus peel)	*Pericarpium Citri Reticulatae*
厚　朴	Hou Po (Magnolia bark)	*Cortex Magnoliae Officinalis*
藿　香	Huo Xiang (Agastache)	*Herba Agastachis*
佩　蘭	Pei Lan (Eupatorium)	*Herba Eupatorii*

Dà Bǔ Yīn Wán　　大補陰丸
(Ta-Pu-Yin-Wan)
(Pills for Replenishing the Yin)

Constituents:

知　母	Zhi Mu (Anemarrhena)	20 gm.	*Rhizoma Anemarrhena*
黄　柏	Huang Bai (Phellodendron)	20 gm.	*Cortex Phellodendri*
熟地黄	Shu Di Huang (Prep. rehmannia)	30 gm.	*Radix Rehmanniae Praeparatae*
龜　板	Gui Ban (Turtle plastron)	30 gm.	*Plastrum Testudinis*
豬脊髓	Zhu Ji Shui (bone marrow of pig)	50 gm.	

Mix the above ingredients into pills.

Action:

1. To replenish the water content in the kidney
2. to subdue the upflaring of fire caused by deficiency of *Yin* (vital essence) of the kidney.

Indication:

For a person with upflaring of fire caused by deficiency of *Yin* (vital essence) of the kidney. The symptoms are: tidal fever, steaming sensation in the bones, night perspiration, lumbago, face red, dizziness or vertigo, tinnitus, cough with blood, restlessness, nocturnal spermatorrhea.

Tongue: red with thin coating
Pulse: rapid and forceful

Application:

Spermatorrhea, lumbago, tuberculosis, diabetes, chronic nephritis, tinnitus, Addison's disease.

Dà Chái Hú Tāng　大柴胡湯
(Ta-Chai-Hu-Tang)
(Major Bupleurum Decoction)

Constituents:

柴　胡	Chai Hu (Bupleurum)	9-12 gm.	*Radix Bupleuri*
黃　芩	Huang Qin (Scutellaria)	9-12 gm.	*Radix Scutellariae*
枳　實	Zhi Shi (Immature bitter orange)	6-9 gm.	*Fructus Aurantii Immaturus*
大　黃	Da Huang (Rhubarb)	6-9 gm.	*Radix et Rhizoma Rhei*
半　夏	Ban Xia (Pinellia)	6-9 gm.	*Rhizoma Pinelliae*
白芍藥	Bai Shao Yao (White peony)	6-9 gm.	*Radix Paeoniae Alba*
生　薑	Sheng Jiang (Fresh ginger)	3-6 gm.	*Rhizoma Zingiberis Recens*
大　棗	Da Zao (Jujube)	3-5 pc.	*Fructus Ziziphus Jujubae*

Action:

1. To mediate the Shao-yang (Minor Yang) channel
2. To purge the interior heat

Indication:

For a person with syndromes of the Shao-yang (Minor Yang) and Yang-ming channels. The symptoms are: alternate chills and fever, mouth bitter, vomiting, fullness and oppression or spasmodic pain in the epigastric region, constipation or diarrhea.

Tongue: with yellow coating
Pulse: wiry/taut and forceful

Application:

Simple intestinal obstruction, acute pancreatitis, acute cholecystitis, biliary calculus.

Modification:

1. With jaundice, add:

茵陳蒿	Yin Chen Hao (Capillaris)	*Herba Artemisiae Capillaris*
梔　子	Zhi Zi (Gardenia fruit)	*Fructus Gardeniae*
黃　柏	Huang Bai (Phellodendron)	*Cortex Phellodendri*

2. With vomiting, add:

黃　連	Huang Lian (Coptis)	*Rhizoma Coptidis*
吳茱萸	Wu Zhu Yu (Evodia fruit)	*Fructus Evodiae*
竹　茹	Zhu Ru (Bamboo shavings)	*Caulus Bambusae in Taenis*

3. With constipation, add:

芒　硝	Mang Xiao (Mirabilitum)	*Natrii Sulfas*

Generic Name:

Major Bupleurum Combination

Dà Chéng Qì Tāng　　大承氣湯
(Ta-Cheng-Chi-Tang)
(Drastic Purgative Decoction)

Constituents:

大 黃	Da Huang (Rhubarb)	9-12 gm.	*Radix et Rhizoma Rhei*
芒 硝	Mang Xiao (Mirabilitum)	6-9 gm.	*Natrii Sulfas*
厚 朴	Hou Po (Magnolia bark)	9-12 gm.	*Cortex Magnoliae Officinalis*
枳 實	Zhi Shi (Immature bitter orange)	9-12 gm.	*Fructus Aurantii Immaturus*

Action:

To purge the true heat in the stomach and intestines

Indication:

1. For excessiveness symptom-complex in the Yang-ming bowels. The symptoms are: constipation, fever, abdominal fullness, delirium, irritability, tongue yellow and prickly, pulse deep and forceful.

2. For accumulation of pathogenic heat and dry stool in the intestines, with symptoms of watery diarrhea, abdominal pain and fullness, mouth and tongue dry, pulse slippery and rapid

3. For syncope and seizures

Application:

Constipation, acute simple intestinal obstruction, acute cholecystitis, acute appendicitis, syncope, seizures.

Method of Preparation:

Decoct Hou Po (Magnolia bark 厚朴) and Zhi Shi (Immature bitter orange 枳實) first, then add Da Huang (Rhubarb 大黃), and add Mang Xiao (Mirabilitum 芒硝) last.

Generic Name:

Major Rhubarb Combination

Dà Dìng Fēng Zhū 大定風珠
(Ta-Ting-Feng-Chu)
(The Big Pearl for Endogenous Wind)

Constituents:

雞子黃	Ji Zi Huang (Egg yolk)	1-2 pc.	
阿 膠	E Jiao (Donkey-hide gelatin)	6-9 gm.	*Colla Corti Asini*
生地黃	Sheng Di Huang (Fresh rehmannia)	10-15 gm.	*Radix Rehmanniae*
麥門冬	Mai Men Dong (Ophiopogon)	10-15 gm.	*Radix Ophiopogonis*
白芍藥	Bai Shao Yao (White peony)	9-12 gm.	*Radix Paeoniae Alba*
龜 板	Gui Ban (Tortoise plastron)	9-12 gm.	*Plastrum Testudinis*
鱉 甲	Bei Jia (Tortoise shell)	9-12 gm.	*Carapax Trionycis*
牡 蠣	Mu Li (Oyster shell)	9-12 gm.	*Concha Ostreae*
五味子	Wu Wei Zi (Schisandra)	6-9 gm.	*Fructus Schisandrae*
火麻仁	Huo Ma Ren (Cannabis seed)	6-9 gm.	*Fructus Cannabis*
炙甘草	Zhi Gan Cao (Baked licorice)	3-6 gm.	*Radix Glycyrrhizae Praeparatae*

Action:

1. To replenish the *Yin* (vital essence)
2. To subdue the endogenous wind

Indication:

For a person with clonic convulsions due to the depletion of *Yin* (vital essence) and thus the hyperactivity of the endogenous wind. The symptoms are: fatigue, clonic convulsion, prostration.

> Tongue: dark red with thin coating
> Pulse: weak and faint

Application:

Prostration, clonic convulsions, encephalitis (type B), muscular atrophy, Wilson's disease (hepatocuticular degeneration), sclerosis of funiculus lateralis, athetosis.

Modification:

1. With spontaneous perspiration, add:

龍 骨	Long Gu (Dragon's bone)	*Os Draconis*
浮小麥	Fu Xiao Mai (Light wheat)	*Fructus Tritici Levis*

2. With palpitation, add:

茯 神	Fu Shen (Poria)	*Poria*
黨 參	Dang Shen (Codonopsis)	*Radix Codonopsis Pilosulae*

3. With panting, add:

人 參	Ren Shen (Ginseng)	*Radix Ginseng*

Dà Huáng Fù Zǐ Tāng　大黃附子湯
(Ta-Huang-Fu-Tzu-Tang)
(Decoction of Rhubarb and Aconite)

Constituents:

大　黃　Da Huang (Rhubarb)	6-9 gm.	*Radix et Rhizoma Rhei*
附　子　Fu Zi (Aconite)	6-9 gm.	*Radix Aconiti Praeparatae*
細　辛　Xi Xin (Asarum)	1-3 gm.	*Herba Asari*

Action:

1. To warm the body and dispel the cold
2. Purgative

Indication:

For a person with excessive accumulation of cold in the body. The symptoms are: constipation, abdominal and unilateral pain in the hypochondrium, cold hands and feet, intolerance of cold.

    Tongue: white coating
    Pulse: wiry/taut and tight

Application:

Hernia

Modification:

1. With abdominal fullness, add:

厚　朴　Hou Po (Magnolia bark)	*Cortex Magnoliae Officinalis*
木　香　Mu Xiang (Saussurea)	*Radix Saussureae*

2. For a person with weak constitution, add:

黨　參　Dang Shen (Codonopsis)	*Radix Codonopsis Pilosulae*
當　歸　Dang Gui (Chinese angelica root)	*Radix Angelicae Sinensis*

Generic Name:

Rhubarb and Aconite Combination

Dà Huáng Mǔ Dān Pí Tāng 大黄牡丹皮湯
(Ta-Huang-Mu-Tan-Pi-Tang)
(Decoction of Rhubarb and Moutan Bark)

Constituents:

大　黄 Da Huang (Rhubarb)	9-12 gm.	*Radix et Rhizoma Rhei*
牡丹皮 Mu Dan Pi (Moutan bark)	6-9 gm.	*Cortex Moutan Radicis*
桃　仁 Tao Ren (Persica seed)	6-9 gm.	*Semen Persicae*
冬瓜仁 Dong Gua Ren (Benincasa seed)	15-30 gm.	*Semen Benincasae*
芒　硝 Mang Xiao (Mirabilitum)	6-9 gm.	*Natrii Sulfas*

Action:

1. To eliminate the stagnant heat in the intestines
2. To disperse lumps and reduce swelling

Indication:

For intestinal abscess. The symptoms are: right lower abdominal pain, refused to be pressed, with hard lumps, prefer to put right leg in flexed posture rather than in extended posture.

Tongue: with white or yellow greasy coating
Pulse: wiry/taut and tight or rapid

Application:

Intestinal abscess, acute appendicitis, adnexitis, pelvic inflammation.

Contraindication:

For a weak, elderly, pregnant person with appendicitis.

Modification:

To enhance the effect for the treatment of acute appendicitis, add:

黄　連 Huang Lian (Coptis)	*Rhizoma Coptidis*
金銀花 Jin Yin Hua (Lonicera flower)	*Flos Lonicerae*
蒲公英 Pu Gong Yin (Dandelion)	*Herba Taraxaci*
敗醬草 Bai Jiang Cao (Thlaspi)	*Herba Thlaspii*
赤芍藥 Chi Shao Yao (Red peony)	*Radix Paeoniae Rubra*

Generic Name:

Rhubarb and Moutan Combination

Dà Jiàn Zhōng Tāng   大建中湯
(Ta-Chien-Chung-Tang)
(Major Decoction for Restoring the Normal Function of the Middle Burner)

Constituents:

花 椒	Hua Jiao (Zanthoxylum)	3-6 gm.	*Pericarpium Zanthoxyli*
乾 薑	Gan Jiang (Dry ginger)	6-9 gm.	*Rhizoma Zingiberis*
人 參	Ren Shen (Ginseng)	6-9 gm.	*Radix Ginseng*
飴 糖	Yi Tang (Maltose)	30-60 gm.	*Oryza Sativa*

Action:

1. To replenish the *Yang* (vital function) of the spleen and stomach
2. To relieve spasmodic pain of the abdomen

Indication:

For a person with deficiency of *Yang* (vital function) of the spleen and stomach, and with severe abdominal pain. The symptoms are: vomit, severe abdominal pain, inability to take in any food.

> Tongue: with white and greasy coating, tongue proper pale
> or dark purple
> Pulse: wiry/taut and slow; or deep and thready

Application:

Severe abdominal pain with spasms, biliary ascariasis, gastric or duodenal ulcer, vomiting.

Modification:

1. With constipation, add:

大 黄	Da Huang (Rhubarb)	*Radix et Rhizoma Rhei*
芒 硝	Mang Xiao (Mirabilitum)	*Natrii Sulfas*

2. With cold hands and feet, add:

桂 枝	Gui Zhi (Cinnamon twig)	*Ramulus Cinnamomi*
細 辛	Xi Xin (Asarum)	*Herba Asari*

3. With blood stasis, add:

三 棱	San Leng (Burreed tuber)	*Rhizoma Sparganii*
莪 术	E Zhu (Zedoary)	*Rhizoma Zedoariae*

4. With stagnancy of flow of vital energy, add:

砂 仁	Sha Ren (Cardamon)	*Fructus Amomi*
檀 香	Tan Xiang (Sandal wood)	*Lignum Santali Albi*

Generic Name:

Major Zanthoxylum Combination

Dà Qīng Lóng Tāng　　大青龍湯

(Ta-Ching-Lung-Tang)
(Major Decoction of Blue Dragon)

Constituents:

麻 黄	Ma Huang (Ephedra)	10-15 gm.	*Herba Ephedrae*
桂 枝	Gui Zhi (Cinnamon twig)	6-9 gm.	*Ramulus Cinnamomi*
杏 仁	Xing Ren (Apricot seed)	9-12 gm.	*Semen Armeniacae Amarum*
石 膏	Shi Gao (Gypsum)	10-20 gm.	*Gypsum Fibrosum*
炙甘草	Zhi Gan Cao (Baked licorice)	3-6 gm.	*Radix Glycyrrhizae Praeparatae*
生 薑	Sheng Jiang (Fresh ginger)	3-6 gm.	*Rhizome Zingiberis Recens*
大 棗	Da Zao (Jujube)	3-5 pc.	*Fructus Ziziphus Jujubae*

Action:

1. To dispel exterior wind and cold
2. To eliminate interior heat

Indication:

For a person with exterior affection of wind and cold, and interior heat. The symptoms are: fever, intolerance of cold, headache, muscle-ache, no perspiration, asthma, thirst, edema, restlessness, and fidgetiness.

> Pulse: floating and tight or rapid
> Tongue: with thin white or yellow coating

Application:

Common cold, influenza, fidgetiness, edema, pleurisy with cough.

Generic Name:

Major Blue Dragon Combination

Dà Xiàn Xiōng Tāng 大陷胸湯
(Ta-Hsien-Hsiung-Tang)
(Major Decoction Sinking into the Chest)

Constituents:

大 黃 Da Huang (Rhubarb)	9-12 gm.	*Radix et Rhizoma Rhei*
芒 硝 Mang Xiao (Mirabilitum)	9-12 gm.	*Natrii Sulfas*
甘 遂 Gan Sui (Kansui root)	1-3 gm.	*Radix Euphorbiae Kansui*

Action:

1. To purge the interior heat
2. To dispel water
3. To disperse lumps or hardening

Indication:

For a person with accumulation of heat and water in the chest and abdomen. The symptoms are: constipation, epigastric and abdominal pain and hard, thirst, afternoon fever.

      Tongue; red and dry
      Pulse: deep and tight

Application:

Acute pancreatitis with edema, acute intestinal obstruction, intercostal neuralgia.

Contraindication:

For a very weak or chronic patient.

Method of Preparation:

Decoct Da Huang (Rhubarb) first, then add the other two ingredients.

Generic Name:

Rhubarb and Kansui Combination

Dá Yuán Yǐn 達原飲 (达原饮)
(Ta-Yuan-Yin)
(Decoction Acting on the Half-exterior & Half-interior Portion of the Body)

Constituents:

檳 榔	Bing Lang (Areca seed)	6-9 gm.	*Semen Arecae*
厚 朴	Hou Po (Magnolia bark)	3-6 gm.	*Cortex Magnoliae Officinalis*
草 果	Cao Guo (Tsao-ko)	1-3 gm.	*Fructus Tsaoko*
黃 芩	Huang Qin (Scutellaria)	3-6 gm.	*Radix Scutellariae*
知 母	Zhi Mu (Anemarrhena)	3-6 gm.	*Rhizoma Anemarrhenae*
白芍藥	Bai Shao (White peony)	6-9 gm.	*Radix Paeoniae Alba*
甘 草	Gan Cao (Licorice)	1-3 gm.	*Radix Glycyrrhizae*

Action:

To eliminate the dirt and turbidity in the half-exterior and half-interior portion of the body.

Indication:

For a person with epidemic diseases or malaria with the pathogenic factors hidden in the half-exterior and half-interior portion of the body. The symptoms are: alternate chills and fever, nausea, stuffiness sensation in the chest, headache, restlessness.

Tongue: dark red along the side, with thick and greasy coating
Pulse: wiry/taut and rapid

Application:

Malaria, epidemic diseases, influenza.

Modification:

1. With dampness greater than heat in the body, add:

佩 蘭	Pei Lan (Eupatorium)	*Herba Eupatorii*
茵陳蒿	Yin Chen Hao (Capillaris)	*Herba Artemisiae capillaris*
	and eliminate:	
白 芍	Bai Shao (White peony)	*Radix Paeoniae Alba*
知 母	Zhi Mu (Anemarrhena)	*Rhizoma Anemarrhenae*

2. With fever higher and longer than chills, add:

白 薇	Bai Wei (Swallowwort)	*Radix Cynanchi Atrati*
梔 子	Zhi Zi (Gardenia fruit)	*Fructus Gardenia*
	and eliminate:	
檳 榔	Bing Lang (Areca seed)	*Semen Arecae*

Dǎn Dào Pái Shí Tāng   膽道排石湯 （胆道排石汤）
(Tan-Tao-Pai-Shih-Tang)
(Biliary Lithagogue Decoction)

Constituents:

金錢草	Jin Qian Cao (Lysimachia)	6-9 gm.	*Herba Lysimachiae*
茵陳蒿	Yin Chen Hao (Capillaris)	6-9 gm.	*Herba Artemisiae Capillaris*
郁 金	Yu Jin (Curcuma root)	6-9 gm.	*Radix Curcumae*
枳 殼	Zhi Ke (Bitter orange)	6-9 gm.	*Fructus Aurantii*
木 香	Mu Xiang (Saussurea)	6-9 gm.	*Radix Saussureae*
大 黄	Da Huang (Rhubarb)	6-9 gm.	*Radix et Rhizoma Rhei*

Action:

1. To eliminate heat and dampness
2. To invigorate the circulation of vital energy and relieve pain
3. To expel the calculi from the bile duct

Indication:

For a person with calculi in the bile duct. The symptoms are: fever, intolerance of cold, mouth bitter, indigestion, nausea and vomiting, distention of the chest and abdomen, severe pain in the upper right abdomen (especially after a meal or after eating greasy food, may radiate to the right shoulder and back), jaundice, constipation, urine color amber.

Tongue: with thin yellow and greasy coating
Pulse: wiry/taut, slippery and rapid

Application:

Cholelithiasis

Dān Shēn Yǐn   丹參飲

(Tan-Sheng-Yin)
(Decoction of Salvia Root)

Constituents:

丹 參 Dan Shen (Salvia root)	15-30 gm.	*Radix Salviae Miltiorrhizae*
檀 香 Tan Xiang (Sandal wood)	3-6 gm.	*Ligmum Santali Albi*
砂 仁 Sha Ren (Cardamon)	3-6 gm.	*Fructus Amomi*

Action:

1. To invigorate the circulation of blood and *Qi* (vital energy)
2. To remove blood stasis and relieve pain

Indication:

For a person with angina pectoris due to stagnancy of both *Qi* (vital energy) and blood. The symptoms are: pain in the epigastric region and abdomen, radiating to the back or scapular, stuffiness sensation in the chest, shortness of breath, hiccup, constipation, loss of appetite.

Tongue: purple with purple spots
Pulse: hesitant, or wiry/taut and tight

Application:

Angina pectoris

Dān Zhī Xiāo Yáo Sàn　　丹栀逍遥散
(Tan-Chi-Hsiao-Yao-San)
(The Ease Powder plus Moutan Bark and Gardenia)

Constituents:

牡丹皮	Mu Dan Pi (Moutan bark)	6-9 gm.	*Cortex Moutan Radicis*
栀 子	Zhi Zi (Gardenia fruit)	3-6 gm.	*Fructus Gardeniae*
柴 胡	Chai Hu (Bupleurum)	6-9 gm.	*Radix Bupleuri*
當 歸	Dang Gui (Chinese angelica)	6-9 gm.	*Radix Angelicae Sinensis*
白芍藥	Bai Shao Yao (White peony)	9-12 gm.	*Radix Paeoniae Alba*
白 术	Bai Zhu (White atractylodes)	6-9 gm.	*Rhizoma Atractylodis Macrocephalae*
茯 苓	Fu Ling (Poria)	9-15 gm.	*Poria*
薄 荷	Bo He (Mentha)	1-3 gm.	*Herba Menthae*
生 薑	Sheng Jiang (Fresh ginger)	1-3 gm.	*Rhizoma Zingiberis Recens*
炙甘草	Zhi Gan Cao (Baked licorice)	3-6 gm.	*Radix Glycyrrhizae Praeparatae*

Action:

1. To relieve the stagnation of liver *Qi* (vital energy)
2. To replenish blood and reinforce the spleen
3. To eliminate heat in the liver

Indication:

For a person with stagnation of liver *Qi* (vital energy), and with heat in the body due to deficiency of blood. The symptoms are: fever or tidal fever, spontaneous or night sweat, headache, blood-shot eyes, restlessness, cheeks red, mouth dry, irregular menstruation, abdominal pain, heavy sensation in the lower abdomen, pain and difficulty in urination.

> Tongue: red
> Pulse: wiry/taut and rapid

Application:

Chronic hepatitis, irregular menstruation, uterine bleeding, climacteric syndromes.

Generic Name:

Bupleurum and Peony Formula

68

Dāng Guī Bǔ Xuè Tāng　當歸補血湯 (当归补血汤)
(Tang-Kuei-Pu-Hsieh-Tang)
(Blood Tonifying Decoction with Chinese Angelica)

Constituents:

| 黃 芪 | Huang Qi (Astragalus) | 30 gm. | Radix Astragali |
| 當 歸 | Dang Gui (Chinese angelica) | 6-9 gm. | Radix Angelicae Sinensis |

Action:

1. To replenish *Qi* and blood
2. To promote the healing of wounds

Indication:

For a person with anemia and high body temperature. The symptoms are: fever, anemia, fatigue, headache, flushed face, thirst but with no desire to drink water, excessive loss of blood, or with purulent abscess.

Tongue: pale
Pulse: gigantic and weak

Application:

Anemia, uterine bleeding, post-partum bleeding, purulent abscesses.

Modification:

1. For a female with common cold and fever with headache during menstruation or after birth, add:

葱 白	Cong Bai (Allium bulb)	Bulbus Allii Fistulosumi
淡豆豉	Dan Dou Chi (Prepared soybean)	Semen Sojae Praepartatum
生 薑	Sheng Jiang (Fresh ginger)	Rhizoma Zingiberis Recens
大 棗	Da Zao (Jujube)	Fructus Ziziphus Jujubae

2. For general anemia, add:

熟地黃	Shu Di Huang (Prep. rehmannia)	Radix Rehmanniae Praeparatae
何首烏	He Shou Wu (Fleeceflower root)	Radix Polygoni Multiflori
桑寄生	Sang Ji Sheng (Mulberry mistletoe)	Ramulus Loranthi
白芍藥	Bai Shao Yao (White peony)	Radix Paeoniae Alba

Generic Name:

Tang-kuei and Astragalus Combination

Dāng Guī Jiàn Zhōng Tāng　當歸健中湯　(当归健中汤)

(Tang-Kuei-Chien-Chung-Tang)
(Decoction for Restoring the Normal Function of the Middle Burner with Chinese Angelica)

Constituents:

當 歸	Dang Gui (Chinese angelica)	6-9 gm.	*Radix Angelicae Sinensis*
飴 糖	Yi Tang (Maltose)	20-30 gm.	*Saccharum Granorum*
桂 枝	Gui Zhi (Cinnamon twig)	6-9 gm.	*Ramulus Cinnamomi*
白 芍	Bai Shao Yao (White peony)	10-15 gm.	*Radix Paeoniae Alba*
炙甘草	Zhi Gan Cao (Baked licorice)	3-6 gm.	*Radix Glycyrrhizae Preparata*
生 薑	Sheng Jiang (Fresh ginger)	3-6 gm.	*Rhizoma Zingiberis Recens*
大 棗	Da Zao (Jujube)	3-5 pc.	*Fructus Ziziphus Jujubae*

Action:

1. To warm and tonify the spleen and stomach
2. To relieve spasmodic pain

Indication:

For a person with spasmodic pain due to deficiency of blood. The symptoms are: face pale, fatigue, anemia, lose of appetite, incessant abdominal pain with spasms, or with radiation to the waist and back.

Tongue: pale with white coating
Pulse: slow and weak

Application:

Postpartum fever, aplastic anemia, gastric and duodenal ulcer, gastric and intestinal spasms.

Generic Name:

Tang-kuei, Cinnamon and Peony Combination

Dāng Guī Liù Huáng Tāng　當歸六黃湯（当归六黄汤）
(Tang-Kuei-Liu-Huang-Tang)
(Decoction of Chinese Angelica and Six Yellow Ingredients)

Constituents:

當　歸	Dang Gui (Chinese angelica)	6-9 gm.	*Radix Angelicae Sinensis*
生地黃	Sheng Di Huang (Fresh rehmannia)	12-15 gm.	*Radix Rehmanniae*
熟地黃	Shu Di Huang (Prep. rehmannia)	12-15 gm.	*Radix Rehmanniae Praeparatae*
黃　芪	Huang Qi (Astragalus)	9-15 gm.	*Rhizoma Astragali*
黃　連	Huang Lian (Coptis)	3-6 gm.	*Rhizoma Coptidis*
黃　芩	Huang Qin (Scutellaria)	6-12 gm.	*Radix Scutellariae*
黃　柏	Huang Bai (Phellodendron)	6-12 gm.	*Cortex Phellodendri*

Action:

1. Anti-hidrotic
2. To replenish both *Qi* (vital energy) and blood
3. To purge the fire
4. To replenish the *Yin* (vital essence)
5. To consolidate the exterior defensive system

Indication:

For a person with deficiency of *Yin* (vital essence) and blood, with hyperactivity of fire. The symptoms are: fever, night sweat, dry mouth, vexation.

Tongue: dark red and dry
Pulse: rapid

Application:

Pulmonary tuberculosis, chronic febrile disease.

Modification:

1. With severe night sweat, add:

麻黃根	Ma Huang Gen (Ephedra root)	*Radix Ephedrae*
浮小麥	Fu Xiao Mai (Light wheat)	*Fructus Tritici Levis*
糯稻根鬚	Nuo Dao Gen Xu (Rice rhizome)	*Rhizoma Oryzae*

2. To replenish *Yin* (vital essence), add:

牡　蠣	Mu Li (Oyster shell)	*Concha Ostreae*
龜　板	Gui Ban (Tortoise plastron)	*Plastrum Testudinis*
鱉　甲	Bie Jia (Tortoise shell)	*Carapax Trionycis*

Dāng Guī Lóng Huì Wán 當歸龍薈丸 (当归龙荟丸)
(Tang-Kuei-Long-Hui-Wan)
(Pills of Chinese Angelica, Gentiana and Aloe)

Constituents:

當 歸	Dang Gui (Chinese angelica)	6-9 gm.	Radix Angelicae Sinensis
蘆 薈	Lu Hui (Aloe)	6-9 gm.	Aloe
龍膽草	Long Dan Cao (Gentiana)	6-9 gm.	Radix Gentianae
黃 連	Huang Lian (Coptis)	9-12 gm.	Rhizoma Coptidis
黃 芩	Huang Qin (Scutellaria)	9-12 gm.	Radix Scutellariae
黃 柏	Huang Bai (Phellodendron)	9-12 gm.	Cortex Phellodendri
栀 子	Zhi Zi (Gardenia fruit)	3-6 gm.	Fructus Gardeniae
大 黃	Da Huang (Rhubarb)	3-6 gm.	Radix et Rhizoma Rhei
青 黛	Qing Dai (Indigo)	3-6 gm.	Indigo Naturalis
木 香	Mu Xiang (Saussurea root)	6-9 gm.	Radix Saussureae
麝 香	She Xiang (Musk)	.3-.5 gm.	Moschus

Action:

To purge the fire of liver and gallbladder (Febrifugal)

Indication:

For a person with true or excessive heat or fire in the liver and gallbladder.
The symptoms are: headache, dizziness, vertigo, face red, eyes red,
irritable, mouth bitter, throat dry, tinnitus, delirium, mania, abdominal
fullness, constipation, urine yellow or amber, chest pain.

> Tongue: red with yellow coating
> Pulse: wiry/taut and rapid

Application:

Hypertension, mania, convulsions, leukemia, hypochondriac pain.

Dāng Guī Sháo Yào Sàn 當歸芍藥散 (当归芍药散)
(Tang-Kuei-Shao-Yao-San)
(Powder of Chinese Angelica and White Peony)

Constituents:

當 歸	Dang Gui (Chinese angelica)	6-9 gm.	*Radix Angelicae Sinensis*
白芍藥	Bai Shao Yao (White peony)	6-9 gm.	*Radix Paeoniae Alba*
白 术	Bai Zhu (White atractylodes)	6-9 gm.	*Rhizoma Atractylodis Macrocephalae*
川 芎	Chuan Xiong (Ligusticum)	6-9 gm.	*Rhizoma Ligustici Chuanxiong*
茯 苓	Fu Ling (Poria)	6-9 gm.	*Poria*
澤 瀉	Ze Xie (Alisma)	6-9 gm.	*Rhizoma Alismatis*

Action:

1. To replenish blood
2. To reinforce the spleen and kidney

Indication:

For a person with anemia and abdominal pain due to spleen and kidney asthenia. The symptoms are: pale face, fatigue, anemia, abdominal pain, heaviness sensation of the head, dizziness, tinnitus, lumbago, palpitation, cold feet, edema.

Tongue: pale with thin coating
Pulse: deep and weak

Application:

Anemia, lumbago, menopause, irregular menstruation, edema, chronic nephritis.

Generic Name:

Tang-kuei and Peony Formula

Dāng Guī Sì Nì Jiā Wú Zhū Yú Shēng Jiāng Tāng

當歸四逆加吳茱萸生薑湯 （当归四逆加吴茱萸生姜汤）

(Tang-Kuei-Si-Ni-Chia-Wu-Chu-Yu-Sheng-Chiang-Tang)

(Decoction with Chinese Angelica, Evodia & Fresh Ginger
for Vital Prostration with Cold Limbs)

Constituents:

當 歸	Dang Gui (Chinese angelica)	9-12 gm.	*Radix Angelicae Sinensis*
吳茱萸	Wu Zhu Yu (Evodia)	3-6 gm.	*Fructus Evodiae*
生 薑	Sheng Jiang (Fresh ginger)	3-6 gm.	*Rhizoma Zingiberis Recens*
桂 枝	Gui Zhi (Cinnamon twig)	9-12 gm.	*Ramulus Cinnamomi*
白芍藥	Bai Shao Yao (White peony)	10-15 gm.	*Radix Paeoniae Alba*
細 辛	Xi Xin (Asarum)	3-6 gm.	*Herba Asari*
木 通	Mu Tong (Akebia)	6-9 gm.	*Caulis Akebiae*
炙甘草	Zhi Gan Cao (Baked licorice)	3-6 gm.	*Radix Glycyrrhizae Praeparatae*
大 棗	Da Zao (Jujube)	3-5 pc.	*Fructus Ziziphus Jujubae*

Action:

1. To warm the channels and collaterals and dispel cold
2. To nourish the blood and the vascular system
3. Anti-emetic

Indication:

For a person with vomiting, retention of fluid, and cold due to deficiency of blood. The symptoms are: cold hands and feet, anemia, vomiting with frothy fluid, retention of fluid in the stomach, and vertical headache.

> Tongue: pale with white coating
> Pulse: soft and weak

Application:

Vomiting with vertical headache, anemia, arthritis, hernia, frostbite, menstrual pain, thromboangiitis obliterans (Buerger's disease).

Generic Name:

Tang-kuei, Evodia and Ginger Combination

Dāng Guī Sì Nì Tāng　當歸四逆湯 (当归四逆汤)
(Tang-Kuei-Szu-Ni-Tang)
(Decoction with Chinese Angelica for Treating Vital Prostration with Cold Limbs)

Constituents:

當　歸	Dang Gui (Chinese angelica)	9-12 gm.	*Radix Angelicae Sinensis*
桂　枝	Gui Zhi (Cinnamon twig)	9-12 gm.	*Ramulus Cinnamomi*
白芍藥	Bai Shao Yao (White peony)	10-15 gm.	*Radix Paeoniae Alba*
細　辛	Xi Xin (Asarum)	3-6 gm.	*Herba Asari*
木　通	Mu Tong (Akebia)	6-9 gm.	*Caulis Akebiae*
炙甘草	Zhi Gan Cao (Baked licorice)	3-6 gm.	*Radix Glycyrrhizae Praeparatae*
大　棗	Da Zao (Jujube)	3-5 pc.	*Fructus Ziziphus Jujubae*

Action:

1. To warm the channels and dispel cold
2. To nourish the blood and invigorate the vascular system.

Indication:

For a person with cold due to deficiency of blood. The symptoms are: anemia, with cold hands and feet.

> Tongue: pale with white coating
> Pulse: deep and thready

Application:

Anemia, arthritis, hernia (due to cold), frostbite, menstrual abdominal pain, thromboangiitis obliterans (Buerger's disease).

Modification:

With vertical headache, vomiting with foams, add:

吳茱萸	Wu Zhu Yu (Evodia)	*Fructus Evodiae*
生　薑	Sheng Jiang (Fresh ginger)	*Rhizoma Zingiberis Recens*

This formula is now called: Dang Gui Si Ni Jia Wu Zhu Yu Sheng Jiang Tang 當歸四逆加吳茱萸生薑湯

Generic Name:

Tang-kuei and Jujube Combination

Dǎo Chì Sàn　　　導赤散　(导赤散)
(Tao-Chih-San)
(Powder to Conduct the Heart Fire Downward)

Constituents:

生地黄	Sheng Di Huang (Fresh rehmannia)	10-15 gm.	*Radix Rehmanniae*
木　通	Mu Tong (Akebia)	9-12 gm.	*Caulis Akebiae*
竹　葉	Zhu Ye (Bamboo leaf)	6-9 gm.	*Folium Bambusae*
甘草梢	Gan Cao Shao (Licorice)	3-6 gm.	*Radix Glycyrrhizae Praeparatae*

Action:

To conduct the heat/fire from the heart channel down to the small intestine and purged through urination. The symptoms are: annoying heat sensation in the heart and chest, face red, thirsty (like to drink cold drink), infection of the oral cavity, urine color amber, urination short, hesitant and painful.

> Tongue: red
> Pulse: rapid

Application:

Acute urinary tract infection, infection of the oral cavity.

Modification:

1. With excessive heart fire, add:

黄　連　Huang Lian (Coptis)　　　　*Rhizoma Coptidis*

2. For hematuria, add:

旱蓮草　Han Lian Cao (Eclipta)　　　*Herba Ecliptae*
小　薊　Xiao Ji (Small thistle)　　　　*Herba Cephalanoploris*

Generic Name:

Rehmannia and Akebia Formula

Dǎo Qì Tāng   導氣湯 (导气汤)

(Tao-Chi-Tang)
(Conducting the Vital Energy Decoction)

Constituents:

川楝子	Chuan Lian Zi (Sichuan chinaberry)	12-16 gm.	*Fructus Meliae Toosendan*
木 香	Mu Xiang (Saussurea)	6-9 gm.	*Radix Saussureae*
茴 香	Hui Xiang (Fennel fruit)	3-6 gm.	*Fructus Foeniculi*
吳茱萸	Wu Zhu Yu (Evodia)	3-6 gm.	*Fructus Evodiae*

Action:

1. To dispel cold in the liver channel
2. To invigorate the circulation of *Qi* (vital energy)
3. To relieve hernia pain

Indication:

For a person with inguinal hernia caused by stagnation of cold and vital energy, with manifestation of pain in the lower lateral abdomen, radiating to the genital region, normal cord structure is palpable.

Tongue: pale with white coating
Pulse: deep, slow or wiry/taut

Application:

Inguinal hernia

Modification:

1. If hernia is caused by cold, add:

肉 桂	Rou Gui (Cinnamon bark)	*Cortex Cinnamomi*
烏 药	Wu Yao (Lindera)	*Radix Linderae*

2. If hernia is caused by heat, add:

龍膽草	Long Dan Cao (Gentiana)	*Radix Gentianae*
黃 芩	Huang Qin (Scutellaria)	*Radix Scutellariae*
梔 子	Zhi Zi (Gardenia)	*Fructus Gardeniae*

3. If hernia is caused by dampness, add:

蒼 术	Cang Zhu (Atractylodes)	*Rhizoma Atractylodis*
薏苡仁	Yi Yi Ren (Coix)	*Semen Coicis*

Dǎo Tán Tāng 導痰湯 (导痰汤)
(Tao-Tan-Tang)
(The Phlegm Resolving Decoction)

Constituents:

制南星	Zhi Nan Xing (Prepared Arisaema)	6-9 gm.	*Rhizoma Arisaematis Praeparatae*
枳實	Zhi Shi (Immature bitter orange)	6-9 gm.	*Fructus Aurantii Immaturus*
半夏	Ban Xia (Pinellia)	6-9 gm.	*Rhizoma Pinelliae*
陳皮	Chen Pi (Citrus peel)	3-6 gm.	*Pericarpium Citri Reticulatae*
茯苓	Fu Ling (Poria)	6-9 gm.	*Poria*
甘草	Gan Cao (Licorice)	3-6 gm.	*Radix Glycyrrhizae*

Action:

1. To resolve phlegm
2. Antitussive

Indication:

For a person with coma due to obstruction of phlegm. The symptoms are: dizziness or vertigo, headache, dyspnea, cough with thick and sticky sputum, vomiting, fullness and oppression in the chest, epigastric and hypochondriac region, restlessness, loss of appetite.

Tongue: white with greasy fur
Pulse: slippery

Application:

Chronic tracheitis, bronchitis, pulmonary emphysema, goiter, obesity, amenorrhea

Dì Huáng Yǐn Zǐ　　地黄飲子

(Ti-Huang-Yin-Tzu)
(Decoction with Rehmannia for Aphasia & Paralysis)

Constituents:

熟地黃	Di Huang (Dry or prepared rehmannia)	6-9 gm.	*Radix Rehmanniae Praeparatae*
山茱萸	Shan Zhu Yu (Cornus)	9-12 gm.	*Fructus Corni*
巴戟天	Ba Ji Tian (Morinda)	6-9 gm.	*Radix Morindae Officinalis*
肉蓯蓉	Rou Cong Rong (Cistanche)	9-12 gm.	*Herba Cistanchis*
肉　桂	Rou Gui (Cinnamon bark)	1-3 gm.	*Cortex Cinnamomi*
附　子	Fu Zi (Aconite)	3-6 gm.	*Radix Aconiti Praeparatae*
石　斛	Shi Hu (Dendrobium)	6-9 gm.	*Herba Dendrobii*
麥門冬	Mai Men Dong (Ophiopogon)	6-9 gm.	*Radix Ophiopogonis*
五味子	Wu Wei Zi (Schisandra)	3-6 gm.	*Fructus Schisandrae*
茯　苓	Fu Ling (Poria)	6-9 gm.	*Poria*
九節菖蒲	Jiu Jie Chang Pu (Altaica)	3-6 gm.	*Rhizoma Anemoni Altaicae*
遠　志	Yuan Zhi (Polygala)	3-6 gm.	*Radix Polygalae*
薄　荷	Bo He (Mentha)	3-6 gm.	*Herba Menthae*
生　薑	Sheng Jiang (Fresh ginger)	3-6 gm.	*Rhizoma Zingiberis Recens*
大　棗	Da Zao (Jujube)	3-5 pc.	*Fructus Ziziphus Jujubae*

Action:

1. To replenish the *Yin* (vital essence) and *Yang* (vital function) of the kidney
2. To resolve phlegm and open the orifices

Indication:

For a person with aphasia and paralysis due to deficiency of both *Yin* (vital essence) and *Yang* (vital function) of the kidney. The symptoms are: aphasia, loss of speech, paralysis of the legs, mouth dry but with no desire to drink.

　　　　Tongue: with greasy coating
　　　　Pulse: deep, slow and thready or weak

Application:

Aphasia, paralysis of the legs.

Modification:

1. With deficiency of *Yin* (vital essence), add:

地骨皮	Di Gu Pi (Lycium bark)	*Cortex Lycii Radicis*
鱉　甲	Bie Jia (Tortoise shell)	*Carapax Trionycis*

2. With deficiency of *Yang* (vital function), add:

淫羊藿	Yin Yang Huo (Epimedium)	*Herba Epimedii*
仙　茅	Xian Mao (Curculigo)	*Rhizoma Curculiginis*

Dìng Chuǎn Tāng 定喘湯

(Ting-Chuan-Tang)
(Decoction for Asthma)

Constituents:

白 果	Bai Guo (Ginkgo seed)	3-7 pc.	*Semen Ginkgo*
麻 黃	Ma Huang (Ephedra)	6-9 gm.	*Herba Ephedrae*
蘇 子	Su Zi (Perilla seed)	9-12 gm.	*Fructus Perillae*
款冬花	Kuan Dong Hua (Tussilago)	9-12 gm.	*Flos Farfarae*
杏 仁	Xing Ren (Apricot seed)	9-12 gm.	*Semen Armeniacae Amarum*
桑白皮	Sang Bai Pi (Mulberry bark)	9-12 gm.	*Cortex Mori Radicis*
黃 芩	Huang Qin (Scutellaria)	6-9 gm.	*Radix Scutellariae*
半 夏	Ban Xia (Pinellia)	9-12 gm.	*Rhizoma Pinelliae*
甘 草	Gan Cao (Licorice)	3-6 gm.	*Radix Glycyrrhizae*

Action:

1. To clear the heat in the lung
2. Expectorant, anti-asthma

Indication:

For a person with asthma due to heat factors. The symptoms are: cough with thick, sticky and yellow sputum, difficult to spit out, dyspnea, wheezing, fidgetiness, face red, spontaneous perspiration, thirst with desire to drink water, headache, fever.

> Tongue: red with yellow and greasy coating
> Pulse: slippery and rapid

Application:

Asthma, chronic bronchitis, bronchial asthma, pulmonary emphysema.

Generic Name:

Ping Chuan Pill;
Ma-huang and Ginkgo Combination

Dīng Xiāng Shì Dì Tāng   丁香柿蒂湯
(Ting-Hsiang-Shih-Ti-Tang)
(Decoction of Cloves and Kaki Calyx)

Constituents:

丁 香	Ding Xiang (Cloves)	1-3 gm.	*Flos Caryophylli*
柿 蒂	Shi Di (Kaki or persimmon calyx)	6-9 gm.	*Calyx Kaki*
人 參	Ren Shen (Ginseng)	3-6 gm.	*Radix Ginseng*
生 薑	Sheng Jiang (Fresh ginger)	6-9 gm.	*Rhizoma Zingiberis Recens*

Action:

1. To warm the spleen and stomach and replenish the *Qi* (vital energy)
2. To reverse the upward flow of stomach *Qi* (anti-hiccup)

Indication:

For a person with hiccup caused by coldness and deficiency of *Qi* in the stomach. The symptoms are: hiccup, vomiting, abdominal fullness, chest distention, loss of appetite.

> Tongue: light with white coating
> Pulse: sinking, slow and weak

Application:

Hiccup, phreno-spasm in post abdominal operation, nervous hiccup.

Modification:

1. If the stomach *Qi* (vital energy) is not deficiency, subtract:
人 參 Ren Shen (Ginseng)   *Radix Ginseng*
This formula is called Shi Di Tang (Kaki Combination) (柿蒂湯)

2. If coldness of abdomen is not severe, subtract:
生 薑 Sheng Jiang (Fresh ginger)   *Rhizoma Zingiberis Recens*
This formula is now called Shi Qian San (柿錢散)

3. If there is stagnanation of *Qi* and phlegm, add:
陳 皮 Chen Pi (Citrus peel)   *Pericarpium Citri Reticulatae*
沉 香 Chen Xiang (Aquilaria wood)   *Lignum Aquilariae Resinatum*
半 夏 Ban Xia (Pinellia tuber)   *Rhizoma Pinelliae*

Generic Name:

Clove and Kaki Combination

Dú Huó Jì Shēng Tāng　獨活寄生湯（独活寄生汤）
(Tu-Huo-Chi-Sheng-Tang)
(Decoction of Pubescent Angelica and Loranthus)

Constituents:

獨　活	Du Huo (Pubescent angelica)	6-9 gm.	*Radix Angelicae Pubescentis*
秦　艽	Qin Jiao (Large leaf gentian)	3-6 gm.	*Radix Gentianae*
防　風	Fang Feng (Ledebouriella)	3-6 gm.	*Radix Ledebouriellae*
細　辛	Xi Xin (Asarum; Wild ginger)	1-3 gm.	*Herba Asari*
桑寄生	Sang Ji Sheng (Mulberry mistletoe)	6-9 gm.	*Ramulus Loranthi*
杜　仲	Du Zhong (Eucommia)	3-6 gm.	*Cortex Eucommiae*
懷牛膝	Huai Niu Xi (Achyranthes)	3-6 gm.	*Radix Achyranthis Bidentatae*
肉　桂	Rou Gui (Cinnamon bark)	1-3 gm.	*Cortex Cinnamomi*
當　歸	Dang Gui (Chinese angelica)	3-6 gm.	*Radix Angelicae Sinensis*
川　芎	Chuan Xiong (Ligusticum)	3-6 gm.	*Rhizoma Ligustici Chuanxiong*
地　黄	Di Huang (Rehmannia)	6-9 gm.	*Radix Rehmanniae*
白芍藥	Bai Shao Yao (White peony)	3-6 gm.	*Radix Paeoniae Alba*
人　參	Ren Shen (Ginseng)	3-6 gm.	*Radix Ginseng*
茯　苓	Fu Ling (Poria)	9-12 gm.	*Poria*
甘　草	Gan Cao (Licorice)	3-6 gm.	*Radix Glycyrrhizae*

Action:

1. To dispel wind, cold and dampness (anti-rheumatic)
2. To tonify the liver and kidney
3. To replenish *Qi* (vital energy) and blood

Indication:

For a person with chronic arthralgia, numbness, weak liver and kidney, deficiency of *Qi* (vital energy) and blood. The symptoms are: pain in the lumbar region and knees with cold sensation and difficulty of joint movements, paralysis, intolerance of cold but preference of heat.

Tongue: light color with white coating
Pulse: weak and feeble

Application:

Chronic rheumatic arthritis, rheumatic sciatica.

Contraindication: For a person with acute arthritis.

Modification:

1. If pain is severe, add:
川烏頭 Chuan Wu Tou (Sichuan aconite)　　*Radix Aconiti*
2. With blood stasis, add:
桃　仁 Tao Ren (Persica seed)　　*Semen Persicae*
紅　花 Hong Hua (Carthamus)　　*Flos Carthami*

Generic Name:

Du Huo Jisheng Tang; Tuhuo and Vaeicum Combination

Dū Qì Wán (Qī Wèi Dū Qì Wán) 都氣丸 (七味都氣丸)
(Tu-Chi-Wan) (Chi-Wei-Tu-Chi-Wan)
(Pills of all Qi)

Constituents:

五味子	Wu Wei Zi (Schisandra)	6-9 gm.	*Fructus Schisandrae*
熟地黃	Shu Di Huang (Prep. rehmannia)	10-15 gm.	*Radix Rehmanniae Praeparatae*
山茱萸	Shan Zhu Yu (Cornus)	9-12 gm.	*Fructus Corni*
山　藥	Shan Yao (Dioscorea)	10-15 gm.	*Rhizoma Dioscoreae*
澤　瀉	Ze Xie (Alisma)	9-12 gm.	*Rhizoma Alismatis*
牡丹皮	Mu Dan Pi (Moutan bark)	6-9 gm.	*Cortex Moutan Radicis*
茯　苓	Fu Ling (Poria)	9-12 gm.	*Poria*

Action:

1. To replenish the *Yin* (vital essence) of kidney
2. Antitussive and anti-asthma

Indication:

For a person with asthma due to deficiency of kidney. The symptoms are: cough, asthma, hiccup, dyspnea.

Tongue: red with thin coating
Pulse: thready and rapid

Application:

Asthma, bronchial asthma, pulmonary emphysema, pulmonary tuberculosis.

Generic Name:

Rehmannia and Schisandra Formula

Èr Chén Tāng　　二陳湯（二陈汤）

(Erh-Chen-Tang)
(Decoction of Two Herbs-Citrus peel and Pinellia)

Constituents:

半 夏	Ban Xia (Pinellia tuber)	6-9 gm.	*Rhizoma Pinelliae*
陳 皮	Chen Pi (Citrus peel)	3-6 gm.	*Pericarpium Citri Reticulate*
茯 苓	Fu Ling (Poria)	6-9 gm.	*Poria*
甘 草	Gan Cao (Licorice)	3-6 gm.	*Radix Glycyrrhizae*

and may add:

生 薑	Sheng Jiang (Fresh ginger)	7 pc.	*Rhizoma Zingiberis Recens*
烏 梅	Wu Mei (Mume; Black plums)	1 pc.	*Fructus Mume*

Action:

1. To resolve phlegm by drying internal dampness
2. To regulate the function of the spleen and stomach

Indication:

For a person with internal damp phlegm and *Qi* (vital energy) deficiency. The symptoms are: profuse watery and foamy sputum of white color, fullness over the epigastric region, nausea, vomiting, dizziness, palpitation.

　　Tongue: white with greasy fur
　　Pulse: Slippery

Application:

Chronic tracheitis, bronchitis, pulmonary emphysema, goiter.

Modification:

1. With heat phlegm and irritability, add:

枳 實	Zhi Shi (Immature bitter orange)	*Fructus Auranti Immaturus*
竹 茹	Zhu Ru (Bamboo shavings)	*Caulus Bambusae in Taenis*
大 棗	Da Zao (Jujube)	*Fructus Ziziphus Jujubae*

This formula is called Wen Dan Tang (Bamboo and Hoelen Combination) (溫胆湯)

2. For an elderly person , with weak lung and kidney, has a common cold with cough and profuse sputum, add:

當 歸	Dang Gui (Chinese angelica)	*Radix Angelicae Sinensis*
熟地黄	Shu Di Huang (Prep. rehmannia)	*Radix Rehmanniae Praeparatae*

This formula is called Jin Shui Liu Jun Jian（金水六君煎）

3. For vomiting due to coldness in the stomach, add:

木 香	Mu Xiang (Saussurea)	*Radix Saussureae*
砂 仁	Sha Ren (Cardamon, Amomum)	*Fructus Amomi*

This formula is called Xiang Sha Er Chen Tang (香砂二陳湯)

Generic Name:

Citrus and Pinellia Combination

Ěr Lóng Zuǒ Cí Wán   耳聾左慈丸

(Er-Lung-Chuo-Chi-Wan)
(Pills for the Deaf)

Constituents:

九節菖蒲	Jiu Jie Chang Pu (Altaica)	6-9 gm.	*Rhizoma Anemoni Altaicae*
磁 石	Ci Shi (Magnetite)	1-3 gm.	*Mangetitum*
五味子	Wu Wei Zi (Schisandra)	6-9 gm.	*Fructus Schisandrae*
熟地黃	Shu Di Huang (Prep. rehmannia)	20-25 gm.	*Radix Rehmanniae Praeparatae*
山茱萸	Shan Zhu Yu (Cornus)	10-15 mg.	*Fructus Corni*
山 藥	Shan Yao (Dioscorea)	10-15 gm.	*Rhizoma Dioscoreae*
澤 瀉	Ze Xie (Alisma)	9-12 gm.	*Rhizoma Alismatis*
牡丹皮	Mu Dan Pi (Moutan bark)	6-9 gm.	*Cortex Moutan Radicis*
茯 苓	Fu Ling (Poria)	9-12 gm.	*Poria*

Action:

1. To replenish the *Yin* (vital essence) of kidney
2. To open the apertures of the ear

Indication:

For a person with hearing difficulty due to kidney *Yin* deficiency. The symptoms are: tinnitus, deaf, vertigo.

> Tongue: red
> Pulse: thready and rapid

Application:

Deaf, tinnitus, Meniere's disease, diabetes.

Generic Name:

Tso-tzu Otic Pills

Èr Miào Sàn   二妙散

(Er-Miao-San)
(Powder of Two Effective Ingredients)

Constituents;

黄　柏	Huang Bai (Phellodendron)	6-9 gm.	*Cortex Phellodendri*
蒼　术	Cang Zhu (Atractylodes)	9-12 gm.	*Rhizoma Atractylodis*

Action:

To eliminate heat and dampness

Indication:

For a person with low back pain caused by heat and dampness. The symptoms are: pain in the knees and low back, eczema, leukorrhea, urination scanty and yellow in color.

Tongue: with yellow and greasy coating
Pulse: soft and rapid

Application:

Low back pain, tinea pedis, eczema, leukorrhea, gonorrhea.

Modification:

1. To reinforce the liver and kidney, add:
懷牛膝　Huai Niu Xi (Achyranthes)　　　*Radix Achyranthis Bidentatae*
This formula is called San Miao San（三妙散）

2. To eliminate dampness, add:
懷牛膝　Huai Niu Xi (Achyranthes)　　　*Radix Achyranthis Bidentatae*
薏苡仁　Yi Yi Ren (Coix)　　　　　　　*Semen Coicis*
This formula is called Si Miao San（四妙散）

3. For tinea pedis, add:
薏苡仁　Yi Yi Ren (Coix)　　　　　　*Semen Coicis*
木　瓜　Mu Gua (Chaenomeles fruit)　*Fructus Chaenomelis*
檳　榔　Bing Lang (Areca seed)　　　*Semen Arecae*

4. For leukorrhea, add:
芡　實　Qian Shi (Euryale seed)　　*Semen Euryales*
椿　皮　Chun Pi (Ailanthus bark)　*Cortex Ailanthi*
白　果　Bai Guo (Ginkgo seed)　　*Semen Ginkgo*

Èr Xiān Tāng　　二仙湯

(Er-Hsian-Tang)
(Decoction of Curculigo and Epimedium)

Constituents:

仙　茅	Xian Mao (Curculigo)	6-15 gm.	*Rhizoma Curculiginis*
仙靈脾	Xian Ling Pi (Epidmedium)	9-15 gm.	*Herba Epimedi*
巴戟天	Ba Ji Tian (Morinda)	6-9 gm.	*Radix Morindae Officinalis*
當　歸	Dang Gui (Chinese angelica)	6-9 gm.	*Radix Angelicae Sinensis*
黃　柏	Huang Bai (Phellodendron)	4-9 gm.	*Cortex Phellodendri*
知　母	Zhi Mu (Anemarrhena)	4-9 gm.	*Rhizoma Anemarrhenae*

Action:

1. To replenish the *Yin* (vital essence) and *Yang* (vital function) of kidney
2. To purge the fire
3. To regulate the Chong (Vital) and Ren (Front Midline) channels.

Indication:

For a person with climacteric syndromes due to deficiency of both *Yin* (vital essence) and *Yang* (vital function) of kidney, and disharmony between the Chong (Vital) and Ren (Front Midline) channels. The symptoms are: irregular menstruation, dizziness, tinnitus, flaccidity of the muscles, feet cold, headache.

Tongue: pale
Pulse: thready and rapid

Application:

Menopause, amenorrhea, hypertension, nephritis, pyonephritis, urinary tract infection.

Fáng Fēng Tōng Shèng Sàn   防風通聖散
(Fang-Feng-Tung-Sheng-San)
(Pills of Ledebouriella with Magical Therapeutic Effects)

Constituents:

防 風	Fang Feng (Ledebouriella)	6-9 gm.	Radix Ledebouriellae
荊 芥	Jing Jie (Schizonepeta)	6-9 gm.	Herba Schizonepetae
麻 黃	Ma Huang (Ephedra)	3-6 gm.	Herba Ephedrae
桔 梗	Jie Geng (Platycodon)	6-9 gm.	Radix Platycodi
薄 荷	Bo He (Mentha)	3-6 gm.	Herba Menthae
連 翹	Lian Qiao (Forsythia)	6-9 gm.	Fructus Forsythiae
黃 芩	Huang Qin (Scutellaria)	3-6 gm.	Radix Scutellariae
梔 子	Zhi Zi (Gardenia)	3-6 gm.	Fructus Gardeniae
大 黃	Da Huang (Rhubarb)	3-6 gm.	Radix et Rhizoma Rhei
石 膏	Shi Gao (Gypsum)	9-12 gm.	Gypsum Fibrosum
芒 硝	Mang Xiao (Mirabilitum)	3-6 gm.	Natrii Sulfas
滑 石	Hua Shi (Talc)	9-12 gm.	Talcum
當 歸	Dang Gui (Chinese angelica)	6-9 gm.	Radix Angelicae Sinensis
川 芎	Chuan Xiong (Ligusticum)	3-6 gm.	Rhizoma Ligustici Chuanxiong
白 术	Bai Zhu (White atractylodes)	6-9 gm.	Rhizoma Atractylodis Macrocephalae
白芍藥	Bai Shao Yao (White peony)	6-9 gm.	Radix Paeoniae Alba
甘 草	Gan Cao (Licorice)	3-6 gm.	Radix Glycyrrhizae
生 薑	Sheng Jiang (Fresh ginger)	3-6 gm.	Rhizoma Zingiberis Recens

Action:

To eliminate intense heat and fire in the exterior and interior system of the body.

Indication:

For a person with intense heat and fire in the body, and with affection of wind and heat. The symptoms are: high body temperature, headache, sore throat, fullness in the chest, constipation, skin rupture or ulcer, obese.

> Tongue: red with yellow coating
> Pulse: forceful and rapid

Application:

Obesity, hypertension, constipation, skin rupture or ulcers.

Generic Name:

Fang Feng Tong Sheng San;
Siler and Platycodon Formula

Fáng Jǐ Fú Líng Tāng　　防己茯苓湯
(Fang-Chi-Fu-Ling-Tang)
(Decoction of Stephania and Poria)

Constituents:

黄 芪	Huang Qi (Astragalus)	10-15 gm.	*Radix Astragali*
防 己	Fang Ji (Stephania)	9-12 gm.	*Radix Stephaniae Tetrandrae*
茯 苓	Fu Ling (Poria)	6-9 gm.	*Poria*
桂 枝	Gui Zhi (Cinnamon twig)	6-9 gm.	*Ramulus Cinnamomi*
甘 草	Gan Cao (Licorice)	3-6 gm.	*Radix Glycyrrhizae*

Action:

1. Diuretic
2. To replenish *Qi* (vital energy)
3. To activate the *Yang* (vital function)

Indication:

For a person with accumulation of water in the skin all over the body. The symptoms are: edema all over the body, especially in the four limbs, heaviness sensation, dysuria, no intolerance of wind.

Tongue: pale with white coating
Pulse: floating and feeble, or soft and thready

Application:

Cardiac and nephritic edema

Generic Name:

Stephania and Hoelen Combination

Fáng Jǐ Huáng Qí Tāng   防己黄芪湯
(Fang-Chi-Huang-Chi-Tang)
(Decoction of Stephania and Astragalus)

Constituents:

黄 芪	Huang Qi (Astragalus)	10-15 gm.	*Radix Astragali*
防 己	Fang Ji (Stephania)	9-12 gm.	*Radix Stephaniae Tetrandrae*
白 术	Bai Zhu (White atractylodes)	6-9 gm.	*Rhizoma Atractylodis Macrocephalae*
生 薑	Sheng Jiang (Fresh ginger)	1-3 gm.	*Rhizoma Zingiberis Recens*
炙甘草	Zhi Gan Cao (Baked licorice)	3-6 gm.	*Radix Glycyrrhizae Praeparatae*
大 棗	Da Zao (Jujube)	3-5 gm.	*Fructus Ziziphus Jujubae*

Action:

1. Diuretic, to reduce edema
2. To strengthen the spleen *Qi* (vital energy)
3. To dispel wind

Indication:

For a person with accumulation of water or dampness and with exterior syndrome of deficiency. The symptoms are: spontaneous perspiration, intolerance of wind, heaviness sensation of the body, dysuria, edema.

Tongue: light color with white coating
Pulse: Floating and feeble, or soft and thready

Application:

For cardiac and nephritic edema.

Modification:

1. With heaviness sensation in lower back and feet, add:

茯 苓	Fu Ling (Poria; Hoelen)	*Poria*
薏苡仁	Yi Yi Ren (Coix)	*Semen Coicis*

2. With abdominal distention, add:

陳 皮	Chen Pi (Citrus peel)	*Pericarpium Citri Reticulatae*
枳 殼	Zhi Ke (Bitter orange)	*Fructus Aurantii*

3. With deficiency of *Qi* (vital energy), add:

黨 參	Dang Shen (Codonopsis)	*Radix Codonopsis Pilosulae*

Generic Name:

Stephania and Astragalus Combination

Fù Guì Lǐ Zhōng Wán   附桂理中丸

(Fu-Kuei-Li-Chung-Wan)
(Decoction to Regulate the Spleen and Stomach with Aconite and Cinnamon Bark)

Constituents:

附　子 Fu Zi (Aconite)	3-6 gm.	*Radix Aconiti Praeparatae*
肉　桂 Rou Gui (Cinnamon bark)	3-6 gm.	*Cortex Cinnamomi*
人　參 Ren Shen (Ginseng)	10-15 gm.	*Radix Ginseng*
白　术 Bai Zhu (White atractylodes)	6-9 gm.	*Rhizoma Atractylodis Macrocephalae*
乾　薑 Gan Jiang (Dry ginger)	6-9 gm.	*Rhizoma Zingiberis*
炙甘草 Zhi Gan Cao (Baked licorice)	3-6 gm.	*Radix Glycyrrhizae Praeparatae*

Action:

1. To dispel cold and replenish the *Yang* (vital function)
2. To warm and tonify the spleen and stomach

Indication:

For a person with deficiency of spleen and stomach with accumulation of cold. The symptoms are: fullness in the epigastric region or abdomen (like to be pressed), loss of appetite, no thirsty sensation, vomiting, diarrhea, loose stools, lock-jaw, hands and feet cold and stiff.

Tongue: pale with white coating
Pulse: deep, slow and weak

Application:

Acute and chronic gastroenteritis, gastroduodenal ulcer, gastrectasis, gastroptosis, chronic colitis, cholera.

Fù Yuán Huó Xuè Tāng　　復元活血湯
(Fu-Yuan-Huo-Hsieh-Tang)
(Decoction to Invigorate Blood Circulation for Recovery)

Constituents:

當 歸	Dang Gui (Chinese angelica)	6-9 gm.	*Radix Angelica Sinensis*
桃 仁	Tao Ren (Persica seed)	6-9 gm.	*Semen Persicae*
紅 花	Hong Hua (Carthamus)	6-9 gm.	*Flos Carthami*
大 黃	Da Huang (Rhubarb)	6-9 gm.	*Radix et Rhizoma Rhei*
穿山甲	Chuan Shan Jia (Anteater scales)	6-9 gm.	*Squama Manitis*
天花粉	Tian Hua Fen (Trichosanthes root)	10-15 gm.	*Radix Trichosanthis*
柴 胡	Chai Hu (Bupleurum)	6-9 gm.	*Radix Bupleuri*
甘 草	Gan Cao (Licorice)	3-6 gm.	*Radix Glycyrrhizae*
酒	Jiu (wine)		

Action:

1. To invigorate blood circulation and remove stasis
2. To relieve stagnation of liver *Qi* (vital energy) in the liver

Indication:

For a person with acute traumatic injury, with severe pain and blood stasis in the hypochondriac region.

Application:

Traumatic injury, intercostal neuralgia, costalgia of the cartilage

Modification:

1. With severe pain, add:

三 七	San Qi (Pseudoginseng)	*Panax Pseudoginseng*
郁 金	Yu Jin (Curcuma root)	*Radix Curcumae*
川 芎	Chuan Xiong (Ligusticum)	*Rhizoma Ligustici Chuanxiong*
乳 香	Ru Xiang (Mastic)	*Resina Olibani*
沒 藥	Mo Yao (Myrrh)	*Resina Myrrhae*

2. With Stagnation of *Qi*, add:

香 附	Xiang Fu (Cyperus tuber)	*Rhizoma Cyperi*
青 皮	Qing Pi (Green tangerine peel)	*Pericarpium Citri Reticulatae Viridae*
枳 殼	Zhi Ke (Bitter orange)	*Fructus Aurantii*

Generic Name:

Tang-kuei and Persica Combination

Fù Zǐ Lǐ Zhōng Wán　　附子理中丸 (湯)

(Fu-Tzu-Li-Chung-Wan)
(Decoction to Regulate the Spleen and Stomach with Aconite)

Constituents:

附　子 Fu Zi (Aconite)	3-6 gm.	*Radix Aconiti Praeparatae*
人　參 Ren Shen (Ginseng)	10-15 gm.	*Radix Ginseng*
白　朮 Bai Zhu (White atractylodes)	6-9 gm.	*Rhizoma Atractylodis acrocephalae*
乾　薑 Gan Jiang (Dry ginger)	6-9 gm.	*Rhizoma Zingiberis*
炙甘草 Zhi Gan Cao (Baked licorice)	3-6 gm.	*Radix Glycyrrhizae Praeparatae*

Action:

1. To warm the abdomen and dispel cold
2. To replenish the *Yang* (vital function) of spleen and stomach.

Indication:

For a person with deficiency and coldness of the spleen and stomach (serious condition). The symptoms are: fullness in the epigastric region or abdomen (like to be pressed), no thirsty sensation, vomiting, diarrhea, coldness of the hands and feet, rigidity, spasms, lockjaw, and may result in syncope.

> Tongue: light red with white coating
> Pulse: deep, slow and fainting

Application:

Acute and chronic gastroenteritis, gastro-duodenal ulcer, gastrectasis, gastroptosis, chronic colitis, cholera.

Modification:

To enhance the effect of replenishing *Yang* (vital function), add:
肉桂 Rou Gui (Cinnamon bark)　　*Cortex Cinnamomi*

This formula is called Fu Gui Li Zhong Wan (附桂理中丸)

Generic Name:

Aconite, Ginseng, and Ginger Combination

Fù Zǐ Tāng   附子湯
(Fu-Tzu-Tang)
(Decoction of Prepared Aconite)

Constituents:

附 子 Fu Zi (Prepared aconite)	6-9 gm.	*Radix Aconiti Praeparatae*
白 术 Bai Zhu (White atractylodes)	9-12 gm.	*Rhizoma Atractylodis Macrocephalae*
人 參 Ren Shen (Ginseng)	3-6 gm.	*Radix Ginseng*
茯 苓 Fu Ling (Poria)	9-12 gm.	*Poria*
白芍藥 Bai Shao Yao (White peony)	6-12 gm.	*Radix Paeoniae Alba*

Action:

1. To dispel cold and reinforce the *Yang* (vital function)
2. To dispel dampness and relieve pain

Indication:

For a person with arthritis due to cold and dampness. The symptoms are: muscle-ache and soreness in the whole body, intolerance of cold, hands and feet cold.

Tongue: with white coating
Pulse: deep and slow or weak

Application:

Arthritis (due to cold and dampness).

Fù Zǐ Xiè Xīn Tāng   附子瀉心湯

(Fu-Tzu-Hsieh-Hsin-Tang)
(The Stomach Purging Decoction with Aconite)

Constituents:

炮附子 Pao Fu Zi (Baked aconite)	3-6 gm.	*Radix Aconiti Praeparatae*
大 黃 Da Huang (Rhubarb)	10-15 gm.	*Radix et Rhizoma Rhei*
黃 連 Huang Lian (Coptis)	3-6 gm.	*Rhizoma Coptidis*
黃 芩 Huang Qin (Scutellaria)	6-9 gm.	*Radix Scutellariae*

Action:

1. To eliminate heat
2. To relieve fullness and distention
3. To replenish the *Yang* (vital function)
4. To consolidate the exterior defensive system

Indication:

For a person with abdominal fullness and oppression due to deficiency of *Yang* (vital function) of spleen and stomach, and accumulation of heat. The symptoms are: indigestion, borborygmus, retch, vexation, restlessness, fullness and distention of the chest and abdomen, intolerance of cold, spontaneous perspiration.

      Tongue: pale with thin white coating
      Pulse: slow and weak

Application:

Acute gastroenteritis

Gān Cǎo Xiè Xīn Tāng 甘草瀉心湯
(Kan-Tsao-Hsieh-Hsin-Tang)
(The Stomach Purging Decoction with Licorice)

Constituents:

半 夏	Ban Xia (Pinellia)	9-12 gm.	*Rhizoma Pinelliae*
黄 連	Huang Lian (Coptis)	3-6 gm.	*Rhizoma Coptidis*
黄 芩	Huang Qin (Scutellaria)	6-9 gm.	*Radix Scutellariae*
乾 薑	Gan Jiang (Dry ginger)	9-12 gm.	*Rhizoma Zingiberis*
人 參	Ren Shen (Ginseng)	6-9 gm.	*Radix Ginseng*
炙甘草	Zhi Gan Cao (Baked licorice)	9-12 gm.	*Radix Glycyrrhizae Praeparatae*
大 棗	Da Zao (Jujube)	3-5 pc.	*Fructus Ziziphus Jujubae*

Action:

1. To disperse lumps or hardening
2. To regulate the spleen and stomach

Indication:

For a person with abdominal fullness and oppression due to asthenia of stomach, thus leading to stagnation of *Qi* (vital energy). The symptoms are: indigestion, borborygmus, retch, vexation, restlessness, fullness and distention of the chest and abdomen.

> Tongue: pale, with thin white coating
> Pulse: slow and weak

Application:

Acute gastroenteritis.

Generic Name:

Pinellia and Licorice Combination

Gān Lù Xiāo Dú Dān　　甘露消毒丹

(Kan-Lu-Hsiao-Tu-Dan)
(Antiphlogistic Pills of Dew)

Constituents:

滑　石	Hua Shi (Talc)	15-20 gm.	*Talcum*
茵陳蒿	Yin Chen Hao (Capillaris)	10-15 gm.	*Herba Artemisiae Capillaris*
木　通	Mu Tong (Akebia)	5-10 gm.	*Caulis Akebiae*
黄　芩	Huang Qin (Scutellaria)	10-15 gm.	*Radix Scutellariae*
連　翹	Lian Qiao (Forsythia)	5-10 gm.	*Fructus Forsythiae*
川貝母	Chuan Bei Mu (Fritillary)	5-10 gm.	*Bulbus Fritillariae Cirrhosae*
射　干	She Gan (Belamcanda)	5-10 gm.	*Rhizoma Belamcandae*
石菖蒲	Shi Chang Pu (Acorus)	6-10 gm.	*Rhizoma Acori Graminei*
藿　香	Huo Xiang (Agastache)	5-10 gm.	*Herba Agastachis*
薄　荷	Bo He (Mentha)	3-6 gm.	*Herba Menthae*
白豆蔻	Bai Dou Kou (Cluster)	5-10 gm.	*Semen Cardamomi Rotundi*

Action:

1. To resolve dampness and turbidity
2. To clear heat and toxin

Indication:

For a person with interior heat and dampness in the *Qi* (secondary defensive) system. The symptoms are: fever, malaise, fullness and distention in the chest and abdomen, sore throat, jaundice, thirst, nausea, vomiting, diarrhea, amber colored urine.

Tongue: with white or yellow and greasy coating
Pulse: soft and rapid

Application:

Acute gastritis, acute diarrhea (especially in the summer season), hepatitis, acute gastroenteritis.

Gān Mài Dà Zǎo Tāng   甘麥大棗湯

(Kan-Mai-Ta-Tsao-Tang)
(Decoction of Licorice, Light Wheat and Jujube)

Constituents:

甘 草	Gan Cao (Licorice)	9-12 gm.	*Radix Glycyrrhizae*
浮小麥	Fu Xiao Mai (Light wheat)	30-50 gm.	*Fructus Tritici Levis*
大 棗	Da Zao (Jujube)	10-15 gm.	*Fructus Ziziphus Jujubae*

Action:

1. Sedative
2. Nourishing
3. Anti-spasmodic

Indication:

For a person with hysteria due to dehydration in the visceras. The symptoms are: absentmindedness, moody, feel like crying, restlessness, cannot sleep well, weird behavior.

Tongue: with thin white coating
Pulse: wiry/taut and thready

Application:

Hysteria, mania, convulsions

Modification:

1. To increase the sedative action, add:

柏子仁	Bai Zi Ren (Biota seed)	*Semen Biotae*
酸棗仁	Suan Zao Ren (Wild jujube seed)	*Semen Ziziphi Spinosae*
茯 神	Fu Shen (Poria)	*Poria*
合歡花	He Huan Hua (Albizzia flower)	*Flos Albizziae*

2. For insomnia, dizziness and irritability, add:

珍珠母	Zhen Zhu Mu (Mother-of-pearl)	*Concha Margaritifera Usta*
龍 齒	Long Chi (Dragon's teeth)	*Dens Draconis*

Generic Name:

Licorice and Jujube Combination

Gān Suì Tōng Jié Tāng 甘遂通結湯
(Kan-Sui-Tung-Chieh-Tang)
(Decoction of Kansui for Intestinal Obstruction)

Constituents:

甘 遂 Gan Sui (Kansui root)	0.5-1 gm.	*Radix Euphorbiae Kansui*
大 黄 Da Huang (Rhubarb)	9-24 gm.	*Radix et Rhizoma Rhei*
桃 仁 Tao Ren (Persica seed)	6-9 gm.	*Semen Persicae*
赤芍藥 Chi Shao (Red peony)	12-15 gm.	*Radix Paeoniae Rubra*
牛 膝 Niu Xi (Cyanthula)	6-9 gm.	*Radix Cyathulae*
厚 朴 Hou Po (Magnolia bark)	15-30 gm.	*Cortex Magnoliae Officinalis*
木 香 Mu Xiang (Saussurea)	6-9 gm.	*Radix Saussureae*

Action:

1. To invigorate the circulation of *Qi* (vital energy) and blood
2. To dispel water

Indication:

For a person with intestinal obstruction. The symptoms are: vomiting, abdominal pain and distention, no gas, no defecation.

Tongue: with yellow, dry, thick or greasy coating
Pulse: slippery and rapid

Application:

Acute intestinal obstruction

Comment:

Decoct the above ingredients except the Gan Sui root powder. Add the powder to the decoction later. And then induce the decoction (through the gastric tube), after the bowels are emptied and the pressure is reduced in the GI tract.

Gé Gēn Huáng Qín Huáng Lián Tāng　葛根黃芩黃連湯

(Ko-Ken-Huang-Chin-Huang-Lien-Tang)
(Decoction of Pueraria, Scutellaria and Coptis)

Constituents:

葛　根	Ge Gen (Pueraria)	10-15 gm.	*Radix Puerariae*
黃　芩	Huang Qin (Scutellaria)	6-9 gm.	*Radix Scutellariae*
黃　連	Huang Lian (Coptis)	3-6 gm.	*Rhizoma Coptidis*
炙甘草	Zhi Gan Cao (Baked licorice)	3-6 gm.	*Radix Glycyrrhizae Praeparatae*

Action:

1. To dispel exterior pathogenic factors
2. To eliminate internal heat in the stomach and intestines (Febrifugal)

Indication:

For a person with exterior symptom-complex and interior heat in the stomach and intestines. The symptoms are: fever, diarrhea, irritating heat sensation in the chest and epigastric region, thirst, mouth dry.

> Tongue: red with yellow coating
> Pulse: rapid

Application:

Diarrhea, bacterial dysentery, amoebic dysentery, acute colitis.

Contraindication:

For a person with diarrhea but no fever due to coldness and deficiency.

Modification:

1. With diarrhea and vomiting, add:

半　夏　Ban Xia (Pinellia)　　　　*Rhizoma Pinelliae*

2. With indigestion, add:

山　楂　Shan Zha (Crataegus fruit)　*Fructus Crataegi*
神　曲　Shen Qu (Medicated leaven)　*Massa Fermentata Medicinalis*

3. With abdominal pain, add:

木　香　Mu Xiang (Saussurea root)　*Radix Saussureae*
白芍藥　Bai Shao Yao (White peony)　*Radix Paeoniae Alba*

4. For acute colitis, add:

金銀花　Jin Yin Hua (Lonicera flower)　*Flos Lonicerae*
車前子　Che Qian Zi (Plantago seed)　*Semen Plantaginis*

Generic Name:

Pueraria, Coptis and Scute Combination

Gé Gēn Tāng　　葛根湯
(Ko-Ken-Tang)
(Decoction of Pueraria)

Constituents:

葛　根	Ge Gen (Pueraria)	6-9 gm.	*Radix Puerariae*
麻　黄	Ma Huang (Ephedra)	6-9 gm.	*Herba Ephedrae*
桂　枝	Gui Zhi (Cinnamon twig)	6-9 gm.	*Ramulus Cinnamomi*
白芍藥	Bai Shao Yao (White peony)	6-9 gm.	*Radix Paeoniae Alba*
乾　薑	Gan Jiang (Ginger)	3 gm.	*Rhizoma Zingiberis*
甘　草	Gan Cao (Licorice)	3 gm.	*Radix Glycyrrhizae*
大　棗	Da Zao (Jujube)	3-5 pc.	*Fructus Ziziphus Jujubae*

Action:

　　1. To dispel exterior wind and cold (Diaphoretic)
　　2. To relieve muscle-ache of the neck

Indication:

For a person with common cold caused by wind and cold factors in the Tai-yang channel. The symptoms are: fever, intolerance of wind, no perspiration, muscle-ache of the neck.

　　　　Tongue: pink with white coating
　　　　Pulse: floating and tight

Application:

Common cold, headache, stiff-neck, frozen shoulder.

Modification:

　　1. With headache, add:

羌　活	Qiang Huo (Notopterygium)	*Rhizoma seu Radix Notopterygii*
白　芷	Bai Zhi (Angelica root)	*Radix Angelicae Dahuricae*

　　2. With interior heat, add:

黄　芩	Huang Qin (Scutellaria)	*Radix Scutellariae*
石　膏	Shi Gao (Gypsum)	*Gypsum Fibrosum*

Generic Name:

Pueraria Combination

Gé Xià Zhú Yū Tāng　　膈下逐瘀湯
(Ke-Chia-Chu-Yu-Tang)
(Decoction to Remove Blood Stasis below the Diaphragm)

Constituents:

當　歸	Dang Gui (Chinese angelica)	6-9 gm.	*Radix Angelicae Sinensis*
川　芎	Chuan Xiong (Ligusticum)	6-9 gm.	*Rhizoma Ligustici Chuanxiong*
桃　仁	Tao Ren (Persica seed)	6-9 gm.	*Semen Persicae*
紅　花	Hong Hua (Safflower)	6-9 gm.	*Flos Carthami*
五靈脂	Wu Ling Zhi (Pteropus excrement)	6-9 gm.	*Faeces Trogopterorum*
烏　葯	Wu Yao (Lindera)	6-9 gm.	*Radix Linderae*
延胡索	Yan Hu Suo (Corydalis)	3-6 gm.	*Rhizoma Corydalis*
香　附	Xiang Fu (Cyperus tuber)	3-6 gm.	*Rhizoma Cyperi*
赤芍藥	Chi Shao Yao (Red peony)	6-9 gm.	*Radix Paeoniae Rubra*
牡丹皮	Mu Dan Pi (Moutan bark)	6-9 gm.	*Cortex Moutan Radicis*
枳　殼	Zhi Ke (Bitter orange)	3-6 gm.	*Fructus Aurantii*
甘　草	Gan Cao (Licorice)	1-3 gm.	*Radix Glycyrrhizae*

Action:

To relieve pain below the diaphragm by invigorating the circulation of *Qi* (vital energy) and blood in liver.

Indication:

For a person with stagnation of *Qi* (vital energy) and blood stasis. The symptoms are: abdominal pain (fixed) with hardening, hypochondriac pain (piercing), irritability, indigestion, constipation.

> Tongue: with purple spots on the side
> Pulse: wiry/taut and hesitant

Application:

Hypochondriac pain, dysmenorrhea, amenorrhea, irregular menstruation, breast distention, abdominal tumors.

Gù Chōng Tāng 固沖湯
(Gu-Chong-Tang)
(Decoction to Reinforce the Chong Channel)

Constituents:

黄 芪	Huang Qi (Astragalus)	15-20 gm.	*Radix Astragali*
白 术	Bai Zhu (White atractylodes)	25-30 gm.	*Rz. Atractylodis Macrocephalae*
白芍藥	Bai Shao (White peony)	12-15 gm.	*Radix Paeoniae Alba*
山茱萸	Shan Zhu Yu (Cornus)	20-25 gm.	*Fructus Corni*
煅龍骨	Duan Long Gu (Cal. Dragon's bone)	20-25 gm.	*Os Draconis*
煅牡蠣	Duan Mu Li (Calcined oyster shell)	20-25 gm.	*Concha Ostreae*
海螵蛸	Hai Piao Xiao (Cuttlefish bone)	12-15 gm.	*Os Sepiae*
棕櫚炭	Zong Lu Tan (Charred palm)	6-9 gm.	*Cortex Trachycarpi*
五倍子	Wu Bei Zi (Nutgall)	1-2 gm.	*Galla Chinenis*
茜 草	Xi Cao (Rubia root)	9-12 gm.	*Radix Rubiae*

Action:

1. To increase *Qi* (vital energy) and strengthen the spleen
2. To reinforce the Chong channel and stop bleeding (Hemostatic)

Indication:

For a person with menorrhagia caused by inconsolidation of the Chong channel. The symptoms are: excessive menstrual bleeding, color light red, heart palpitation, shortness of breath.

> Tongue: pale pink
> Pulse: weak and soft, or feeble and hollow

Application:

Metrorrhagia, metrostaxis, functional uterine bleeding, ulcerous bleeding, post-partum bleeding.

Gù Jīng Wán 固經丸

(Ku-Ching-Wan)
(Pills for Menorrhagia)

Constituents:

龜 板 Gui Ban (Tortoise plastron)	9-12 gm.	*Plastrum Testudinis*
赤芍藥 Chi Shao Yao (Red peony)	6-9 gm.	*Radix Paeoniae Rubra*
黃 芩 Huang Qin (Scutellaria)	6-9 gm.	*Radix Scutellariae*
黃 柏 Huang Bai (Phellodendron)	6-9 gm.	*Cortex Phellodendri*
椿 皮 Chun Pi (Ailanthus bark)	3-6 gm.	*Cortex Ailanthi*
香 附 Xiang Fu (Cyperus)	6-9 gm.	*Rhizoma Cyperi*

Action:

1. To eliminate the heat caused by deficiency of *Yin* (vital essence)
2. To stop bleeding (hemostatic)

Indication:

For a person with menorrhagia due to deficiency of *Yin* and hyperactivity of fire. The symptoms are: increased blood flow in menstruation, color dark red or purple, very thick and sticky, may have blood clots, period delayed, face red, mouth dry, urine yellow, difficulty in defecation, leukorrhea.

> Tongue: red with yellow coating
> Pulse: slippery and rapid

Application:

Menorrhagia, leukorrhea, uterine bleeding.

Guā Dì Sàn 瓜蒂散

(Kua-Ti-San)
(Powder of Melon Pedicle)

Constituents:

瓜 蒂 Gua Di (Melon pedicle)	1-3 gm.	*Pedicellus Cucumis*
赤小豆 Chi Xiao Dou (Phaseolus seed)	1-3 gm.	*Semen Phaseoli*
淡豆豉 Dan Dou Chi (Prepared soybean)	6-9 gm.	*Semen Sojae Praepartatae*

Grind Gua Di (melon pedicle) and Chi Xiao Dou (phaseolus seed) into powder. Decoct Dan Dou Chi (prepared soybean) separately and drink it with the powder.

Action:

Emetic

Indication:

For a person with stagnation of phlegm or food due to indigestion or food poisoning. The symptoms are: epigastric fullness or obstruction, air-way obstruction, irritability, abdominal fullness.

Tongue: with spongy and curdy coating
Pulse: slippery

Application:

Crapulence, indigestion, food poisoning, acute jaundice, mushroom poisoning.

Contraindication:

For a person of weak constitution.

Modification:

1. With heat and phlegm in the febrile disease of the Taiyin channel, add:
栀 子 Zhi Zi (Gardenia)　　　　*Fructus Gardeniae*
This formula is also called Gua Di San (瓜蒂散)

2. For acute jaundice, subtract:
淡豆豉 Dan Dou Chi (Prepared soybean)　　*Semen Sojae Praepartatum*
This formula is also called Gua Di San (瓜蒂散)

Generic Name:

Melon Pedicle Formula

Guā Lóu Xiè Bái Bái Jiŭ Tāng　瓜蔞薤白白酒湯
(Kua-Lou-Hsieh-Pai-Pai-Chiu-Tang)
(Decoction of Trichosanthes, Macrostem Onion & White Wine)

Constituents:

瓜蔞子 Gua Lou Zi (Trichosanthes fruit)	10-15 gm.	*Fructus Trichosanthis*
薤　白 Xie Bai (Macrostem onion)	6-9 gm.	*Bulbus Allii*
白　酒 Bai Jiu (White wine)	30-60 c.c.	

Decoct with water and wine; or with water first and add wine later.

Action:

1. To regulate the flow of *Qi* (vital energy) & *Yang* (vital function)
2. To resolve phlegm and hardening

IIndication:

For a person with chest pain due to obstruction of phlegm and flow of vital energy. The symptoms are: chest pain radiating to the back, cough, spitting saliva, shortness of breath, asthma.

Tongue: white with greasy coating
Pulse: sinking and wiry or tight

Application:

Chest pain, angina pectoris, chronic bronchitis, intercostal neuralgia.

Contraindication: For a person that is allergic to alcohol.

Modification:

1. For a person with severe chest pain, profuse expectoration, add:
半　夏 Ban Xia (Pinellia tuber)　　*Rhizoma Pinelliae*
This is now called Gua Lou Xie Bai Ban Xia Tang (Trichosanthes, Bakeri and Pinellia Combination)（瓜蔞薤白半夏湯）

2. For angina pectoris, add:

丹　參 Dan Shen (Salvia root)	*Radix Salviae Miltiorrhizae*
紅　花 Hong Hua (Carthamus)	*Flos Carthami*
赤芍藥 Chi Shao Yao (Red peony)	*Radix Paeoniae Rubra*
川　芎 Chuan Xiong (Chuanxiong)	*Rhizoma Ligustici Chuanxiong*

3. For intercostal neuralgia, use it together with

柴　胡 Chai Hu (Bupleurum)	*Radix Bupleuri*
枳　實 Zhi Shi (Immature bitter orange)	*Fructus Aurantii Immaturus*
白芍藥 Bai Shao Yao (White peony)	*Radix Paeoniae Alba*
甘　草 Gan Cao (Licorice)	*Radix Glycyrrhizae*

Which is the formula called Si Ni San (Bupleurum and Chih-shih Formula) （四逆散）

Generic Name:

Trichosanthes, Bakeri and White Wine Combination

Guā Lóu Zhǐ Shí Tāng 瓜蔞枳實湯
(Kua-Lou-Chih-Shih-Tang)
(Decoction of Trichosanthes Seed and Immature Bitter Orange)

Constituents:

瓜蔞仁	Gua Lu Ren (Trichosanthes seed)	6-9 gm.	*Semen Trichosanthis*
枳實	Zhi Shi (Imm. bitter orange)	3-6 gm.	*Fructus Aurantii Immaturus*
桔梗	Jie Geng (Platycodon)	6-9 gm.	*Radix Platycodi*
茯苓	Fu Ling (Poria)	6-9 gm.	*Poria*
貝母	Bei Mu (Fritillaria)	6-9 gm.	*Bulbus Fritillariae*
黃芩	Huang Qin (Scutellaria)	6-9 gm.	*Radix Scutellariae*
梔子	Zhi Zi (Gardenia fruit)	6-9 gm.	*Fructus Gardeniae*
當歸	Dang Gui (Chinese angelica)	6-9 gm.	*Radix Angelicae Sinensis*
竹瀝	Zhu Li (Bamboo sap)	6-9 gm.	*Saccus Bambusae*
砂仁	Sha Ren (Cardamon)	3-6 gm.	*Fructus Amomi*
木香	Mu Xiang (Saussurea)	3-6 gm.	*Radix Saussureae*
陳皮	Chen Pi (Citrus peel)	3-6 gm.	*Pericarpium Citri Reticulatae*
生薑	Sheng Jiang (Fresh ginger)	3-6 gm.	*Rhizoma Zingiberis Recens*
甘草	Gan Cao (Licorice)	3-6 gm.	*Radix Glycyrrhizae*

Action:

1. To eliminate heat in liver and kidney
2. To relieve the dry cough by moistening (Antitussive)
3. To resolve the obstruction of phlegm in the chest

Indication:

For a person with phlegm and dry cough, especially in the morning. The symptoms are: cough, dry sputum, dyspnea, chest pain, urine color dark yellow.

Tongue: red with dry yellow coat
Pulse: slippery

Application:

Coma with difficulty of speech, smoker's dry cough, dyspnea.

Modification:

1. With coma, caused by obstruction of phlegm in the orifices, add:
石菖蒲 Shi Chang Pu (Acorus)   *Rhizoma Acori Graminei*
2. With asthma, add:
桑白皮 Sang Bai Pi (Morus bark)   *Cortex Mori Radicis*
蘇子 Su Zi (Perilla seed)   *Fructus Perillae*

Generic Name:

Trichosanthes and Chih-shih Combination

Guī Lù Ěr Xiān Jiāo   龜鹿二仙膠
(Kuei-Lu-Er-Hsian-Chiao)
(Magic Glue of Tortoise Plastron and Antler Horn)

Constituents:

龜 板 Gui Ban (Tortoise plastron)	5-10 gm.	*Plastrum Testudinis*
鹿 角 Lu Jiao (Antler horn)	10-20 gm.	*Cornus Cervi*
枸杞子 Gou Qi Zi (Lycium fruit)	3-6 gm.	*Fructus Lycii*
人 參 Ren Shen (Ginseng)	3-6 gm.	*Radix Ginseng*

Action:

1. To replenish both *Yin* (vital essence) and *Yang* (vital function) of the kidney
2. To replenish both *Qi* and blood

Indication:

For a person with deficiency of both kidney *Yin* and Yang. The symptoms are: emaciation, fatigue, nocturnal emission, impotence, lumbago, weakness of the knees.

Tongue: pale with white coating
Pulse: deep, slow and weak

Application:

Impotence, nocturnal seminal emission, lumbago.

Guī Pí Tāng　　歸脾湯 (归脾汤)
(Kuei-Pi-Tang)
(Decoction to Strengthen the Heart and the Spleen)

Constituents:

人 參	Ren Shen (Ginseng)	6-9 gm.	Radix Ginseng
黃 芪	Huang Qi (Astragalus)	9-12 gm.	Radix Astragali
當 歸	Dang Gui (Chinese angelica)	6-9 gm.	Radix Angelicae Sinensis
龍眼肉	Long Yan Rou (Longan aril)	9-12 gm.	Arillus Longan
白 术	Bai Zhu (White atractylodes)	6-9 gm.	Rhizoma Atractylodis Macrocephalae
木 香	Mu Xiang (Saussurea)	3-6 gm.	Radix Saussureae
茯 苓	Fu Ling (Poria)	9-12 gm.	Poria
遠 志	Yuan Zhi (Polygala)	6-9 gm.	Radix Polygalae
酸棗仁	Suan Zao Ren (Ziziphus)	9-12 gm.	Semen Ziziphi Spinosae
炙甘草	Zhi Gan Cao (Baked licorice)	3-6 gm.	Radix Glycyrrhizae Praeparatae
生 薑	Sheng Jiang (Fresh ginger)	1-3 gm.	Rhizoma Zingiberis Recens
大 棗	Da Zao (Jujube)	3-5 pc.	Fructus Ziziphus Jujubae

Action:

1. To replenish Qi (vital energy) and blood
2. To strength the heart and the spleen

Indication:

For a person with heart and spleen deficiency. The symptoms are:
palpitation, insomnia, forgetfulness, nightmares, fatigue, lack of appetite,
face sallow or pale, uterine bleeding or menorrhagia.

Tongue: pale, plump, with thin white coating
Pulse: thready and weak

Application:

Neurasthenia, gastric and duodenal ulcer, functional uterine bleeding,
thrombocytopenic purpura, aplastic anemia, general anemia, chronic
bleeding, menorrhagia, uterine bleeding.

Modification:

1. To enhance the effect of blood tonification, add:
熟地黃 Shu Di Huang (Prep. rehmannia)　　*Radix Rehmanniae Praeparatae*
2. Irregular menstruation with increased blood volume but light in color,
add:
阿 膠 E Jiao (Donkey-hide gelatin)　　*Colla Corii Asini*
桑寄生 Sang Ji Sheng (Mulberry mistletoe)　*Ramulus Loranthi*
何首烏 He Shou Wu (Fleece flower root)　　*Radix Polygoni Multiflori*

Generic Name:

Kwei Be Wan; Ginseng and Longan Combination

Guì Zhī Fú Líng Wán   桂枝茯苓丸
(Kuei-Chih-Fu-Ling-Wan)
(Pills of Cinnamon and Poria)

Constituents:

桂　枝	Gui Zhi (Cinnamon twig)	6-9 gm.	Ramulus Cinnamomi
茯　苓	Fu Ling (Poria)	6-9 gm.	Poria
牡丹皮	Mu Dan Pi (Moutan bark)	6-9 gm.	Cortex Moutan Radicis
桃　仁	Tao Ren (Persica seed)	6-9 gm.	Semen Persicae
赤芍藥	Chi Shao Yao (Red peony)	6-9 gm.	Radix Paeoniae Rubra

Action:

1. To remove stagnant blood
2. To soften hard lumps

Indication:

For a person with hard lumps in the lower abdomen. The symptoms are: hard lumps in the lower abdomen, painful and spasmodic, difficulty in menstruation, dysmenorrhea; or retention of lochia with abdominal pain (refused to be pressed) after childbirth.

Application:

Endometritis, adnexitis, hysteromyoma, ovarian cyst, dysmenorrhea, infertility, post-partum bleeding, retention of lochia, irregular menstruation.

Generic Name:

Cinnamon and Hoelen Formula

Guì Zhī Sháo Yào Zhī Mǔ Tāng   桂枝芍藥知母湯
(Kuei-Chih-Shao-Yao-Chi-Mu-Tang)
(Decoction of Cinnamon Twig, Paeonia and Anemarrhena)

Constituents:

桂　枝	Gui Zhi (Cinnamon twig)	6-9 gm.	*Ramulus Cinnamomi*
白芍藥	Bai Shao Yao (White peony)	6-9 gm.	*Radix Paeonae Alba*
知　母	Zhi Mu (Anemarrhena)	6-9 gm.	*Rhizoma Anemarrhenae*
麻　黄	Ma Huang (Ephedra)	6-9 gm.	*Herba Ephedrae*
防　風	Fang Feng (Ledebouriella)	6-9 gm.	*Radix Ledebouriellae*
白　术	Bai Zhu (White atractylodes)	6-9 gm.	*Rhizoma Atractylodis acrocephalae*
附　子	Fu Zi (Aconite)	6-9 gm.	*Radix Aconiti Praeparatae*
炙甘草	Zhi Gan Cao (Baked licorice)	3-6 gm.	*Radix Glycyrrhiae Praeparatae*
生　薑	Sheng Jiang (Fresh ginger)	3-5 pc.	*Rhizoma Zingigeris Recens*

Action:

1. To dispel wind and dampness
2. To eliminate heat and relieve pain

Indication:

For a person with arthritis due to wind, cold and dampness. The symptoms are: pain in the joints, swollen and with burning sensation, no increase of body temperature, edema.

   Tongue: with yellow coating
   Pulse: slippery and rapid

Application:

Arthralgia

Guì Zhī Tāng　桂枝湯
(Kuei-Chih-Tang)
(Decoction of Cinnamon Twig)

Constituents:

桂　枝	Gui Zhi (Cinnamon twig)	6-9 gm.	*Ramulus Cinnamomi*
白芍藥	Bai Shao Yao (White peony)	6-9 gm.	*Radix Paeoniae Alba*
生　薑	Sheng Jiang (Fresh ginger)	3-6 gm.	*Rhizoma Zingiberis Recens*
炙甘草	Zhi Gan Cao (Baked licorice)	3-6 gm.	*Radix Glycyrrhizae Praeparatae*
大　棗	Da Zao (Jujube)	3-5 pc.	*Fructus Ziziphus Jujubae*

Action:

1. Diaphoretic
2. Regulate the *Ying* (nutrient) and Wei (defensive system).

Indication:

For a person with deficiency in the exterior caused by attack of wind and cold. The symptoms are: fever, headache, intolerance of wind, spontaneous perspiration, decreased body resistance.

> Tongue: with thin white coating
> Pulse: floating, tardy

Application:

Common cold, influenza, postpartum care, morning sickness, skin diseases (eczema, frostbite, tinea, etc.)

Modification:

1. With arthritis caused by wind, cold and dampness, add:

薑　黃	Jiang Huang (Tumeric rhizome)	*Rhizoma Curcumae Longae*
細　辛	Xi Xin (Asarum)	*Herba Asari*
威靈仙	Wei Ling Xian (Clematis)	*Radix Clematidis*

2. With stiff neck and shoulder, add:

葛　根	Ge Gen (Pueraria)	*Radix Puerariae*

This formula is called Gui Zhi Jia Ge Gen Tang　桂枝加葛根湯

3. With nocturnal emission, excessive dreams, cold sensation in the lower part of the body, dizziness, loss of hair, add:

龍　骨	Long Gu (Dragon's bone)	*Os Draconis*
牡　蠣	Mu Li (Oyster shell)	*Concha Ostreae*

This formula is called Gui Zhi Jia Long Gu Mu Li Tang　桂枝加龍骨牡蠣湯

4. With dyspnea, asthma and sputum, add:

厚　朴	Hou Po (Magnolia bark)	*Cortex Magnoliae Officinalis*
杏　仁	Xing Ren (Apricot seed)	*Semen Armeniacae Amarum*

This formula is called Gui Zhi Jia Hou Po Xing Ren Tang　桂枝加厚朴杏仁湯

Generic Name: Cinnamon Combination

Hǎi Zǎo Yù Hú Tāng   海藻玉壺湯

(Hai-Chao-Yu-Hu-Tang)
(The Seaweed Decoction)

Constituents:

海 藻	Hai Zao (Sargassum)	6-9 gm.	*Sargassum*
昆 布	Kun Bu (Ecklonia)	6-9 gm.	*Thallus Eckloniae*
海 帶	Hai Dai (Kelp)	6-9 gm.	*Thallus Laminariae*
浙貝母	Zhe Bei Mu (Fritillaria)	6-9 gm.	*Bulbus Fritillariae Thunbergii*
半 夏	Ban Xia (Pinellia)	6-9 gm.	*Rhizoma Pinelliae*
陳 皮	Chen Pi (Citrus peel)	3-6 gm.	*Pericarpium Citri Reticulatae*
青 皮	Qing Pi (Green tangerine peel)	3-6 gm.	*Pericarpium Citri Reticulatae Viridae*
連 翹	Lian Qiao (Forsythia)	6-9 gm.	*Fructus Forsythiae*
當 歸	Dang Gui (Chinese angelica)	6-9 gm.	*Radix Angelicae Sinensis*
川 芎	Chuan Xiong (Ligusticum)	3-6 gm.	*Rhizoma Ligustici Chuanxiong*
獨 活	Du Huo (Pubescent angelica)	6-9 gm.	*Radix Angelicae Pubescentis*
甘 草	Gan Cao (Licorice)	3-6 gm.	*Radix Glycyrrhizae*

Action:

To resolve phlegm and hardening

Indication:

For a person with goiter caused by stagnation of *Qi* and blood in the liver, or caused by deficiency of iodine. The symptoms are: hard lumps or nodules anterior or posterior to the ear, soft and not painful, fullness in the chest, hypochondriac pain, like to sigh or take deep breathing.

Tongue: with thin greasy coating
Pulse: wiry and slippery

Application:

Goiter, hyperthyroidism, acute simple lymphadenitis.

Modification:

If the swelling is hard and with nodules, add:

桃 仁	Tao Ren (Persica seed)	*Semen Persicae*
紅 花	Hong Hua (Safflower)	*Flos Carthami*

Hāo Qín Qīng Dǎn Tāng　蒿芩清膽湯
(Hao-Chin-Ching-Tan-Tang)
(Febrifugal Decoction with Sweet Wormwood and Scutellaria)

Constituents:

青 蒿	Qing Hao (Sweet wormwood)	6-9 gm.	*Herba Artemisiae Chinghao*
黃 芩	Huang Qin (Scutellaria)	9-12 gm.	*Radix Scutellariae*
竹 茹	Zhu Ru (Bamboo shavings)	6-9 gm.	*Caulus Bambusae in Taenis*
半 夏	Ban Xia (Pinellia)	9-12 gm.	*Radix Pinelliae*
枳 殼	Zhi Ke (Bitter orange)	6-9 gm.	*Fructus Aurantii*
陳 皮	Chen Pi (Citrus peel)	6-9 gm.	*Pericarpium Citri Reticulatae*
赤茯苓	Chi Fu Ling (Red poria)	12-15 gm.	*Poria*
碧玉散	Bi Yu San:	9-12 gm.	
	滑石 Hua Shi (Talc)		*Talcum*
	青黛 Qing Dai (Indigo)		*Indigo Naturalis*
	甘草 Gan Cao (Licorice)		*Radix Glycyrrhizae*

Action:

1. To eliminate the heat and dampness in gallbladder
2. To resolve the phlegm in the stomach

Indication:

For a person with heat and dampness in the gallbladder of the Shao-yang channel. The symptoms are: alternate fever and chills (fever more severe than chills), pain and distention in the chest and costal region, nausea, dry vomiting or with yellow and sticky saliva, bitterness in the mouth, acid regurgitation.

Tongue: white and greasy, or yellow and greasy
Pulse: wiry/taut and rapid, or soft and rapid

Application:

Acute cholecystitis, acute gastritis, acute icteric hepatitis, chronic pancreatitis, malaria

Modification:

1. With vomiting, add:

黃 連	Huang Lian (Coptis)	*Rhizoma Coptidis*
吳茱萸	Wu Zhu Yu (Evodia fruit)	*Fructus Evodiae*

2. With jaundice, add:

茵陳蒿	Yin Chen Hao (Capillaris)	*Herba Artemisiae Capillaris*
梔 子	Zhi Zi (Gardenia fruit)	*Fructus Gardeniae*

3. With dampness, add:

白豆蔻	Bai Dou Kou (Round cardamon)	*Semen Cardamomi Rotundi*
草 果	Cao Guo (Tsao-ko)	*Fructus Tsao-ko*

Hé Chē Dà Zào Wán   河車大造丸

(Ho-Che-Ta-Chao-Wan)
(Pills of Human Placenta)

Constituents:

紫河車	Zi He Che (Human placenta)	1 pc.	*Placenta Hominis*
人 參	Ren Shen (Ginseng)	6-9 gm.	*Radix Ginseng*
熟地黃	Shu Di Huang (Prep. rehmannia)	12-15 gm.	*Radix Rehmanniae Praeparatae*
杜 仲	Du Zhong (Eucommia)	6-9 gm.	*Cortex Eucommiae*
天門冬	Tian Men Dong (Asparagus)	6-9 gm.	*Radix Asparagi*
麥門冬	Mai Men Dong (Ophiopogon)	6-9 gm.	*Radix Ophiopogonis*
龜 板	Gui Ban (Tortoise plastron)	6-9 gm.	*Plastrum Testudinis*
黃 柏	Huang Bai (Phellodendron)	6-9 gm.	*Cortex Phellodendri*
茯 苓	Fu Ling ((Poria)	6-9 gm.	*Poria*
懷牛膝	Huai Niu Xi (Achyranthes)	6-9 gm.	*Radix Achyranthis Bidentatae*

Action:

1. To replenish the *Yin* (vital essence) of kidney and lung.
2. To subdue the fire

Indication:

For a person with weak fire due to the deficiency of *Yin* (vital essence) of the kidney and lung. The symptoms are: dizziness, tinnitus, lumbago, cough, tidal fever, retarded growth in children (physically and mentally).

    Tongue: red
    Pulse: thready and rapid

Application:

Lumbago, tinnitus, chronic cough, tuberculosis retarded growth in children.

Generic Name:

Restorative Pills

Hóng Huā Táo Rén Jiān   紅花桃仁煎
(Hung-Hua-Tao-Ren-Chian)
(Decoction of Carthamus and Persica Seed)

Constituents:

紅 花	Hong Hua (Carthamus)	6-9 gm.	*Flos Carthami*
桃 仁	Tao Ren (Persica seed)	6-9 gm.	*Semen Persicae*
丹 參	Dan Shen (Salvia)	6-9 gm.	*Radix Salviae Miltiorrhizae*
當 歸	Dang Gui (Chinese angelica)	6-9 gm.	*Radix Angelicae Sinensis*
川 芎	Chuan Xiong (Ligusticum)	3-6 gm.	*Rhizoma Ligustici Chuanxiong*
生地黃	Sheng Di Huang (Fresh rehmannia)	9-12 gm.	*Radix Rehmanniae*
赤芍藥	Chi Shao Yao (Red peony)	6-9 gm.	*Radix Paeoniae Rubra*
香 附	Xiang Fu (Cyperus)	3-6 gm.	*Rhizoma Cyperi*
延胡索	Yan Hu Suo (Corydalis)	6-9 gm.	*Rhizoma Corydalis*
青 皮	Qing Pi (Green tangerine peel)	3-6 gm.	*Pericarpium Citri Reticulatae Viridae*

Action:

1. To invigorate the circulation of blood
2. To remove blood stasis

Indication:

For a person with blood stasis and stagnation of *Qi* (vital energy). The symptoms are: abdominal pain and distention (more severe if pressed), hypochondriac distention, irregular menstruation (delayed or with sluggish flow), mental depression.

Tongue: with purple spots, thin coating
Pulse: deep and hesitant, or deep and wiry/taut

Application:

Amenorrhea, dysmenorrhea.

Hòu Pò Wēn Zhōng Tāng　　厚朴温中湯
(Hou-Pu-Wen-Chung-Tang)
(Decoction of Magnolia to warm the Spleen and Stomach)

Constituents:

厚 朴	Hou Po (Magnolia bark)	20-30 gm.	*Cortex Magnoliae Officinalis*
草豆蔻	Cao Dou Kou (Katsumadai seed)	12-15 gm.	*Semen Alpiniae Katsumadai*
乾 薑	Gan Jiang (Dry ginger)	2-3 gm.	*Rhizoma Zingiberis*
木 香	Mu Xiang (Saussurea)	12-15 gm.	*Radix Saussureae*
陳 皮	Chen Pi (Citrus peel)	20-30 gm.	*Pericarpium Citri Reticulatae*
茯 苓	Fu Ling (Poria)	12-15 gm.	*Poria*
炙甘草	Zhi Gan Cao (Baked licorice)	12-15 gm.	*Radix Glycyrrhizae Praeparatae*

Action:

1. To warm the spleen and stomach, and regulate the flow of *Qi*
2. To eliminate dampness and distention by drying method

Indication:

For a person with symptoms of cold and dampness in the spleen and stomach. The symptoms are: malaise, poor appetite, abdominal pain and distention, preference of heat over the abdomen, loose stools.

Tongue: Pale white with greasy coating
Pulse: Slippery and thready

Application:

Chronic colitis, leukorrhea

117

Hŭ Qián Wán 虎潛丸
(Hu-Chian-Wan)
(The Tiger Pills)

Constituents:

熱地黃	Shu Di Huang (Prep. rehmannia)	9-12 gm.	*Radix Rehmanniae Preparatae*
龜 版	Gui Ban (Tortoise plastron)	9-12 gm.	*Plastrum Testudinis*
黃 柏	Huang Bai (Phellodendron)	6-9 gm.	*Cortex Phellodendri*
知 母	Zhi Mu (Anemarrhena)	6-9 gm.	*Rhizoma Anemarrhenae*
虎 骨	Hu Gu (Tiger's bone)	6-9 gm.	*Os Tigridis*
鎖 陽	Suo Yang (Cynomorium)	6-9 gm.	*Herba Cynomorii*
懷牛膝	Huai Niu Xi (Achyranthes)	6-9 gm.	*Radix Achyranthi Bidentatae*
當 歸	Dang Gui (Chinese angelica)	6-9 gm.	*Radix Angelicae Sinensis*
白芍藥	Bai Shao Yao (White peony)	6-9 gm.	*Radix Angelicae Sinensis*
陳 皮	Chen Pi (Citrus peel)	4-6 gm.	*Pericarpium Citri Reticulatae*
乾 薑	Gan Jiang (Dry ginger)	3-6 gm.	*Rhizoma Zingiberis*
羊 肉	Yang Rou (Lamb)		

Take 6-9 gm. of the pills made, 1-2 times daily with salt water.

Action:

1. To purge the fire
2. To nourish the *Yin* (Vital essence)
3. To strengthen the bones and sinews

Indication:

For a person with flaccidity of muscles and bones due to asthenia of liver and kidney. The symptoms are: dizziness, tinnitus, flaccidity of the muscles and bones, difficulty in walking, lumbago.

Tongue: red
Pulse: thready and rapid

Application:

Lumbago, flaccidity of muscles and bones, with difficulty in walking.

Generic Name:

Chien Pu Hu Chien Wan

Huái Huā Sàn 槐花散

(Huai-Hua-San)
(Powder of Sophora Flower)

Constituents:

槐　花	Huai Hua (Sophora flower)	10-15 gm.	*Flos Sophorae*
側柏葉	Ce Bai Ye (Biota tops)	6-9 gm.	*Cacumen Biotae*
荊芥穗	Jing Jie Sui (Schizonepeta spikes)	6-9 gm.	*Herba Schizonepetae*
枳　殼	Zhi Ke (Bitter orange)	6-9 gm.	*Fructus Aurantii*

Action:

1. Hemostatic
2. To dispel wind, heat and toxin in the intestines

Indication:

For a person with bleeding disorders in the lower part of the body. The symptoms are: stool with blood, color bright red or dark red.

Tongue: red
Pulse: wiry and rapid

Application:

Hemorrhoids, bleeding from the anus, rectum or the intestines

Modification:

1. If heat in the intestines is intense, add:

黃　連	Huang Lian (Coptis)	*Rhizoma Coptidis*
黃　柏	Huang Bai (Phellodendron)	*Cortex Phellodendri*

2. For hemorrhoid, add:

地　瑜	Di Yu (Sanguisorba)	*Radix Sanguisorbae*

Huái Jiǎo Wán   槐角丸
(Huai-Chiao-Wan)
(Pills of Sophora Fruit)

Constituents:

槐 角	Huai Jiao (Sophora fruit)	10-15 gm.	*Fructus Sophorae*
地 瑜	Di Yi (Sanguisorba)	6-9 gm.	*Radix Sanguisorbae*
防 風	Fang Feng (Ledebouriella)	6-9 gm.	*Radix Ledebouriellae*
當 歸	Dang Gui (Chinese angelica)	6-9 gm.	*Radix Angelicae Sinensis*
枳 殼	Zhi Ke (Bitter orange)	6-9 gm.	*Fructus Aurantii*
黃 芩	Huang Qin (Scutellaria)	6-9 gm.	*Radix Scutellariae*

Action:

1. To eliminate the heat in the intestines
2. To stop bleeding (Hemostatic)

Indication:

For a person with hemorrhoid bleeding. The symptoms are: bloody stool, color red, hemorrhoid.

Tongue: red
Pulse: wiry/taut and rapid

Application:

Hemorrhoid, fresh bloody stool.

Contraindication:

For a person with chronic bloody stool or the color of blood is dark purplish.

Generic Name:

Fructus Sophorae

Huáng Lián É Jiāo Tāng　黄連阿膠湯

(Huang-Lien-Ah-Chiao-Tang)
(Decoction of Coptis and Gelatin)

Constituents:

黄　連	Huang Lian (Coptis)	3-6 gm.	*Rhizoma Coptidis*
阿　膠	E Jiao (Donkey-hide gelatin)	9-12 gm.	*Colla Corii Asini*
黄　芩	Huang Qin (Scutellaria)	9-12 gm.	*Radix Scutellariae*
白芍藥	Bai Shao Yao (White peony)	9-12 gm.	*Radix Paeoniae Alba*
雞子黄	Ji Zi Huang (Egg yolk)	2 yolks	

Action:

1. To purge the fire
2. To replenish the *Yin* (vital essence)

Indication:

For a person with excessive fire due to deficiency of *Yin* (vital essence) of the kidney and heart. The symptoms are: restlessness, insomnia, mouth and throat dry, fidgetiness.

Tongue: red or dark red, dry
Pulse: deep, thready and rapid

Application:

Insomnia, neurasthenia.

Modification:

1. For dry throat, add:

玄　參	Xuan Shen (Scrophularia)	*Radix Scrophulariae*
麥門冬	Mai Men Dong (Ophiopogon)	*Radix Ophiopogonis*
石　斛	Shi Hu (Dendrobium)	*Herba Dendrobii*

2. For restlessness, add:

梔　子	Zhi Zi (Gardenia fruit)	*Fructus Gardeniae*
竹　葉	Zhu Ye (Bamboo leaf)	*Folium Bambusae*

3. With tendency to be awakened easily, add:

珍珠母	Zhen Zhu Mu (Mother-of-pearl)	*Concha Margaritifera Usta*
牡　蠣	Mu Li (Oyster shell)	*Concha Ostreae*

Generic Name:

Coptis and Gelatin Combination

Huáng Lián Jiě Dú Tāng　黃連解毒湯
(Huang-Lien-Chieh-Tu-Tang)
(Antiphlogistic Decoction of Coptis)

Constituents:

黄 連	Huang Lian (Coptis)	9-12 gm.	*Rhizoma Coptidis*
黄 芩	Huang Qin (Scutellaria)	9-12 gm.	*Radix Scutellariae*
黄 柏	Huang Bai (Phellodendron)	9-12 gm.	*Cortex Phellodendri*
梔 子	Zhi Zi (Gardenia fruit)	3-6 gm.	*Fructus Gardeniae*

Action:

To dispel noxious heat and toxin from all three burners.

Indication:

For a person with heat in all three burners. The symptoms are: high fever, irritability, mouth and throat dry, insomnia, spitting blood, epistaxis, macula, boils, suppurative infections.

Tongue: red with yellow coating
Pulse: rapid and forceful

Application:

Septicemia, dysentery, pneumonia, acute infection of the urinary tract, carbuncle or furuncle, boils.

Contraindication:

For a person with disappearance of the fur on tongue, indicating deficiency of vital essence in the stomach.

Modification:

1. With spitting blood, epistaxis, add:

玄 參	Xuan Shen (Scrophularia)	*Radix Scrophulariae*
生地黄	Sheng Di Huang (Fresh rehmannia)	*Radix Rehmanniae*
牡丹皮	Mu Dan Pi (Moutan bark)	*Cortex Moutan Radicis*

2. With jaundice, add:

茵陳蒿	Yin Chen Hao (Capillaris)	*Herba Artemisiae Capillaris*
大 黄	Da Huang (Rhubarb)	*Radix et Rhizoma Rhei*

Generic Name:

Coptis and Scute Combination

Huáng Lián Tāng　黄連湯

(Huang-Lien-Tang)
(The Coptis Decoction)

Constituents:

黄 連	Huang Lian (Coptis)	3-6 gm.	*Rhizoma Coptidis*
乾 薑	Gan Jiang (Dry ginger)	3-6 gm.	*Rhizoma Zingiberis*
桂 枝	Gui Zhi (Cinnamon)	6-9 gm.	*Ramulus Cinnamomi*
半 夏	Ban Xia (Pinellia)	6-9 gm.	*Rhizoma Pinelliae*
人 參	Ren Shen (Ginseng)	3-6 gm.	*Radix Ginseng*
大 棗	Da Zao (Jujube)	3-5 pc.	*Fructus Ziziphus Jujubae*
炙甘草	Zhi Gan Cao (Baked licorice)	3-6 gm.	*Radix Glycyrrhizae Praeparatae*

Action:

1. To eliminate the heat in the upper body
2. To warm the lower part of the body
3. To oppress the ascending flow of stomach *Qi* (vital energy).

Indication:

For a person with heat in the upper part of the body and coldness in the lower part. The symptoms are: irritable heat in the chest, hiccough, vomiting, diarrhea, abdominal pain, fullness and oppression in the chest.

Tongue: with white slippery coating
Pulse: wiry/taut

Application:

Hiccough, acute gastroenteritis.

Generic Name:

Coptis Combination

Huáng Lóng Tāng 黄龍湯 (黄龙汤)
(Huang-Lung-Tang)
(The Yellow Dragon Decoction)

Constituents:

大 黃	Da Huang (Rhubarb)	9-12 gm.	*Radix et Rhizoma Rhei*
芒 硝	Mang Xiao (Mirabilitum)	6-9 gm.	*Natrii Sulfas*
枳 實	Zhi Shi (Immature bitter orange)	6-9 gm.	*Fructus Aurantii Immaturus*
厚 朴	Hou Po (Magnolia bark)	6-9 gm.	*Cortex Magnoliae Officinalis*
人 參	Ren Shen (Ginseng)	3-6 gm.	*Radix Ginseng*
當 歸	Dang Gui (Chinese angelica)	6-9 gm.	*Radix Angelicae Sinensis*
桔 梗	Jie Geng (Platycodon)	3-6 gm.	*Radix Platycodi*
生 薑	Sheng Jiang (Fresh ginger)	1-3 gm.	*Rhizoma Zingiberis Recens*
甘 草	Gan Cao (Licorice)	1-3 gm.	*Radix Glycyrrhizae*
大 棗	Da Zao (Jujube)	3-5 pc.	*Fructus Ziziphus Jujubae*

Action:

1. To eliminate the true heat in the Yang-ming visceras (the stomach and the intestines)
2. To replenish blood and vital energy

Indication:

For a person with deficiency of *Qi* (vital energy) and blood, but with true heat in the stomach and intestines. The symptoms are: constipation, abdominal distention, pain and fullness in the epigastric region, watery diarrhea, hot and thirsty sensation, delirium, lassitude.

Tongue: yellow and dry or prickly
Pulse: thready and weak

Application:

Diarrhea or constipation in chronic bacteria dysentery, intestinal tuberculosis, hemorrhoids.

Huáng Qí Guì Zhī Wǔ Wù Tāng　黄芪桂枝五物湯
(Huang-Chi-Kuei-Chih-Wu-Wu-Tang)
(Five Ingredients Decoction with Astragalus and Cinnamon)

Constituents:

黄　芪 Huang Qi (Astragalus)	10-15 gm.	*Radix Astragali*
桂　枝 Gui Zhi (Cinnamon)	9-12 gm.	*Ramulus Cinnamomi*
白芍藥 Bai Shao Yao (White peony)	9-12 gm.	*Radix Paeoniae Alba*
生　薑 Sheng Jiang (Fresh ginger)	10-15 gm.	*Rhizoma Zingiberis Recens*
大　棗 Da Zao (Jujube)	12-15 pc.	*Fructus Ziziphus Jujubae*

Action:

1. To warm the channels and collaterals
2. To replenish *Qi* (vital energy) and blood
3. To dispel cold

Indication:

For a person with arthralgia due to deficiency of blood. The symptoms are: arthralgia, migratory pain, intolerance of wind, with numbness sensation in the body.

> Tongue: with white and greasy coating
> Pulse: faint, hesitant and tight

Application:

Arthritis (migratory) with numbness

Generic Name:

Astragalus and Cinnamon Five Herb Combination

Huáng Qí Jiàn Zhōng Tāng   黃芪建中湯
(Huang-Chi-Chien-Chung-Tang)
(Decoction for Restoring the Normal Function of the Middle Burner with Astragalus)

Constituents:

黃 芪	Huang Qi (Astragalus)	10-15 gm.	*Radix Astragali*
飴 糖	Yi Tang (Maltose)	20-30 gm.	*Saccharum Granorum*
桂 枝	Gui Zhi (Cinnamon twig)	6-9 gm.	*Ramulus Cinnamomi*
白芍藥	Bai Shao Yao (White peony)	10-15 gm.	*Radix Paeoniae Alba*
炙甘草	Zhi Gan Cao (Baked licorice)	3-6 gm.	*Radix Glycyrrhizae*
生 薑	Sheng Jiang (Fresh ginger)	3-6 gm.	*Rhizoma Zingiberis Recens*
大 棗	Da Zao (Jujube)	3-5 pc.	*Fructus Ziziphus Jujubae*

Action:

1. To warm and tonify the spleen and stomach
2. To replenish *Qi* (vital energy)

Indication:

For a person with cold and deficiency symptoms of the spleen and stomach, or impaired exterior defensive system. The symptoms are: dyspnea, spontaneous perspiration, abdominal pain due to cold, face colour pale, fatigue.

Tongue: pale with white coating
Pulse: deep and slow

Application:

Gastric and duodenal ulcer, neurasthenia, aplastic anemia, postpartum fever, chronic hepatitis.

Generic Name:

Astragalus Combination

Huáng Tǔ Tāng 黄土湯

(Huang-Tu-Tang)
(Decoction of Ignited Yellow Earth)

Constituents:

伏龍肝	Fu Long Gan (Zao Xin Tu) (灶心土)	30-50 gm.	*Terra Flava Usta*
白　术	Bai Zhu (White atractylodes)	6-9 gm.	*Rhizoma Atractylodis Macrocephalae*
附　子	Fu Zi (Aconite)	3-6 gm.	*Radix Aconiti Praeparatae*
生地黄	Sheng Di Huang (Fresh rehmannia)	9-12 gm.	*Radix Rehmanniae*
阿　膠	E Jiao (Donkey-hide gelatin)	9-12 gm.	*Colla Corii Asini*
黄　芩	Huang Qin (Scutellaria)	6-9 gm.	*Radix Scutellariae*
甘　草	Gan Cao (Licorice)	6-9 gm.	*Radix Glycyrrhizae*

Action:

1. To strengthen the spleen and reinforce the *Yang* (vital function)
2. To nourish blood and stop bleeding (Hemostatic)

Indication:

For a person with bleeding disorders due to deficiency of spleen *Yang* (vital function). The symptoms are: face pale, cold sensation in the four limbs, vomiting blood, nose-bleeding, bloody stool (stool first, blood later), uterine bleeding, color of blood dull red.

Tongue: light red with white coating
Pulse: sinking, thready or weak

Application:

Chronic GI-tract bleeding, functional uterine bleeding

Modification:

1. If bleeding is excessive, add:

三　七	San Qi (Pseudoginseng)	*Radix Pseudoginseng*
艾　葉	Ai Ye (Artemisia)	*Folium Artemisiae Argyi*
炮　薑	Pao Jiang (Stir-baked ginger)	*Radix Zingiberis*

2. With deficiency of *Qi* (vital energy), add:

人　參	Ren Shen (Ginseng)	*Radix Ginseng*

Generic Name:

Fu-lung-kan Combination

Huò Xiāng Zhèng Qì Sàn　薑香正氣散
(Huo-Hsiang-Cheng-Chi-San)
(Powder for Dispelling Turbidity with Agastache)

Constituents:

薑　香	Huo Xiang (Agastache)	6-9 gm.	*Herba Agastachis*
厚　朴	Hou Po (Magnolia bark)	6-9 gm.	*Cortex Magnoliae Officinalis*
紫蘇葉	Zi Su Ye (Perilla leaf)	6-9 gm.	*Folium Perillae*
白　芷	Bai Zhi (Angelica root)	3-6 gm.	*Radix Angelicae Dahuricae*
陳　皮	Chen Pi (Citrus peel)	3-6 gm.	*Pericarpium Citri Reticulatae*
茯　苓	Fu Ling (Poria)	6-9 gm.	*Poria*
白　术	Bai Zhu (White atractylodes)	6-9 gm.	*Rhizoma Atractylodis Macrocephalae*
大腹皮	Da Fu Pi (Areca peel)	6-9 gm.	*Pericarpium Arecae*
桔　梗	Jie Geng (Platycodon)	6-9 gm.	*Radix Platycodi*
半　夏	Ban Xia (Pinellia)	6-9 gm.	*Rhizoma Pinelliae*
甘　草	Zhi Gan Cao (Baked licorice)	3-6 gm.	*Radix Glycyrrhizae Praeparatae*
生　薑	Sheng Jiang (Fresh ginger)	1-3 gm.	*Rhizoma Zingiberis Recens*
大　棗	Da Zao (Jujube)	3-5 pc.	*Fructus Ziziphus Jujubae*

Action:

1. To resolve damp-turbidity in spleen and stomach
2. To dispel pathogenic factors from the exterior of the body

Indication:

For a person with accumulation of dampness in the interior and affection of wind and cold in the exterior. The symptoms are: fever with headache, aversion to cold, chest distention, abdominal pain, nausea and vomiting, borborygmus and diarrhea.

> Tongue: white with greasy coating
> Pulse: Moderate, or floating and tight

Application:

Acute gastritis, acute diarrhea (especially in the summer season)

Contraindication:

For a person with dampness and heat syndrome with manifestations of thirst, dry throat, fever but is not afraid of cold, tongue with yellow and greasy coating.

Modification:

If acute diarrhea is very severe, add:

炒扁豆	Cao Bian Dou (Stir-fried dolichos seed)	*Semen Dolichi*
炒薏米	Cao Yi Yi Ren (Stir-fried coix seed)	*Semen Coicis*

Generic Name:

Agastache Formula

Jì Chuān Jiān 濟川煎

(Chi-Chuan-Chian)
(The Blood Replenishing Decoction)

Constituents:

肉苁蓉	Rou Cong Rong (Cistanche)	6-9 gm.	*Herba Cistanchis*
當 歸	Dang Gui (Chinese angelica)	9-15 gm.	*Radix Angelicae Sinensis*
懷牛膝	Huai Niu Xi (Achyranthes)	6-9 gm.	*Radix Achyranthis Bidentatae*
澤 瀉	Ze Xie (Alisma)	6-9 gm.	*Rhizoma Alismatis*
枳 殼	Zhi Ke (Bitter orange)	3-6 gm.	*Fructus Aurantii*
升 麻	Sheng Ma (Cimicifuga)	3-6 gm.	*Rhizoma Cimicifugae*

Action:

1. Emollient
2. To replenish blood and strengthen the kidney

Indication:

For a person with constipation due to anemia and kidney deficiency. The symptoms are: constipation, anemia, urination prolonged and color is clear, low back pain, cold sensation in the back.

Tongue: pale with thin white coating
Pulse: thready

Application:

Constipation

Contraindication:

For a person with constipation due to excessive fire or heat in the body.

Modification:

1. With deficiency of vital energy, add:
人 參 Ren Sheng (Ginseng) *Radix Ginseng*
2. With kidney deficiency, add:
熟地黃 Shu Di Huang (Prep. rehmannia) *Radix Rehmanniae Preparata*
3. With internal fire in the body, add:
黃 芩 Huang Qin (Scutellaria) *Radix Scutellariae*
4. With chronic constipation, add:
火麻仁 Huo Ma Ren (Cannabis seed) *Fructus Cannabis*
鎖 陽 Suo Yang (Cynomorium) *Herba Cynomorii*

Jǐ Jiāo Lì Huáng Wán 己椒塵黄丸
(Chi-Chiao-Li-Huang-Wan)
(Pills of Stephania, Zanthoxylum, Lepidium Seed and Rhubarb)

Constituents:

防 己 Fang Ji (Stephania)	9-15 gm.	*Radix Stephaniae Tetrandrae*
椒 目 Jiao Mu (Zanthoxylum)	3-6 gm.	*Pericarpium Zanthoxylii*
葶塵子 Ting Li Zi (Lepidium seed)	9-15 gm.	*Semen Lepidii*
大 黄 Da Huang (Rhubarb)	6-9 gm.	*Radix et Rhizoma Rhei*

Action:

1. To dispel water
2. Diuretic

Indication:

For a person with retention of fluid in the body. The symptoms are: distention and fullness sensation in the chest, cough and asthma with profuse sputum, face swollen, pedal edema.

> Tongue: with thick, slippery or greasy coating
> Pulse: slow and uneven, or intermittent

Application:

Cor pulmonale, pericarditis, pleuritis, asthma.

Modification:

1. With cough and asthma, use in combination with San Niu Tang （三拗湯）

2. With profuse phlegm and fluid in lung, use in combination with San Zi Yang Qing Tang
（三子養親湯）

3. With edema, use in combination with:
Wu Pi Yin (Hoelen and Areca Combination)（五皮飲）
or Wu Ling San (Hoelen Five Herb Formula)（五苓散）

Jī Míng Sàn 雞鳴散 （鸡鸣散）

(Chi-Ming-San)
(Cock-a-doodle-doo Powder)

Constituents:

檳 榔	Bing Lang (Areca seed)	9-12 gm.	*Semen Arecae*
木 瓜	Mu Gua (Chaenomeles fruit)	6-9 gm.	*Fructus Chaenomelis*
陳 皮	Chen Pi (Citrus peel)	6-9 gm.	*Pericarpium Citri Reticulatae*
紫蘇葉	Zi Su Ye (Perilla leaf)	3-6 gm.	*Folium Perillae*
桔 梗	Jie Geng (Platycodon)	3-6 gm.	*Radix Platycodi*
吳茱萸	Wu Zhu Yu (Evodia fruit)	3-6 gm.	*Fructus Evodiae*
生 薑	Sheng Jiang (Fresh ginger)	1-3 gm.	*Rhizoma Zingiberis Recens*

Action:

1. To dispel cold and dampness by warming
2. To invigorate the circulation of vital energy (Carminative)
3. To clear the channels and collaterals

Indication:

For a person with beriberi. The symptoms are: fever, intolerance of cold, legs and feet feel painful, swollen and heavy, edema, difficulty of movement, may have spasms or numbness sensation, chest fullness, nausea.

Tongue: with white and greasy coating
Pulse: soft and slow

Application:

Beriberi, edema.

Modification:

1. If there is wind and dampness, with spontaneous perspiration, intolerance of wind, pulse floating and slow, add:

桂 枝	Gui Zhi (Cinnamon twig)	*Ramulus Cinnamomi*
防 風	Fang Feng (Ledebouriellae)	*Radix Ledebouriellae*

2. With cold and dampness, add:

肉 桂	Rou Gui (Cinnamon bark)	*Cortex Cinnamomi*
附 子	Fu Zi (Aconite)	*Radix Aconiti Praeparatae*

3. With nausea, vomiting, chest fullness, add:

沉 香	Chen Xiang (Aquilaria)	*Lignum Aquilariae Resinatum*
肉 桂	Rou Gui (Cinnamon bark)	*Cortex Cinnamomi*
附 子	Fu Zi (Aconite)	*Radix Aconiti Praeparatae*
制半夏	Zhi Ban Xia (Pinellia)	*Rhizoma Pinelliae*

and eliminate Zi Su Ye (Perilla), Chen Pi (Citrus peel) and Jie Geng (Platycodon). 去紫蘇葉、陳皮與桔梗。

Generic Name:

Areca Seed and Chaenomeles Formula

Jiā Jiǎn Fù Mài Tāng 加減復脈湯
(Chia-Chian-Fu-Mai-Tang)
(Modified Baked Licorice Decoction)

Constituents:

炙甘草	Zhi Gan Cao (Baked licorice)	9-12 gm.	Radix Glycyrrhizae Praeparatae
生地黃	Sheng Di Huang (Fresh rehmannia)	15-20 gm.	Radix Rehmanniae
白芍藥	Bai Shao Yao (White peony)	6-9 gm.	Radix Paeoniae Alba
麥門冬	Mai Men Dong (Ophiopogon)	6-9 gm.	Radix Ophiopogonis
火麻仁	Huo Ma Ren (Cannabis seed)	9-12 gm.	Fructus Cannabis
阿　膠	E Jiao (Donkey-hide gelatin)	6-9 gm.	Colla Corii Asini

Action:

1. To replenish the *Yin* (vital essence)
2. To eliminate heat and dryness
3. To increase the secretion of body fluids

Indication:

For a person with deficiency of *Yin* (vital essence) and blood. The symptoms are: chronic fever, face red, mouth dry, restlessness, palpitation.

Tongue: red, dry, with no coating
Pulse: weak and forceful

Application:

Coronary heart disease, viral myocarditis, arrhythmia, rheumatic heart disease, tuberculosis, neurasthenia.

Jiā Jiǎn Wēi Ruí Tāng 加減葳蕤湯
(Chia-Chian-Wei-Rui-Tang)
(Decoction of Polygonatum Rhizome)

Constituents:

葳 蕤	Wei Rui (Yu Zhu) (Polygonatum)(玉竹)	6-9 gm.	*Rhizoma Polygonati Odorati*
葱 白	Cong Bai (Allium bulb)	2-3 pc.	*Bulbus Allii Fistulosumi*
桔 梗	Jie Geng (Platycodon)	3-6 gm.	*Radix Platycodi*
白 薇	Bai Wei (Swallowwort)	1-3 gm.	*Radix Cynanchi Atrati*
淡豆豉	Dan Dou Chi (Prepared soya)	9-12 gm.	*Semen Sojae Praeparatae*
薄 荷	Bo He (Mentha)	3-6 gm.	*Herba Menthae*
炙甘草	Zhi Gan Cao (Baked licorice)	1-3 gm.	*Radix Glycyrrhizae Praeparatae*
大 棗	Da Zao (Jujube)	3-5 pc.	*Fructus Ziziphus Jujubae*

Actions:

1. To dispel exterior wind and heat (Diaphoretic)
2. To replenish the *Yin* (vital essence)

Indication:

For a person with common cold caused by wind and heat factors, but with deficiency of *Yin* (vital essence) constitution. The symptoms are: fever, headache, slightly intolerance to wind and cold, throat dry and thirsty, cough with sticky sputum, with no or slight perspiration, irritability.

Tongue: red
Pulse: rapid and weak

Application:

Common cold, influenza

Contraindication:

For a person with common cold but with deficiency of *Yang* (vital function) constitution.

Modification:

1. With thick and sticky sputum, add:

牛蒡子	Niu Bang Zi (Arctium)	*Fructus Arctii*
瓜蔞皮	Gua Lou Pi (Trichosanthes peel)	*Pericarpium Trichosanthis*

2. With thirst and irritability, add:

竹 葉	Zhu Ye (Bamboo leaf)	*Folium Bambusae*
天花粉	Tian Hua Fen (Trichosanthes root)	*Radix Trichosanthis*

Jiā Wèi Èr Miào Sàn　　加味二妙散

(Chia-Wei-Er-Miao-San)
(Modified Decoction of Two Effective Ingredients)

Constituents:

黄　柏	Huang Bai (Phellodendron)	6-9 gm.	*Cortex Phellodendri*
蒼　术	Cang Zhu (Atractylodes)	9-12 gm.	*Rhizoma Atractylodis*
防　己	Fang Ji (Stephania)	6-9 gm.	*Radix Stephaniae Tetrandrae*
草　薢	Bi Xie (Hypoglauca)	6-9 gm.	*Rhizoma Dioscoreae*
當　歸	Dang Gui (Chinese angelica)	6-9 gm.	*Radix Angelicae Sinensis*
牛　膝	Niu Xi (Achyranthes)	6-9 gm.	*Radix Achyranthis*
龜　版	Gui Ban (Tortoise plastron)	6-9 gm.	*Plastrum Testudinis*

Action:

1. To eliminate heat and dampness
2. To invigorate the blood circulation in the channels and collaterals

Indication:

For a person with low back pain due to heat and dampness. The symptoms are: low back pain, with heat and burning sensation, mouth bitter and dry, irritability, urine color amber and duration short.

Tongue: with yellow greasy coating
Pulse: soft and rapid

Application:

Low back pain, eczema, leukorrhea, chronic nephritis.

Jiàn Pí Wán　　健脾丸
(Chien-Pi-Wan)
(Spleen and Stomach Tonic Pill)

Constituents:

人 參 Ren Shen (Ginseng)	45 gm.	Radix Ginseng
白 术 Bai Zhu (White Atractylodes)	75 gm.	Rz. Atractylodis Macrocephalae
山 藥 Shan Yao (Dioscorea)	30 gm.	Rhizoma Dioscoreae
茯 苓 Fu Ling (Poria)	60 gm.	Poria
肉豆蔻 Rou Dou Kou (Nutmeg)	30 gm.	Semen Myristicae
山 楂 Shan Zha (Crataegus)	30 gm.	Fructus Crataegi
麥 芽 Mai Ya (Malt)	30 gm.	Fructus Hordei Germinatus
神 曲 Shen Qu (Medicated leaven)	30 gm.	Massa Fermentata Medicinalis
砂 仁 Sha Ren (Cardamon)	30 gm.	Fructus Amomi
木 香 Mu Xiang (Saussurea)	22.5 gm.	Radix Saussureae
陳 皮 Chen Pi (Citrus peel)	30 gm.	Pericarpium Citri Reticulatae
黃 連 Huang Lian (Coptis)	22.5 gm.	Rhizoma Coptidis
甘 草 Gan Cao (Licorice)	22.5 gm.	Radix Glycyrrhizae

Take 6-9 gm. each time, twice daily.

Action:

To strengthen the digestive function of the spleen (Digestive)

Indication:

For a person with interior accumulation of food, and with weak digestive function of the spleen and stomach. The symptoms are: indigestion, abdominal distention, decreased food intake and appetite, loose stools.

> Tongue: with greasy and yellow coating
> Pulse: weak

Modification:

1. If there is no symptoms of heat, eliminate:
   黃 連 Huang Lian (Coptis)　　　Rhizoma Coptidis
2. With asthenia and cold symptoms, add:
   乾 薑 Gan Jiang (Dry ginger)　　Rhizoma Zingiberis
   附 子 Fu Zi (Aconite)　　　Radix Aconiti Praeparatae

Generic Name:

Ginseng Stomachic Pills

Jiāo Ài Tāng　膠艾湯　(胶艾汤)
(Chiao-Ai-Tang)
(Decoction of Artemisia and Donkey-hide Gelatin)

Constituents:

熱地黃	Shu Di Huang (Prep. rehmannia)	9-12 gm.	Radix Rehmanniae Praeparatae
當　歸	Dang Gui (Chinese angelica)	6-9 gm.	Radix Angelicae Sinensis
川　芎	Chuan Xiong (Ligusticum)	3-6 gm.	Rhizoma Ligustici Chuanxiong
白芍藥	Bai Shao Yao (White peony)	6-9 gm.	Radix Paeoniae Alba
阿　膠	E Jiao (Donkey-hide gelatin)	6-9 gm.	Colla Corii Asini
艾　葉	Ai Ye (Artemisia)	6-9 gm.	Folium Artemisiae Argyi
甘　草	Gan Cao (Licorice)	3-6 gm.	Radix Glycyrrhizae
酒	Jiao (Wine)		

Action:

1. To stop bleeding by warming and nourishing (Hemostatic)
2. To regulate menstruation
3. To prevent miscarriage

Indication:

For a person with bleeding due to deficiency and coldness in the Chong (Vital) and Ren (Conception) channels. The symptoms are: menorrhagia, abdominal pain, bleeding after abortion, delivery or during pregnancy.

Application:

Threatened abortion, uterine bleeding, vaginal bleeding during pregnancy or after childbirth, menorrhagia.

Contraindication:

For a person with bleeding disorders due to heat and random flow of blood in the body.

Modification:

1. With deficiency of Qi (vital energy), add:

黨　參	Dang Shen (Codonopsis)	Radix Codonopsis Pilosulae
黃　芪	Huang Qi (Astragalus)	Radix Astragali

2. With lumbago, add:

杜　仲	Du Zhong (Eucommia bark)	Cortex Eucommiae
桑寄生	Sang Ji Sheng (Mulberry mistletoe)	Ramulus Loranthi

Generic Name:

Tang-kuei and Gelatin Combination

Jīn Kuì Shèn Qì Wán (Bā Wèi Dì Huáng Wán)
金匱腎氣丸 （八味地黄丸）
(Chin-Kuei-Shen-Chi-Wan) (Pa-Wei-Ti-Huang-Wan)
(Pills for Restoring the Vital Energy and Function of the Kidney)

Constituents:

炮附子	Pao Fu Zi (Aconite)	10-15 gm.	*Radix Aconiti Praeparatae*
肉 桂	Rou Gui (Cinnamon bark)	6-9 gm.	*Cortex Cinnamomi*
熟地黄	Shu Di Huang (Prep. rehmannia)	20-30 gm.	*Radix Rehmanniae Pareparatae*
山茱萸	Shan Zhu Yu (Cornus)	10-20 gm.	*Fructus Corni*
山 藥	Shan Yao (Dioscorea)	10-15 gm.	*Rhizoma Dioscoreae*
澤 瀉	Ze Xie (Alisma)	10-15 gm.	*Rhizoma Alismatis*
茯 苓	Fu Ling (Poria)	10-15 gm.	*Poria*
牡丹皮	Mu Dan Pi (Moutan bark)	10-15 gm.	*Cortex Moutan Radicis*

Action:

1. To replenish the kidney *Yang* (vital function)
2. To warm the lower part of the body.

Indication:

For a person with kidney *Yang* (vital function) deficiency. The symptoms are: lumbago, coldness sensation in the lower part of the body, spasmodic pain in the lower abdomen, dysuria, frequent urination, nocturia, cough, asthma, edema, persistent diarrhea.

Tongue: whitish
Pulse: deep, slow and weak

Application:

Diabetes mellitus and insipidus, hyperaldosteronism, hypothyroidism, neurasthenia, chronic nephritis, chronic bronchitis, asthma, pulmonary emphysema, urinary retention, climacteric syndromes.

Modification:

1. With edema and dysuria, add:

川牛膝	Chuan Niu Xi (Cyathula root)	*Radix Cyathulae*
車前子	Che Qian Zi (Plantago seed)	*Semen Plantaginis*

2. Lumbago with cold feet, edema, tinnitus, deafness, dysuria, add:

鹿 茸	Lu Rong (Pilose antler)	*Cornu Cervi Pantotrichum*
五味子	Wu Wei Zi (Schisandra fruit)	*Fructus Schisandrae*

This prescription is called Shi Bu Wan (十補丸)

Generic Name:

Sexoton Pills;
Rehmannia Eight Formula.

Jīn Suǒ Gù Jīng Wán 金鎖固經丸

(Chin-Sou-Ku-Ching-Wan)
(Pills for Spermatorrhea)

Constituents:

金櫻子	Jin Ying Zi (Rosa fruit)	10-15 gm.	*Fructus Rosae Laevigatae*
鎖　陽	Suo Yang (Cynomorium)	10-15 gm.	*Herba Cynomorii*
沙苑蒺藜	Sha Yuan Ji Li (Chinese milk vetch)	20-30 gm.	*Semen Astragali*
芡　實	Qian Shi (Euryale)	10-15 gm.	*Semen Euryales*
連　肉	Lian Rou (Lotus seed)	10-15 gm.	*Semen Nelumbinis*
蓮　鬚	Lian Xu (Lotus stamen)	10-15 gm.	*Stamen Nelumbinis*
龍　骨	Long Gu (Dragon bone)	10-15 gm.	*Os Draconis*
牡　蠣	Mu Li (Oyster shell)	10-15 gm.	*Concha Ostreae*

Action:

1. To consolidate the kidney and the essence of life
2. Astringent

Indication:

For a person with kidney asthenia and unconsolidated vital energy. The symptoms are: nocturnal and spontaneous emission, fatigue, loss of muscle strength, low back pain, tinnitus.

> Tongue: light color with white coating
> Pulse: deep and weak

Application:

Neurasthenia, nocturnal and spontaneous emission, enuresis, insomnia, leukorrhea.

Contraindication:

1. For nocturnal emission due to hyperactivity of ministerial fire of liver or kidney

2. For spermatorrhea due to heat and dampness in the liver

Modification:

1. With loose stool or diarrhea, add:

補骨脂	Bu Gu Zhi (Psoralea)	*Fructus Psoraleae*
五味子	Wu Wei Zi (Schisandra fruit)	*Fructus Schisandrae*

2. With impotence, add:

淫羊藿	Yin Yang Huo (Epimedium)	*Herba Epimedii*

3. With lumbago, add:

杜　仲	Du Zhong (Eucommia bark)	*Cortex Eucommiae*
續　斷	Xu Duan (Dipsacus root) Radix Dipsaci	

Generic Name:

Chin So Ku Ching Wan; Lotus Stamen Formula

Jīng Fáng Bài Dú Sàn   荆防敗毒散

(Ching-Fang-Pai-Tu-San)
(Antiphlogistic Powder of Schizonepeta and Ledebouriella)

Constituents:

荆 芥	Jing Jie (Schizonepeta)	6-9 gm.	*Herba Schizonepetae*
防 風	Fang Feng (Ledebouriellae)	6-9 gm.	*Radix Ledebouriellae*
羌 活	Qiang Huo (Notopterygium)	6-9 gm.	*Radix Notopterygii*
獨 活	Du Huo (Pubescent angelica)	6-9 gm.	*Radix Angelicae Pubescentis*
川 芎	Chuan Xiong (Ligusticum)	6-9 gm.	*Rhizoma Ligustici*
柴 胡	Chai Hu (Bupleurum)	6-9 gm.	*Radix Bupleuri*
前 胡	Qian Hu (Peucedanum)	6-9 gm.	*Radix Peucedani*
桔 梗	Jie Geng (Platycodon)	6-9 gm.	*Radix Platycodi*
枳 殼	Zhi Ke (Bitter orange)	6-9 gm.	*Fructus Aurantii*
茯 苓	Fu Ling (Poria)	6-9 gm.	*Poria*
薄 荷	Bo He (Mentha)	3-6 gm.	*Herba Menthae*
甘 草	Gan Cao (Licorice)	3-6 gm.	*Radix Glycyrrhizae*

Action:

1. To dispel exterior wind, cold and dampness (Diaphoretic)
2. Anti-inflammatory

Indication:

For a person with exterior affection of wind, cold and dampness. The symptoms are: fever, intolerance of cold, headache, muscle-ache, no perspiration, stuffy-nose, blood-shot eyes.

Tongue: with thin white coating
Pulse: floating and rapid

Application:

Common cold, influenza, parotitis, inflammations, dysentery, tonsillitis.

Modification:

1. For tonsillitis, add:

牛蒡子	Niu Bang Zi (Arctium fruit)	*Fructus Arctii*
射 干	She Gan (Belamcanda rhizome)	*Rhizoma Belamcandae*

2. For testitis, add:

川楝子	Chuan Lian Zi (Sichuan chinaberry)	*Fructus Meliae Toosendan*
茴 香	Hui Xiang (Fennel fruit)	*Fructus Foeniculi*

Generic Name:

Schizonepeta and Siler Formula

Jiŭ Wèi Qiāng Huó Tāng   九味羌活湯
(Chiu-Wei-Chiang-Huo-Tang)
(Decoction of Nine Ingredients with Notopterygium)

Constituents:

羌 活	Qiang Huo (Notopterygium)	6-9 gm.	*Radix Notopterygii*
防 風	Fang Feng (Ledebouriella)	6-9 gm.	*Radix Ledebouriellae*
蒼 术	Cang Zhu (Atractylodes)	6-9 gm.	*Rhizoma Atractlodis*
細 辛	Xi Xin (Asarum)	3-6 gm.	*Herba Asari*
白 芷	Bai Zhi (Angelica)	6-9 gm.	*Radix Angelicae Dahuricae*
川 芎	Chuan Xiong (Ligusticum)	6-9 gm.	*Rhizoma Ligustici*
生地黃	Sheng Di Huang (Raw rehmannia)	6-9 gm.	*Radix Rehmanniae*
黃 芩	Huang Qin (Scutellaria)	6-9 gm.	*Radix Scutellariae*
甘 草	Gan Cao (Licorice)	3-6 gm.	*Radix Glycyrrhizae*

Action:

1. Diaphoretic
2. To dispel dampness
3. To eliminate interior heat

Indication:

For a person with exterior affection of wind, cold and dampness, and with interior heat. The symptoms are: fever, no perspiration, intolerance of cold, headache, muscle-ache, stiff neck, mouth bitter, thirst.

    Tongue: with thin white coating
    Pulse: floating

Application:

Common cold, influenza, rheumatic arthritis.

Jú Hé Wán 橘核丸

(Chu-Ho-Wan)
(Pills of Tangerine Seed)

Constituents:

橘 核	Ju He (Tangerine seed)	9-12 gm.	*Semen Citri Reticulatae*
川楝子	Chuan Lian Zi (Sichuan chinaberry)	3-6 gm.	*Fructus Meliae Toosendan*
延胡索	Yan Hu Suo (Corydalis tuber)	6-9 gm.	*Rhizoma Corydalis*
厚 朴	Hou Po (Magnolia bark)	6-9 gm.	*Cortex Magnoliae Officinalis*
枳 實	Zhi Shi (Immature bitter orange)	6-9 gm.	*Fructus Aurantii Immaturus*
肉 桂	Rou Gui (Cinnamon bark)	1-3 gm.	*Cortex Cinnamomi*
昆 布	Kun Bu (Ecklonia)	6-9 gm.	*Thallus Eckloniae*
海 藻	Hai Zao (Sargassum)	*6-9 gm.*	*Sargassum*
海 帶	Hai Dai (Kelp)	6-9 gm.	*Thallus Laminariae*
桃 仁	Tao Ren (Persica seed)	3-6 gm.	*Semen Persicae*
木 通	Mu Tong (Akebia stem)	6-9 gm.	*Caulis Akebiae*
木 香	Mu Xiang (Saussurea)	3-6 gm.	*Radix Saussureae*

Action:

1. To relieve pain by invigorating the circulation of vital energy
   (Carminative)
2. To soften lumps and hardening

Indication:

For a person with stagnation or depression of vital energy in the small
intestine. The symptoms are: distention and spasmodic pain in the lower
abdomen, with tenesmus, swollen testis, hernia, radiating pain to the
lower spine.

> Tongue: with white coating
> Pulse: deep and wiry/taut

Application:

Testitis, orchidiptosis, hernia

Jú Pí Zhú Rú Tāng   橘皮竹茹湯
(Chu-Pi-Chu-Ju-Tang)
(Decoction of Citrus Peel and Bamboo Shavings)

Constituents:

陳 皮 Chen Pi (Citrus peel)	6-9 gm.	*Pericarpium Citri Reticulatae*
竹 茹 Zhu Ru (Bamboo shavings)	6-9 gm.	*Caulus Bambusae in Taenis*
人 參 Ren Shen (Ginseng)	6-9 gm.	*Radix Ginseng*
炙甘草 Zhi Gan Cao (Baked licorice)	3-6 gm.	*Radix Glycyrrhizae Praeparatae*
生 薑 Sheng Jiang (Fresh ginger)	3-6 gm.	*Rhizoma Zingiberis Recens*
大 棗 Da Zao (Jujube)	3-5 pc.	*Fructus Ziziphus Jujubae*

Action:

1. To regulate the stomach and the flow of vital energy
2. To tonify the body

Indication:

For a person with hiccough due to heat and weakness of the stomach. The symptoms are: hiccough, nausea, retch, mouth dry, thirst.

> Tongue: red and dry
> Pulse: thready and rapid

Application:

Hiccough

Modification:

1. With increased sputum, add:

茯 苓 Fu Ling (Poria)	*Poria*
半 夏 Ban Xia (Pinellia)	*Rhizoma Pinelliae*

2. With deficiency of stomach *Yin* (vital essence), add:

麥門冬 Mai Men Dong (Ophiopogon)	*Radix Ophiopogonis*
石 斛 Shi Hu (Dendrobium)	*Herba Dendrobii*

Generic Name:

Aurantium and Bamboo Combination

Juān Bì Tāng(I)　　　蠲痺湯(I)

(Juan-Pi-Tang)
(Decoction for Arthralgia) (I)

Constituents:

羌 活	Qiang Huo (Notopterygium)	6-9 gm.	*Rhizoma Seu Radix Notopterygii*
薑 黃	Jiang Huang (Tumeric rhizome)	6-9 gm.	*Rhizoma Curcumae Longae*
黃 芪	Huang Qi (Astragalus)	9-12 gm.	*Radix Astragali*
當 歸	Dang Gui (Chinese angelica)	6-9 gm.	*Radix Angelicae Sinensis*
赤芍藥	Chi Shao Yao (Red peony)	6-9 gm.	*Radix Paeoniae Rubra*
防 風	Fang Feng (Siler; Ledebouriella)	6-9 gm.	*Radix Ledebouriellae*
生 薑	Sheng Jiang (Fresh ginger)	3-6 gm.	*Rhizoma Zingiberis Recens*
甘 草	Gan Cao (Licorice)	3-6 gm.	*Radix Glycyrrhizae*
大 棗	Da Zao (Jujube)	3-5 pc.	*Fructus Ziziphus Jujubae*

Action:

1. To dispel wind, cold and dampness
2. Anti-rheumatic

Indication:

For a person with arthralgia due to wind, cold and dampness. The symptoms are: arthralgia (migratory), pain in the neck, back, shoulder and arms, difficulty in movements, numbness in the hands and feet.

Tongue: with white or greasy coating
Pulse: floating or wiry/taut and tight

Application:

Arthralgia in the neck, back, arms and shoulder.

Juān Bì Tāng(II) 蠲痺湯(II)

(Juan-Pi-Tang)
(Decoction for Arthralgia) (II)

Constituents:

羌 活	Qiang Huo (Notopterygium)	6-9 gm.	*Rhizoma Seu Radix Notopterygii*
獨 活	Du Huo (Pubescent angelica)	6-9 gm.	*Radix Angelicae Pubescentis*
桂 枝	Gui Zhi (Cinnamon twig)	6-9 gm.	*Ramulus Cinnamomi*
秦 艽	Qin Jiao (Large leaf gentian)	6-9 gm.	*Radix Gentianae*
海風藤	Hai Feng Teng (Kadsura)	20-30 gm.	*Caulis Piperis*
桑 枝	Sang Zhi (Mulberry twig)	20-30 gm.	*Ramulus Mori*
當 歸	Dang Gui (Chinese angelica)	6-9 gm.	*Radix Angelicae Sinensis*
川 芎	Chuan Xiong (Ligusticum)	6-9 gm.	*Rhizoma Ligustici Chuanxiong*
木 香	Mu Xiang (Saussurea)	3-9 gm.	*Radix Saussureae*
乳 香	Ru Xiang (Mastic)	3-6 gm.	*Resina Olibani*
炙甘草	Zhi Gan Cao (Baked licorice)	3-6 gm.	*Radix Glycyrrhizae Praeparatae*

Action:

To dispel wind, cold and dampness (Anti-rheumatic)

Indication:

For a person with arthralgia due to wind, cold and dampness. The symptoms are: pain in the joints, especially in the wrist, ankle, knee, elbow, difficulty of movements, local inflammations, intolerance of wind, migratory pain, heavy sensation in the body, numbness in hands and feet or body.

> Tongue: with white or greasy coating
> Pulse: floating; wiry/taut and tight; or soft and slow

Application:

Arthralgia

Modification:

1. If arthralgia is caused by wind, add:

防 風 Fang Feng (siler; Ledebouriella)   *Radix Ledebouriellae*

2. If pain is severe, with difficulty of flexion and extension, add:

附 子 Fu Zi (Aconite)   *Radix Aconiti Praeparatae*

3. If pain is fixed, with numbness, heavy sensation, add:

防 己 Fang Ji (Stephania)   *Radix Stephaniae Tetrandrae*
蒼 术 Cang Zhu (Atractylodes)   *Rhizoma Atractylodis*
薏苡仁 Yi Yi Ren (Coix)   *Semen Coicis*

Ké Xuè Fāng　　咳血方

(Ke-Hsieh-Fang)
(Formula for Hemoptysis)

Constituents:

青 黛	Qing Dai (Indigo)	3-6 gm.	*Indigo Naturalis*
栀 子	Zhi Zi (Gardenia)	6-9 gm.	*Fructus Gardeniae*
瓜蔞仁	Gua Lou Ren (Trichosanthes)	6-9 gm.	*Fructus Trichosanthis*
海浮石	Hai Fu Shi (Pumice)	6-9 gm.	*Pumice*
訶 子	He Zi (Chebula fruit)	3-6 gm.	*Fructus Chebulae*

Action:

1. To eliminate heat and phlegm
2. Anti-tussive
3. Stop bleeding

Indication:

For a person with liver fire attacking the lung. The symptoms are: cough with blood and thick mucus, thirst, face red, irritability, constipation.

Tongue: red with yellow coating
Pulse: wiry and rapid

Application:

Cough with blood, nose-bleeding, bronchiectasis, tuberculosis.

Modification:

1. With cough and excessive sputum, add:

杏 仁	Xing Ren (Apricot kernel)	*Semen Armeniacae Amarum*
浙貝母	Zhe Bei Mu (Fritillary bulb)	*Bulbus Fritillarieae Thunbergii*

2. With depletion of *Yin* fluid and excessive fire, add:

沙 參	Sha Shen (Glehnia root)	*Radix Glehniae*
麥門冬	Mai Men Dong (Ophiopogon root)	*Radix Ophiopogonis*

Lǐ Zhōng Wán (Rén Shēn Tāng)理中丸 (人參湯)
(Li-Chung-Wan) (Jen-Sheng-Tang)
(Decoction to Regulate the Spleen and Stomach)
or (Decoction of Ginseng)

Constituents:

人 參	Ren Shen (Ginseng)	10-15 gm.	*Radix Ginseng*
白 术	Bai Zhu (White atractylodes)	6-9 gm.	*Rhizoma Atractylodis Macrocephalae*
乾 薑	Gan Jiang (Dry ginger)	6-9 gm.	*Rhizoma Zingiberis*
炙甘草	Zhi Gan Cao (Baked licorice)	3-6 gm.	*Rhizoma Glycyrrhizae Praeparatae*

Action:

1. To dispel cold
2. To warm and tonify the spleen and stomach

Indication:

For a person with cold and deficiency of the spleen and stomach. The symptoms are: fullness sensation in the epigastric region or abdomen (like to be pressed), loss of appetite, no thirsty sensation, vomiting, diarrhea or with loose stools.

Tongue: light with white coating
Pulse: deep, slow and weak

Application:

Acute and chronic gastroenteritis, gastroduodenal ulcer, gastrectasis, gastroptosis, chronic colitis, cholera, vomiting, anemia, fright in children.

Modification:

1. With coldness in the four limbs, add:
附 子 Fu Zi (Aconite)   *Radix Aconiti Praeparatae*
This formula is called Fu Zi Li Zhong Wan (附子理中丸)

With addition of:
肉 桂 Rou Gui (Cinnamon bark)   *Cortex Cinnamomi*
This formula is called Fu Gui Li Zhong Wan (附桂理中丸)

2. With upset stomach and vomiting, add:

半 夏	Ban Xia (Pinellia)	*Rhizoma Pinelliae*
生 薑	Sheng Jiang (Fresh ginger)	*Rhizoma Zingiberis Recens*
白豆蔻	Bai Dou Kou (Round cardamon)	*Semen Cardamomi Rotundi*
丁 香	Ding Xiang (Cloves)	*Flos Caryophylli*

3. With edema, add:

茯 苓	Fu Ling (Poria)	*Poria*
澤 瀉	Ze Xie (Alisma)	*Rhizoma Alismatis*

Generic Name:

Li Chung Wan; Ginseng and Ginger Combination

Liáng Fù Wán   良附丸
(Liang-Fu-Wan)
(Pills of Galanga and Cyperus)

Constituents:

高良姜 Gao Liang Jiang (Galanga)	10-15 gm.	*Rhizoma Alpiniae Officinarum*
香 附 Xiang Fu (Cyperus tuber)	10-15 gm.	*Rhizoma Cyperi*

Action:

1. To warm the spleen and stomach
2. To dispel cold
3. To relieve abdominal pain

Indication:

For a person with abdominal pain due to stagnation of vital energy and accumulation of cold in the spleen and stomach. The symptoms are: abdominal pain, relieved by warmth and pressure, no thirst, prefer to drink warm liquid.

    Tongue: white
    Pulse: wiry/taut and tight; or deep and slow

Application:

Gastro-intestinal disease, gastric or duodenal ulcer, chronic gastritis.

Contraindication:

For a person with abdominal pain due to fire or depletion of body fluid in the stomach or liver, with tongue proper dark red color.

Liáng Gé Sàn 涼膈散

(Liang-Ke-San)
(The Diaphragm Cooling Powder)

Constituents:

大 黃	Da Huang (Rhubarb)	6-9 gm.	*Radix et Rhizoma Rhei*
芒 硝	Mang Xiao (Mirabilitum)	6-9 gm.	*Natrii Sulfas*
栀 子	Zhi Zi (Gardenia)	3-6 gm.	*Fructus Gardeniae*
黃 芩	Huang Qin (Scutellaria)	3-6 gm.	*Radix Scutellariae*
連 翹	Lian Qiao (Forsythia)	12-15 gm.	*Fructus Forsythiae*
薄 荷	Bo He (Mentha)	3-6 gm.	*Herba Menthae*
甘 草	Gan Cao (Licorice)	3-6 gm.	*Radix Glycyrrhizae*

Grind the above ingredients into powder, mix with bamboo leaves and honey.

Action:

1. To clear the intense heat and fire of the upper burner
2. To purge the heat of the middle burner through excretion.
   (Febrifugal and Purgative)

Indication:

For a person with intense heat and fire in both the upper and middle burner of the body. The symptoms are: irritable heat in the chest and diaphragm region, thirst, face red, lips dry and chapped, oral ulceration, sore throat, toothache, nose-bleeding, constipation, urine color amber.

Tongue: red on the sides, with yellow and greasy coating
Pulse: slippery and rapid

Application:

Acute cholecystitis, cholelithiasis, encephalitis B, epidemic meningitis, measles.

Modification:

1. With cholelithiasis, add:

金錢草	Jin Qian Cao (Lysimachia)	*Herba Lysimachiae*

2. With jaundice, add:

茵陳蒿	Yin Chen Hao (Capillaris)	*Herba Artemisiae Capillaris*
郁 金	Yu Jin (Curcuma)	*Radix Curcumae*

3. With chest pain, add:

柴 胡	Chai Hu (Bupleurum)	*Radix Bupleuri*
川楝子	Chuan Lian Zi (Sichuan chinaberry)	*Fructus Meliae Toosendan*
延胡索	Yan Hu Suo (Corydalis)	*Rhizoma Corydalis*

Líng Gān Wǔ Wèi Jiāng Xīn Tāng   苓甘五味薑辛湯

(Ling-Kan-Wu-Wei-Chiang-Hsin-Tang)
(Decoction of Poria, Licorice, Schisandra, Ginger & Asarum)

Constituents:

乾 薑	Gan Jiang (Dry ginger)	6-9 gm.	*Rhizoma Zingiberis*
細 辛	Xi Xin (Asarum)	1-3 gm.	*Herba Asari*
茯 苓	Fu Ling (Poria)	6-9 gm.	*Poria*
五味子	Wu Wei Zi (Schisandra)	6-9 gm.	*Fructus Schisandrae*
甘 草	Gan Cao (Licorice)	3-6 gm.	*Radix Glycyrrhizae*

Action:

1. To resolve retention of phlegm
2. To warm the lung

Indication:

For a person with cough and retention of phlegm in the lung due to cold. The symptoms are: cough with thin white sputum, salivation, hiccough, fullness sensation in the chest.

Tongue: with white and slippery coating
Pulse: deep and slow

Application:

Chronic tracheitis, bronchitis, pulmonary emphysema

Modification:

1. With vomiting or profuse sputum, add:

制半夏　Zhi Ban Xia (Prepared pinellia)　　*Rhizoma Pinellia Praeparatae*

2. With severe cough, add:

杏 仁	Xing Ren (Apricot seed)	*Semen Armeniacae Amarum*
紫 菀	Zi Wan (Aster root)	*Radix Asteris*
款冬花	Kuan Dong Hua (Tussilago flower)	*Flos Farfarae*

3. With chest distention, add:

陳 皮	Chen Pi (Citrus peel)	*Pericarpium Citri Reticulatae*
砂 仁	Sha Ren (Cardamon)	*Fructus Amomi*

4. With loss of appetite, add:

黨 參	Dang Shen (Codonopsis)	*Radix Codonopsis Pilosulae*
白 术	Bai Zhu (White atractylodes)	*Rhizoma Atractylodis Macrocephalae*

Generic Name:

Hoelen and Schizandra Combination

Líng Guì Zhú Gān Tāng   苓桂术甘湯

(Ling-Kuei-Chu-Kan-Tang)
(Decoction of Poria, Cinnamon, Atractylodes and Licorice)

Constituents:

茯 苓 Fu Ling (Poria)	9-12 gm.	*Poria*
桂 枝 Gui Zhi (Cinnamon twig)	6-9 gm.	*Ramulus Cinnamomi*
白 术 Bai Zhu (White atractylodes)	6-9 gm.	*Rhizoma Atractylodis Macrocephalae*
炙甘草 Zhi Gan Cao (Baked licorice)	3-6 gm.	*Radix Glycyrrhizae Praeparatae*

Action:

1. To strengthen the spleen and resolve dampness (diuretic)
2. To resolve phlegm stagnation by herbs with warm property

Indication:

For a person with stagnation of phlegm due to deficiency of spleen and stomach *Yang* (vital function). The symptoms are: chest distention, vertigo, palpitation, dyspnea.

> Tongue: with white and slippery coating
> Pulse: wiry and slippery, or sinking and tight

Application:

Chronic bronchitis, bronchial asthma, pulmonary emphysema, cardiac or nephritic edema.

Modification:

1. If vomiting with water and sputum, add:

半 夏 Ban Xia (Pinellia)	*Rhizoma Pinelliae*
陳 皮 Chen Pi (Citrus peel)	*Pericarpium Citri Reticulatae*

2. If deficiency of spleen *Qi* (vital energy) is severe, add:

黨 參 Dang Shen (Codonopsis)	*Radix Codonopsis Pilosulae*

Generic Name:

Atractylodes and Hoelen Combination

Líng Yáng Gōu Téng Tāng　羚羊鉤藤湯
(Ling-Yang-Kou-Teng-Tang)
(Decoction of Antelope Horn and Uncaria)

Constituents:

羚羊角	Ling Yang Jiao (Antelope horn)	1-3 gm.	*Cornu Antelopis*
鉤　藤	Gou Teng (Uncaria)	9-12 gm.	*Ramulus Uncariae cum Uncis*
桑　葉	Sang Ye (Mulberry leaf)	6-9 gm.	*Folium Mori*
菊　花	Ju Hua (Chrysanthemum flower)	9-12 gm.	*Flos Chrysanthemi*
白芍藥	Bai Shao Yao (White peony)	6-9 gm.	*Radix Paeoniae Alba*
生地黃	Sheng Di Huang (Fresh rehmannia)	9-15 gm.	*Radix Rehmanniae*
川貝母	Chuan Bei Mu (Tendrilled fritillary)	9-12 gm.	*Bulbus Fritillariae Cirrhosae*
竹　茹	Zhu Ru (Bamboo shavings)	6-9 gm.	*Caulus Bambusae in Taenis*
茯　神	Fu Shen (Poria)	9-12 gm.	*Poria*
甘　草	Gan Cao (Licorice)	1-3 gm.	*Radix Glycyrrhizae*

Action:

1. To subdue the endogenous wind in liver channel (Anti-hypertensive)
2. To eliminate heat and convulsions (Anti-convulsive)

Indication:

For a person with intensive heat and endogenous wind in the liver channel. The symptoms are: high fever, stiff-neck, with convulsion, restlessness, opisthotonos, coma.

> Tongue: red with yellow coating, dry
> Pulse: wiry/taut and rapid

Application:

Hypertension, puerperal eclampsia, chromaffinoma, mania with convulsion.

Modification:

1. With depletion of body fluid, add:

玄　參	Xuan Shen (Scrophularia)	*Radix Scrophulariae*
麥門冬	Mai Men Dong (Ophiopogon)	*Radix Ophiopogonis*
阿　膠	E Jiao (Donkey-hide gelation)	*Colla Corii Asini*

2. With hypertensive headache and dizziness, add:

龍膽草	Long Dan Cao (Gentiana)	*Radix Gentianae*
夏枯草	Xia Ku Cao (Prunella spike)	*Spica Prunellae*
牡　蠣	Mu Li (Oyster shell)	*Concha Ostreae*
珍珠母	Zhen Zhu Mu (Mother-of-pearl)	*Concha Margaritifera Usta*
天　麻	Tian Ma (Gastrodia)	*Rhizoma Gastrodiae*

Liù Jūn Zǐ Tāng   六君子湯
(Liu-Chun-Tzu-Tang)
(The Six Noble Ingredients Decoction)

Constituents:

人 參	Ren Shen (Ginseng)	6-9 gm.	*Radix Ginseng*
白 术	Bai Zhu (White atractylodes)	6-9 gm.	*Radix Atractylodis Macrocephalae*
茯 苓	Fu Ling (Poria)	6-9 gm.	*Poria*
陳 皮	Chen Pi (Citrus peel)	3-6 gm.	*Pericarpium Citri Reticulatae*
半 夏	Ban Xia (Pinellia)	6-9 gm.	*Rhizoma Pinelliae*
炙甘草	Zhi Gan Cao (Baked licorice)	3-6 gm.	*Radix Glycyrrhizae Praeparatae*

Action:

1. To replenish *Qi* (vital energy)
2. To eliminate phlegm and dampness
3. To tonify the spleen and stomach

Indication:

For a person with weakness and asthenia of spleen and stomach, with accumulation of phlegm and dampness. The symptoms are: decreased intake of food, loss of appetite, watery diarrhea, cough with increased amount of thin white sputum, dyspnea, vomiting, acid regurgitation, chest fullness.

Tongue: pale with white and greasy coating
Pulse: soft and weak

Application:

Chronic gastritis, gastric and duodenal ulcer, acid regurgitation, indigestion.

Modification:

1. With decreased appetite, malaise, retention of phlegm, vomiting, chest fullness, add:

木 香	Mu Xiang (Saussurea root)	*Radix Saussureae*
砂 仁	Sha Ren (Cardamon)	*Fructus Amomi*
生 薑	Sheng Jiang (Fresh ginger)	*Rhizoma Zingiberis Recens*

This formula is called Xiang Sha Liu Jin Zi Tang (Saussurea and Cardamon Combination) (香砂六君子湯)

Generic Name:

Liu Jun Zi Wan;
Six Major Herb Combination

Liù Shén Wán   六神丸

(Liu-Shen-Wan)
(Pills of Six Miraculous Drugs)

Constituents:

牛 黄 Niu Huang (Bos calculus)   *Calculus Bovis*
麝 香 She Xiang (Musk)   *Moschus*
蟾 酥 Chan Su (Toad venom)   *Venenum Bufonis*
冰 片 Bing Pian (Borneol)   *Borneolum*
雄 黄 Xiong Huang (Realgar)   *Arsenic Disulfide*
珍 珠 Zhen Zhu (Mother-of-pearl)   *Concha Margaritifera Usta*
樟 腦 Zhang Nao (Camphor)   *Camphor*

Action:

1. To eliminate heat and toxin
2. Anti-phlogistic
3. Analgesic

Indication:

For a person with acute tonsillitis, sore throat, boils, carbuncles and furnacles, dipheria, and all kinds of abscesses.

Contraindication:

For a pregnant woman.

Generic Name:

Liu Shen Wan

Liù Wèi Dì Huáng Wán   六味地黄丸
(Liu-Wei-Ti-Huang-Wan)
(Pills of Six Ingredients with Rehmannia)

Constituents:

熟地黃	Shu Di Huang (Prep. rehmannia)	20-25 gm.	*Radix Rehmanniae Praeparatae*
山茱萸	Shan Zhu Yu (Cornus)	10-15 gm.	*Fructus Cornus*
山 藥	Shan Yao (Dioscorea)	10-15 gm.	*Rhizoma Dioscoreae*
澤 瀉	Ze Xie (Alisma)	*9-12 gm.*	*Rhizoma Alismatis*
牡丹皮	Mu Dan Pi (Moutan bark)	6-9 gm.	*Cortex Moutan Radicis*
茯 苓	Fu Ling (Poria)	9-12 gm.	*Poria*

Action:

To reinforce the *Yin* (vital essence) of liver and kidney.

Indication:

For a person with liver and kidney *Yin* (vital essence) deficiency. The symptoms are: dizziness, tinnitus, sore throat, tidal fever, nocturnal emission, night perspiration, heat sensation in the palm and soles, toothache, mouth dry.

> Tongue: red with thin coating, dry
> Pulse: thready and rapid

Application:

Retarded growth of children, lumbago, optic neuritis, central retinitis, pulmonary tuberculosis, diabetes, hyperthyroidism, Addison's disease, hypertension, neurasthenia, functional anovular uterine bleeding, chronic urinary tract infection, deafness.

Modification:

1. For diabetes, add:

天花粉	Tian Hua Fen (Trichosanthes root)	*Radix Trichosanthis*

2. For deficiency of *Yang* (vital function), add:

肉 桂	Rou Gui (Cinnamon bark)	*Cortex Cinnamomi*
附 子	Fu Zi (Aconite)	*Radix Aconiti Praeparatae*

3. With extreme thirst, add:

石 膏	Shi Gao (Gypsum)	*Gypsum Fibrosum*
石 斛	Shi Hu (Dendrobium stem)	*Herba Dendrobii*

4. For severe deficiency of *Yin* (vital essence), add:

天門冬	Tian Men Dong (Asparagus root)	*Radix Asparagi*
麥門冬	Mai Men Dong (Ophiopogon root)	*Radix Ophiopogonis*
玄 參	Xuan Shen (Scrophularia root)	*Radix Scrophulariae*

Generic Name:

Liu Wei Di Huang Wan; Rehmannia Six Formula

Liù Yī Sàn 六一散

(Liu-I-San)
(Powder of Ingredients Six to One in Ratio)

Constituents:

滑 石 Hua Shi (Talc)	18 gm.	*Talcum*
甘 草 Gan Cao (Licorice)	3 gm.	*Radix Glycyrrhizae*

Mix these two ingredients with honey.

Action:

To clear the summer heat and dampness (Febrifugal)

Indication:

For a person with affection of summer heat and dampness. The symptoms are: high temperature of the body, fidgetiness, thirst, difficulty in urination, vomiting or diarrhea.

> Tongue: with thin greasy coating
> Pulse: forceful and rapid

Application:

Summer diarrhea, summer fever in children, febrile disease in the summer.

Modification:

1. For febrile disease in the summer, add:

西瓜翠衣 Xi Gua Cui Yi (Watermelon peel)   *Exocarpium Citrulli*
絲 瓜 絡 Si Gua Luo (Luffa sponge)   *Fasculus Vascularia Luffae*

2. For urolithiasis with burning sensation in urination, add:

海金砂 Hai Jin Sha (Lygodium Spores)   *Spora Lugodii*
金錢草 Jin Qian Cao (Lysimachia)   *Herba Lysimachiae*

3. For hematuria, add:

側柏葉 Ce Bai Ye (Biota tops)   *Cacumen Biotae*
小 薊 Xiao Ji (Small thistle)   *Herba Cephalanoploris*

4. With sore throat, blood-shot eyes and cold sores, add:

青 黛 Qing Dai (Indigo)   *Indigo Naturalis*

This formula is called Bi Yu San (碧玉散)

Lóng Dăn Xiè Gān Tāng   龍膽瀉肝湯 (龙胆泻肝汤)
(Lung-Tan-Hsieh-Kan-Tang)
(Decoction to Purge the Liver Fire with Gentiana)

Constituents:

龍膽草	Long Dan Cao (Gentiana)	3-6 gm.	*Radix Gentianae*
黄 芩	Huang Qin (Scutellaria)	9-12 gm.	*Radix Scutellariae*
栀 子	Zhi Zi (Gardenia)	6-9 gm.	*Fructus Gardeniae*
澤 瀉	Ze Xie (Alisma)	6-9 gm.	*Rhizoma Alismatis*
車前子	Che Qian Zi (Plantago seed)	6-9 gm.	*Semen Plantaginis*
木 通	Mu Tong (Akebia)	6-9 gm.	*Caulis Akebiae*
生地黄	Sheng Di Huang (Fresh rehmannia)	9-12 gm.	*Radix Rehmanniae*
當歸尾	Dang Gui Wei (Chinese angelica)	6-9 gm.	*Radix Angelicae Sinensis*
柴 胡	Chai Hu (Bupleurum)	6-9 gm.	*Radix Bupleuri*
甘 草	Gan Cao (Licorice)	1-3 gm.	*Radix Glycyrrhizae*

Action:

1. To purge the intense heat or fire from the liver and gallbladder (Febrifugal)
2. To clear the heat and dampness of the three burners.

Indication:

1. For a person with upward flaring of liver fire. The symptoms are: headache, chest pain, mouth with bitterness, blood-shot eyes, ear swollen or deaf, throat dry, urine yellow, constipation.

> Tongue: red with yellow coating
> Pulse: wiry/taut and rapid

2. For a person with dampness and heat in the liver channel.

The symptoms are: urine turbid, swelling or itchiness in the genital region, leukorrhea, hypochondriac pain.

> Tongue: with yellow greasy coating
> Pulse: wiry/taut and rapid

Application:

Acute conjunctivitis, acute otitis media, boils and carbuncles of the vestibular and external auditory canal, hypertension, acute icteric hepatitis, acute cholecystitis, herpes zoster, acute pyelitis, acute cystitis, urethritis, acute pelvic inflammation, acute prostatitis, scrotal eczema, swollen testis.

Generic Name:

Lung Tan Xie Gan Pill;
Gentiana Combination

Má Huáng Fù Zǐ Xì Xīn Tāng 麻黄附子細辛湯
(Ma-Huang-Fu-Tzu-Hsi-Hsin-Tang)
(Decoction of Ephedra, Aconite and Asarum)

Constituents:

麻 黄	Ma Huang (Ephedra)	6-9 gm.	*Herba Ephedrae*
附 子	Fu Zi (Aconite)	3-6 gm.	*Radix Aconiti Praeparatae*
細 辛	Xi Xin (Asarum)	1-3 gm.	*Herba Asari*

Action:

1. To dispel exterior wind and cold (Diaphoretic)
2. To replenish the *Yang* (vital function)

Indication:

For a person with deficiency of *Yang* (vital function) and affection of wind and cold. The symptoms are: fever (high or slightly high), severe intolerance of cold, face pale, weak, hands and feet cold.

Tongue: pale and plump
Pulse: deep

Application:

Common cold, influenza

Contraindication:

For a person with deficiency of *Yin* (vital essence)

Generic Name:

Ma-huang and Asarum Combination

Má Huáng Tāng　　麻黄湯

(Ma-Huang-Tang)
(Decoction of Ephedra)

Constituents:

麻　黄 Ma Huang (Ephedra)	6-9 gm.	*Herba Ephedrae*
桂　枝 Gui Zhi (Cinnamon twig)	6-9 gm.	*Ramulus Cinnamomi*
杏　仁 Xing Ren (Apricot seed)	6-9 gm.	*Semen Armeniacae Amarum*
炙甘草 Zhi Gan Cao (Baked licorice)	3-6 gm.	*Radix Glycyrrhizae Praeparatae*

Action:

1. Diaphoretic
2. To dispel cold
3. Anti-asthmatic

Indication:

For a person with excessiveness syndrome in the exterior caused by external attack of wind and cold. The symptoms are: fever, intolerance of cold, general aching, headache, no perspiration, asthma.

　　Tongue: with thin white coating
　　Pulse: floating and tight

Application:

Common cold, asthma, cough

Modification:

1. With arthritic pain, add:
白　术 Bai Zhu (White atractylodes)　　　*Radix Atractylodis Macrocephalae*
This formula is called Ma Huang Jia Zhu Tang (麻黄加术湯)

2. With common cold, but has perspiration, headache, nasal obstruction, cough with profuse sputum, eliminate:
桂　枝 Gui Zhi (Cinnamon twig)　　　*Ramulus Cinnamomi*
This formula is called San Niu Tang (三拗湯)

Contraindication:

For common cold due to external attack of wind and heat.

Generic Name:

Ma-huang Combination

Má Xìng Shí Gān Tāng　麻杏石甘湯

(Ma-Hsing-Shih-Kan-Tang)

(Decoction of Ephedra, Apricot Seed, Gypsum and Licorice)

Constituents:

麻 黄	Ma Huang (Ephedra)	6-9 gm.	*Herba Ephedrae*
杏 仁	Xing Ren (Apricot Seed)	6-9 gm.	*Semen Armeniacae Amarum*
石 膏	Shi Gao (Gypsum)	15-30 gm.	*Gypsum Fibrosum*
炙甘草	Zhi Gan Cao (Baked licorice)	3-6 gm.	*Radix Glycyrrhizae Praeparatae*

Action:

1. To dispel exterior wind and heat factors (Diaphoretic)
2. Anti-asthmatic

Indication:

For a person with exterior affection of wind and heat and interior accumulation of heat in the lung. The symptoms are: fever, with or with no perspiration, asthma, dry throat, thirsty.

Tongue: with thin white or yellow coating
Pulse: floating, rapid and slippery

Application:

Measles, acute tracheitis, pneumonia, upper respiratory tract infection, acute and chronic bronchitis

Contraindication:

For a person with asthma due to wind and cold factors.

Modification:

1. With dyspnea, add:

葶藶子	Ting Li Zi (Lepidium seed)	*Semen Lepidii*
枇杷葉	Pi Pa Ye (Loquat leaf)	*Folium Eriobotryae*

2. With yellow and thick sputum, add:

瓜蔞子	Gua Lou Zi (Trichosanthes fruit)	*Fructus Trichosanthis*
浙貝母	Zhe Bei Mu (Fritillary bulb)	*Bulbus Fritillariae*

3. With high temperature, asthma and cough, add:

知 母	Zhi Mu (Anemarrhena)	*Rhizoma Anemarrhenae*
黄 芩	Huang Qin (Scutellaria)	*Radix Scutellariae*
瓜蔞子	Gua Lou Zi (Trichosanthes fruit)	*Fructus Trichosanthis*

Generic Name:

Ma Xing Shi Gan Tang (or Ma Xing Chih Ke Pian);
Ma-huang and Apricot Seed Combination

Má Zǐ Rén Wán   麻子仁丸
(Ma-Tzu-Jen-Wan)
(The Cannabis Seed Pills)

Constituents:

麻子仁 Ma Zi Ren (Cannabis seed)	20-30 gm.	*Fructus Cannabis*
白芍藥 Bai Shao Yao (White peony)	10-15 gm.	*Radix Paeoniae Alba*
杏 仁 Xing Ren (Apricot seed)	6-9 gm.	*Semen Armeniacae Amarum*
枳 實 Zhi Shi (Immature bitter orange)	6-9 gm.	*Fructus Aurantii Immaturus*
大 黃 Da Huang (Rhubarb)	6-9 gm.	*Radix et Rhizoma Rhei*
厚 朴 Hou Po (Magnolia bark)	6-9 gm.	*Cortex Magnoliae Officinalis*

Action:

Emollient

Indication:

For a person with very dry heat in the stomach and the intestines due to insufficiency of body fluids. The symptoms are: dry stool, constipation, frequent urination.

> Tongue: yellow and dry
> Pulse: floating and rapid

Application:

Constipation in the elderly and weak person, habitual constipation, hemorrhoid.

Contraindication:

For a pregnant woman.

Modification:

For hemorrhoid hemorrhage, add:

| 槐 花 Huai Hua (Sophora flower) | *Flos Sophorae* |
| 地 瑜 Di Yu (Sanguisorba root) | *Radix Sanguisorbae* |

Generic Name:

Apricot Seed and Linus Formula

Mài Mén Dōng Tāng   麥門冬湯

(Mai-Men-Tung-Tang)
(Decoction of Ophiopogon Root)

Constituents:

麥門冬	Mai Men Dong (Ophiopogon)	15-20 gm.	*Radix Ophiopogonis*
半 夏	Ban Xia (Pinellia)	6-9 gm.	*Rhizoma Pinelliae*
人 參	Ren Shen (Ginseng)	3-6 gm.	*Radix Ginseng*
粳 米	Jing Mi (Rice, Oryza)	15-20 gm.	*Semen Oryzae*
甘 草	Gan Cao (Licorice)	3-6 gm.	*Radix Glycyrrhizae*
大 棗	Da Zao (Jujube)	5 pc.	*Fructus Ziziphus Jujubae*

Action:

1. To replenish the body fluids in the stomach
2. To reverse the flow of *Qi* (vital energy)

Indication:

For a person with depletion of *Yin* (vital essence) in the lung and stomach, with reverse flow of *Qi* (flushing up). The symptoms are: cough with thin sputum, hiccup, dry throat, thirst.

> Tongue: red in the tip
> Pulse: weak and rapid

Application:

Consumptive pulmonary disease due to deficiency of *Yin*, cough, hiccup, pulmonary atelectasis, bronchitis.

Contraindication:

For a person with cough and hiccup due to affection of wind, cold or heat.

Modification:

1. For deficiency of *Yin* in lung, add:

沙 參	Sha Shen (Glehnia)	*Radix Glehniae*
玉 竹	Yu Zhu (Polygonatum rhizome)	*Rhizoma Polygonati Odorati*
天門冬	Tian Men Dong (Asparagus root)	*Radix Asparagi*

2. For deficiency of *Yin* in stomach, add:

石 斛	Shi Hu (Dendrobium stem)	*Herba Dendrobii*
天花粉	Tian Hua Fen (Trichosanthes root)	*Radix Trichosanthis*

Generic Name:

Ophiopogon Combination

Míng Mù Dì Huáng Wán　　明目地黄丸

(Ming-Mu-Ti-Huang-Wan)
(Improving Eyesight Formula with Pills of Six Herbs with Rehmannia)

Constituents:

枸杞子 Gou Qi Zi (Lycium fruit)	6-9 gm.	*Fructus Lycii*
菊 花 Ju Hua (Chrysanthemum flower)	6-9 gm.	*Flos Chrysanthemi*
白蒺藜 Bai Ji Li (Tribulus fruit)	6-9 gm.	*Fructus Tribuli*
石决明 Shi Jue Ming (Abalone shell)	20-30 gm.	*Concha Haliotidis*
熟地黄 Shu Di Huang (Prep. rehmannia)	10-15 gm.	*Radix Rehmanniae Praeparatae*
山茱萸 Shan Zhu Yu (Cornus)	9-12 gm.	*Fructus Corni*
山 藥 Shan Yao (Dioscorea)	9-12 gm.	*Rhizoma Dioscorea*
澤 瀉 Ze Xie (Alisma)	9-12 gm.	*Rhizoma Alismatis*
牡丹皮 Mu Dan Pi (Moutan bark)	6-9 gm.	*Cortex Moutan Radicis*
茯 苓 Fu Ling (Poria)	9-12 gm.	*Poria*

Action:

1. To replenish the *Yin* fluid of liver and kidney
2. To disperse wind and heat, and brighten the eyes

Indication:

For a person with decreased acuity of vision due to liver and kidney deficiency, and with exterior affection of wind and heat. The symptoms are: blurry vision, eyes dry and painful, night-blindness.

> Tongue: red with thin coating
> Pulse: thready and rapid

Application:

Diabetes, glaucoma, hypertension, ophthalmia, ophthalmalgia.

Generic Name:

Ming Mu Di Huang Wan

Mǔ Lì Sàn   牡蠣散

(Mu-Li-San)
(Oyster Shell Powder)

Constituents:

牡　蠣	Mu Li (Oyster shell)	20-30 gm.	*Concha Ostreae*
黄　芪	Huang Qi (Astragalus)	20-30 gm.	*Radix Astragali*
麻黄根	Ma Huang Gen (Ephedra root)	20-30 gm.	*Radix Ephedrae*
浮小麥	Fu Xiao Mai (Light wheat)	20-30 gm.	*Fructus Tritici Levis*

Action:

1. To consolidate the exterior defensive system
2. Anti-hidrotic

Indication:

For a person with profuse perspiration due to body weakness and lowered body resistance. The symptoms are: either spontaneous or night perspiration, palpitation, shortness of breath, fatigue.

Application:

Spontaneous or night perspiration

Modification:

1. For deficiency of *Yang* (vital function), add:

| 附　子 | Fu Zi (Aconite) | *Radix Aconiti Praeparatae* |
| 白　术 | Bai Zhu (White atractylodes) | *Rhizoma Atractylodis Macrocephalae* |

2. For deficiency of *Yin* (vital essence) of liver and kidney, add:

| 乾地黄 | Gan Di Huang (Dried rehmannia) | *Radix Rehmanniae* |
| 白芍藥 | Bai Shao Yao (White peony) | *Radix Paeoniae Alba* |

3. For deficiency of vital energy in spleen and stomach, add:

| 黨　參 | Dang Shen (Codonopsis) | *Radix Codonopsis Pilosulae* |
| 白　术 | Bai Zhu (White atractylodes) | *Rhizoma Atractylodis Macrocephalae* |

4. For blood deficiency, add:

| 熟地黄 | Shu Di Huang (Prep. rehmannia) | *Radix Rehmanniae Praeparatae* |
| 何首烏 | He Shou Wu (Fleeceflower root) | *Radix Polygoni Multiflori* |

Mù Xiāng Bīng Láng Wán　木香檳榔丸
(Mu-Hsiang-Ping-Lang-Wan)
(Pills of Saussurea and Areca Seed)

Constituents:

木 香	Mu Xiang (Saussurea)	9-12 gm.	*Radix Saussureae*
檳 榔	Bing Lang (Areca seed)	9-12 gm.	*Semen Arecae*
香 附	Xiang Fu (Cyperus)	6-9 gm.	*Rhizoma Cyperi*
莪 术	E Zhu (Zedoary)	6-9 gm.	*Rhizoma Zedoariae*
青 皮	Qing Pi (Green tangerine peel)	3-6 gm.	*Pericarpium Citri Reticulatae Viridae*
陳 皮	Chen Pi (Citrus peel)	3-6 gm.	*Pericarpium Citri Reticulatae*
牽牛子	Qian Niu Zi (Pharbitis seed)	6-9 gm.	*Semen Pharbitidis*
大 黃	Da Huang (Rhubarb)	9-12 gm.	*Radix et Rhizoma Rhei*
黄 連	Huang Lian (Coptis)	1-3 gm.	*Rhizoma Coptidis*
黄 柏	Huang Bai (Phellodendron)	3-6 gm.	*Cortex Phellodendri*

Action:

1. To increase the circulation of vital energy (Carminative)
2. To purge the interior heat

Indication:

For a person with accumulation of food in the body, thus leading to stagnation of heat and flow of vital energy. The symptoms are: fullness and distention inn the epigastric region and abdomen, constipation, dysentery, tenesmus.

> Tongue: with yellow and greasy coating
> Pulse: forceful

Application:

Constipation, abdominal fullness, indigestion, gastro-intestinal diseases.

Modification:

To enhance the carminative effect, add:

枳 殼	Zhi Ke (Bitter orange)	*Fructus Aurantii*
三 棱	San Leng (Burreed tuber)	*Rhizoma Sparganii*
芒 硝	Mang Xiao (Mirabilitum)	*Natrii Sulfas*

This formula is also called Mu Xiang Bing Lang Wan (木香檳榔丸)

Niú Huáng Jiĕ Dú Piàn　　牛黄解毒片

(Niu-Huang-Chieh-Tu-Pian)
(Antiphlogistic Pills with Bos Calculus)

Constituents:

牛 黄	Niu Huang (Bos calculus)	*Calculus Bovis*
雄 黄	Xiong Huang (Realgar)	*Arsenic Disulfide*
冰 片	Bing Pian (Borneol)	*Borneolum*
大 黄	Da Huang (Rhubarb)	*Radix et Rhizoma Rhei*
石 膏	Shi Gao (Gypsum)	*Gypsum Fibrosum*
黄 芩	Huang qin (Scutellaria)	*Radix Scutellariae*
桔 梗	Jie Geng (Platycodon)	*Radix Platycodi*
甘 草	Gan Cao (Licorice)	*Radix Glycyrrhizae*

Action:

1. To purge the intense fire
2. Antiphlogistic

Indication:

For a person with intense heat or fire in the liver and stomach. The symptoms are: headache, dizziness, red eyes, tinnitus, oral ulcers, periodontitis, constipation.

> Tongue: red with yellow coating
> Pulse: rapid and forceful

Application:

Tonsillitis, periodontitis, pharyngitis, oral ulcers, boils, furuncle, constipation.

Generic Name:

Niu Huang Chieh Tu Pien

Nuǎn Gān Jiān   暖肝煎
(Nuan-Tan-Chian)
(Decoction for Warming the Liver Channel)

Constituents:

當 歸	Dang Gui (Chinese angelica)	6-9 gm.	*Radix Angelicae Sinensis*
枸杞子	Gou Qi Zi (Lycium fruit)	6-9 gm.	*Fructus Lycii*
肉 桂	Rou Gui (Cinnamon bark)	3-6 gm.	*Cortex Cinnamomi*
茴 香	Hui Xiang (Fennel)	3-6 gm.	*Fructus Foeniculi*
烏 葯	Wu Yao (Lindera)	6-9 gm.	*Radix Linderae*
沉 香	Chen Xiang (Aquilaria wood)	2-3 gm.	*Lignum Aquilariae Resinatum*
茯 苓	Fu Ling (Poria)	6-9 gm.	*Poria*
生 薑	Sheng Jiang (Fresh ginger)	3-5 pc.	*Rhizoma Zingiberis Recens*

Action:

1. To eliminate cold in the liver channel
2. To circulate the flow of *Qi* (vital energy) and alleviate pain

Indication:

For a person with weak constitution and deficiency of liver *Yang* (vital function), and affection of external cold. The symptoms are: hernia, lower abdominal (lateral) pain, coldness in the abdomen and lower extremities.

    Tongue: pale with thin white coat
    Pulse: deep, slow or wiry/taut

Application:

Hernia, inguinal hernia, scrotal hernia, hernia of vagina or testis, abdominal pain.

Píng Wèi Sàn 平胃散
(Ping-Wei-San)
(The Stomach Neutralizing Powder)

Constituents:

蒼 术	Cang Zhu (Atractylodes)	6-9 gm.	*Rhizoma Atractylodis*
厚 朴	Hou Po (Magnolia bark)	6-9 gm.	*Cortex Magnoliae Officinalis*
陳 皮	Chen Pi (Citrus peel)	3-6 gm.	*Pericarpium Citri Reticulatae*
甘 草	Gan Cao (Licorice)	3-6 gm.	*Radix Glycyrrhizae*
生 薑	Sheng Jiang (Fresh ginger)	1-3 gm.	*Rhizoma Zingiberis Recens*
大 棗	Da Zao (Jujube)	3-5 pc.	*Fructus Ziziphus Jujubae*

Action:

1. To dispel the dampness in the spleen by drying method
2. To regulate the circulation of stomach *Qi* (vital energy)

Indication:

For a person with dampness accumulated in the spleen and stomach. The symptoms are: abdominal fullness, loss of taste and appetite, nausea and vomiting, belching, acid regurgitation, heaviness sensation in the body, malaise, diarrhea.

Tongue: white with greasy coating, plumply
Pulse: moderate

Application:

Chronic gastritis, functional gastric neurosis

Modification:

with the addition of
藿 香	Huo Xiang (Agastache)	*Herba Agastachis*
半 夏	Ban Xia (Pinellia)	*Rhizoma Pinelliae*

This formula is now called Bu Huan Jing Zheng Qi San (Pinellia, Atractylodes, and Agastache Formula) (不換金正氣散)

1. With indigestion, add:
神 曲	Shen Qu (Medicated leaven)	*Massa Fermentata Medicinalis*
麥 芽	Mai Ya (Germinated barley)	*Fructus Hordei Germinatus*

2. With indigestion, add:
檳 榔	Bing Lang (Areca seed)	*Semen Arecae*
萊菔子	Lai Fu Zi (Radish seed)	*Semen Raphani*

3. With cold and dampness syndromes, abdominal distention, prefers heat to cold, add:
乾 薑	Gan Jiang (Dry ginger)	*Rhizoma Zingiberis*
肉 桂	Rou Gui (Cinnamon bark)	*Cortex Cinnamomi*
草豆蔻	Cao Dou Kou (Katsumadai seed)	*Semen Alpiniae Katsumadai*

Generic Name:

Magnolia and Ginger Formula

Pǔ Jì Xiāo Dú Yǐn 普濟消毒飲

(Pu-Chi-Hsiao-Tu-Yin)
(Universal Antiphlogistic Decoction)

Constituents:

黃 芩	Huang Qin (Scute)	6-9 gm.	Radix Scutellariae
黃 連	Huang Lian (Copis)	3-6 gm.	Rhizoma Coptidis
連 翹	Lian Qiao (Forsythia)	9-12 gm.	Fructus Forsythiae
牛蒡子	Niu Bang Zi (Arctium fruit)	6-9 gm.	Fructus Arctii
薄 荷	Bo He (Mentha)	3-6 gm.	Herba Menthae
僵 蠶	Jiang Can (White-stiff silkworm)	1-3 gm.	Bombys Batryticatus
玄 參	Xuan Shen (Scrophularia)	6-9 gm.	Radix Scrophulariae
馬 勃	Ma Bo (Lasiosphaera)	6-9 gm.	Lasiosphaera Seu Calvatia
板藍根	Ban Lang Gen (Isatis root)	6-9 gm.	Radix Isatidi
桔 梗	Jie Geng (Platycodon)	6-9 gm.	Radix Platycodi Grandiflorum
陳 皮	Chen Pi (Citrus peel)	3-6 gm.	Pericarpium Citri Reticulatae
柴 胡	Chai Hu (Bupleurum)	6-9 gm.	Radix Bupleuri
升 麻	Sheng Ma (Cimicifuga)	3-6 gm.	Rhizoma Cimicifugae
甘 草	Gan Cao (Licorice)	1-3 gm.	Radix Glycyrrhizae

Action:

1. To dispel pathogenic heat and toxin (Febrifugal)
2. To disperse wind and evil factors

Indication:

For a person with epidemic disease with swelling and redness of the face. The symptoms are: fever, aversion to cold, face red and swollen, sore throat, thirsty.

> Tongue: red with dry and yellow or white coating
> Pulse: floating, rapid and forceful

Application:

Carbuncles, boils, parotitis, acute tonsillitis, lymphadenitis, obstructed backflow of lymphducts, purulent inflammation of the face and head, testitis together with parotitis.

Modification:

1. For testitis together with parotitis, add:

川楝子	Chuan Lian Zi (Sichuan chinaberry)	Fructus Meliae Toosendan
龍膽草	Long Dan Cao (Gentiana)	Radix Gentianae

2. In the serious case of the epidemic disease with swelling and redness of face, add:

金銀花	Jin Yin Hua (Lonicera flower)	Flos Lonicerae
荊 芥	Jing Jie (Schizonepeta)	Herba Schizonepetae

Generic Name:

Scute and Cimicifuga Combination

Qǐ Jú Dì Huáng Wán   杞菊地黄丸

(Chi-Chu-Ti-Huang-Wan)
(Lycium fruit, Chrysanthemum and Pills of Six Herbs with Rehmannia)

Constituents:

枸杞子 Gou Qi Zi (Lycium fruit)	6-9 gm.	*Fructus Lycii*
菊 花 Ju Hua (Chrysanthemum)	3-6 gm.	*Flos Chrysanthemi*
熟地黄 Shu Di Huang (Prep. rehmannia)	10-15 gm.	*Radix Rehmanniae Praeparatae*
山茱萸 Shan Zhu Yu (Cornus)	9-12 gm.	*Fructus Corni*
山 藥 Shan Yao (Dioscorea)	9-12 gm.	*Rhizoma Dioscorea*
澤 瀉 Ze Xie (Alisma)	9-12 gm.	*Rhizoma Alismatis*
牡丹皮 Mu Dan Pi (Moutan bark)	6-9 gm.	*Cortex Moutan Radicis*
茯 苓 Fu Ling (Poria)	9-12 gm.	*Poria*

Action:

1. To replenish the *Yin* (vital essence) of kidney
2. To nourish the liver and brighten the eyes

Indication:

For a person with difficulty of vision due to kidney deficiency. The symptoms are: blurry vision, eyes dry and painful, dizziness, vertigo, high blood pressure.

Tongue: red with thin coating
Pulse: thready and rapid

Application:

Diabetes, glaucoma, hypertension, ophthalmalgia.

Generic Name:

Lycium Rehmannia Tea Pills;
Lycium, Chrysanthemum and Rehmannia Formula

Qī Lí Sàn 七釐散 (七厘散)
(Chi-Li-San)
(Anti-bruises Powder)

Constituents:

血 竭	Xue Jie (Dragon's blood)	30 gm.	Sanguis Draconis	
麝 香	She Xiang (Musk)	0.4 gm.	Moschus	
冰 片	Bing Pian (Borneol)	0.4 gm.	Borneolum	
乳 香	Ru Xiang (Mastic)	5 gm.	Resina Olibani	
沒 藥	Mo Yao (Myrrh)	5 gm.	Resina Myrrhae	
紅 花	Hong Hua (Carthamus)	5 gm.	Flos Carthami	
硃 砂	Zhu Sha (Cinnabar)	4 gm.	Cinnabaris	
兒 茶	Er Cha (Catechu)	7.5 gm.	Catechu	

Grind the above ingredients into powder. Take 0.22-1.5 gm. each time with warm water or yellow wine.

Action:

1. To invigorate the blood circulation and remove stasis
2. To relieve pain and stop bleeding

Indication:

For a person with external or internal injury, bruise, wounds, burns, cut, or traumatic wound with ecchymosis.

Application:

External or internal injury of all kinds.

Contraindication:

For a pregnant woman.

Comment:

For external use, mix the powder with wine.

Generic Name:

Musk and Catechu Formula

Qiān Zhèng Sàn　牽正散

(Chian-Cheng-San)
(Restoring to the Normal Position Powder)

Constituents:

白附子 Bai Fu Zi (Typhonium)	12-16 gm.	*Rhizoma typhonii*
僵 蠶 Jiang Can (White-stiff silkworm)	6-9 gm.	*Bombyx Batryticatus*
全 蠍 Quan Xie (Scorpion)	3 pc.	*Scorpio*

Action:

1. To eliminate wind and phlegm
2. Anti-spasmodic

Indication:

For a person with deviation of the mouth and eyes due to apoplexy. The symptoms are: sudden deviation of the eyes and mouth, paralysis of the skin, difficulty of speech, continuous uncontrolled salivation, hemiplegia, intolerance of cold, fever, spasms of the limbs, joints sore and painful.

Tongue: with thin white coating
Pulse: wiry/taut and thready; or floating and rapid

Application:

Facial paralysis, trigeminal neuralgia, hemiplegia, apoplexy.

Contraindication:

For a person with deviation of mouth and eyes due to deficiency of *Qi* and stasis of blood, or due to endogenous wind in the liver.

Modification:

1. To eliminate wind, add:

荆 芥 Jing Jie (Schizonepeta)	*Herba Schizonepetae*
防 風 Fang Feng (Ledebouriella)	*Radix Ledebouriellae*
白 芷 Bai Zhi (Angelica)	*Radix Angelicae Dahuricae*

2. With blood stasis, add:

紅 花 Hong Hua (Carthamus)	*Flos Carthami*

3. For trigeminal neuralgia, add:

蜈 蚣 Wu Gong (Centipede)	*Scolopendra*

Qiāng Huó Shèng Shī Tāng   羌活勝濕湯

(Chiang-Huo-Sheng-Shi-Tang)
(Decoction of Notopterygium to Dispel Dampness)

Constituents:

羌 活	Qiang Huo (Notopterygium root)	3-6 gm.	*Radix Notopterygii*
獨 活	Du Huo (Tuhuo)	3-6 gm.	*Radix Angelicae Pubescentis*
防 風	Fang Feng (Ledebouriella)	3-6 gm.	*Radix Ledebouriellae*
藁 本	Gan Ben (Straw seed)	3-6 gm.	*Rhizoma et Radix Ligustici*
川 芎	Chuan Xiong (Ligusticum)	1-3 gm.	*Rhizoma Ligustici Chuanxiong*
蔓荆子	Man Jing Zi (Vitex fruit)	3-6 gm.	*Fructus Viticis*
炙甘草	Zhi Gan Cao (Baked licorice)	1-3 gm.	*Radix Glycyrrhizae Praeparatae*

Action:

To dispel wind and dampness

Indication:

For a person with wind and dampness in the superficial. The symptoms are: headache, muscle-ache all over the body with difficulty of motion, aversion to cold, slight increase of body temperature, no perspiration.

> Tongue: with white coating
> Pulse: Floating and tight

Contraindication:

For a person with weak and deficiency syndromes.

Application:

Common cold, rheumatic arthritis, neurotic headache, sciatica.

Modification:

If the cold and dampness is accumulated in the Taiyang channel, with fever and stiff-neck, add:

防 己	Fang Ji (Stephania root)	*Radix Stephaniae Tetrandrae*
附 子	Fu Zi (Aconite root)	*Radix Aconiti Praeparatae*
or	(川烏頭)	
	Chuan Wu Tou (Sichuan aconite)	*Radix Aconitii*

Qiāng Lán Tāng　　羌籃湯
(Chiang-Lan-Tang)
(Decoction of Notopterygium and Isatis Root)

Constituents:

羌　活 Qiang Huo (Notopterygium)	9-12 gm.	*Radix Notopterygii*
板藍根 Ban Lan Gen (Isatis root)	20-30 gm.	*Radix Isatidis*

Action:

1. To dispel heat and toxin
2. Diaphoretic

Indication:

For a person with mumps. The symptoms are: fever, intolerance of cold, headache, muscle-ache, sore throat.

Tongue: red
Pulse: slippery and rapid

Application:

Mumps, epidemic parotitis, upper respiratory tract infection, acute tonsillitis, pharyngitis.

Modification:

1. With stuffy nose, add:
蒼耳子 Cang Er Zi (Xanthium fruit)　　*Fructus Xanthii*
薄　荷 Bo He (Mentha)　　*Herba Menthae*

2. With cough and sore throat, add:
前　胡 Qian Hu (Peucedanum)　　*Radix Peucedani*
牛蒡子 Niu Bang Zi (Arctium fruit)　　*Fructus Arctii*

3. With severe sore throat, add:
山豆根 Shan Dou Gen (Pigeon pea)　　*Radix Sophorae Subprostratae*
馬　勃 Ma Bo (Lasiosphaera)　　*Lasiosphaera seu Calvatia*

4. With cough and sputum, difficulty to spit, add:
桔　梗 Jie Geng (Platycodon)　　*Radix Platycodi*
甘　草 Gan Cao (Licorice)　　*Radix Glycyrrhizae*

5. With cough and dyspnea, add:
麻　黄 Ma Huang (Ephedra)　　*Herba Ephedrae*
杏　仁 Xing Ren (Apricot seed)　　*Semen Armeniacae Amarum*

Qīng É Wán　　青娥丸

(Ching-O-Wan)
(The Blue Fairy Lady Pills for Lumbago)

Constituents:

補骨脂 Bu Gu Zhi (Psoralea)	120 gm.	*Fructus Psoraleae*
杜　仲 Du Zhong (Eucommia bark)	120 gm.	*Cortex Eucommiae*
胡桃肉 Hu Tao Rou (Walnut)	120 gm.	*Semen Juglandis*
大　蒜 Da Suan (Garlic)	120 gm.	*Bulbus Allii*

Grind the above ingredients into powder and made into pills

Take 9 gm. each time, twice daily.

Action:

1. To tonify the kidney
2. To relieve low back pain

Indication:

For a person with lumbago due to kidney deficiency. The symptoms are: low back pain, spermatorrhea, flaccidity of muscles and bones.

Application:

Lumbago

Qīng Gŭ Sàn　　清骨散

(Ching-Ku-San)
(Powder to Clear the Heat in the Bone)

Constituents:

銀柴胡	Yin Chai Hu (Stellaria)	6-9 gm.	*Radix Stellariae*
秦 艽	Qin Jiao (Large leaf gentian)	6-9 gm.	*Radix Gentianae*
青 蒿	Qing Hao (Sweet wormwood)	3-6 gm.	*Herba Artemisiae Chinghao*
地骨皮	Di Gu Pi (Lycium bark)	6-9 gm.	*Cortex Lycii Radicis*
胡黃連	Hu Huang Lian (Picrorhiza)	3-6 gm.	*Radix Picrorhizae*
知 母	Zhi Mu (Anemarrhena)	3-6 gm.	*Rhizoma Anemarrhenae*
鱉 甲	Bie Jia (Tortoise shell)	6-9 gm.	*Carapax Trionycis*
甘 草	Gan Cao (Licorice)	1-3 gm.	*Radix Glycyrrhizae*

Action:

1. To clear the heat caused by deficiency symptom-complex
2. To reduce afternoon fever and bone-steaming sensation

Indication:

For a person with tidal fever in the afternoon and steaming sensation in the bone due to deficiency of *Yin* (vital essence). The symptoms are: afternoon fever, sensation of heat in the bones, center of hand and feet, cheek red, malaise, lips red, night sweat.

> Tongue: red with thin coating
> Pulse: thready and rapid; soft and rapid; or weak and rapid

Application:

Pulmonary tuberculosis

Qīng Hāo Biē Jiǎ Tāng　　青蒿鱉甲湯
(Ching-Hao-Pieh-Chia-Tang)
(Decoction of Sweet Wormwood and Tortoise Shell)

Constituents:

青 蒿	Qing Hao (Sweet wormwood)	6-9 gm.	*Herba Artemisiae Chinghao*
鱉 甲	Bie Jia (Tortoise shell)	10-15 gm.	*Carapax Trionycis*
生地黃	Sheng Di Huang (Fresh rehmannia)	9-12 gm.	*Radix Rehmanniae*
知 母	Zhi Mu (Anemarrhena)	6-9 gm.	*Rhizoma Anemarrhenae*
牡丹皮	Mu Dan Pi (Moutan bark)	6-9 gm.	*Cortex Moutan Radicis*

Action:

To nourish the *Yin* (vital essence) and dispel the heat.

Indication:

For a person with deficiency of *Yin* (vital essence) in the later period of a febrile disease. The symptoms are: low graded body temperature, or tidal fever in the afternoon, emaciation, no loss of appetite.

>Tongue: red with little coating
>Pulse: rapid

Application:

Phthisis, summer fever in children, chronic pyelonephritis, kidney tuberculosis.

Modification:

1. For fever of unknown origin, add:

白 薇	Bai Wei (Swallowwort)	*Radix Cynanchi Atrati*
石 斛	Shi Hu (Dendrobium stem)	*Herba Dendrobii*
地骨皮	Di Gu Pi (Lycium bark)	*Cortex Lycii Radicis*

2. For pulmonary tuberculosis, add:

沙 參	Sha Shen (Glehnia)	*Radix Glehniae*
旱蓮草	Han Lian Cao (Eclipta)	*Herba Ecliptae*

3. For pyelonephritis, kidney tuberculosis, add:

白茅根	Bai Mao Gen (Imperata rhizome)	*Rhizoma Imperatae*

Qīng Qì Huà Tán Wán　　清氣化痰丸
(Ching-Chi-Hua-Tan-Wan)
(The Expectorant Pills)

Constituents:

胆南星	Dan Nan Xing (Arisaema)	1-3 gm.	*Radix Arisaematis Praeparatae*
黄 芩	Huang Qin (Scutellaria)	3-6 gm.	*Radix Scutellariae*
瓜蔞仁	Gua Lou Ren (Trichosanthes fruit)	6-9 gm.	*Fructus Trichosanthis*
半 夏	Ban Xia (Pinellia)	3-6 gm.	*Rhizoma Pinelliae*
枳 實	Zhi Shi (Immature bitter orange)	3-6 gm.	*Fructus Aurantii Immaturus*
陳 皮	Chen Pi (Citrus peel)	3-6 gm.	*Pericarpium Citri Reticulatae*
杏 仁	Xing Ren (Apricot seed)	6-9 gm.	*Semen Armeniacae Amarum*
茯 苓	Fu Ling (Poria)	9-12 gm.	*Poria*

Action:

1. Anti-tussive and expectorant
2. To eliminate heat and phlegm

Indication:

For a person with interior accumulation of heat and phlegm. The symptoms are: cough with yellow sputum (thick and difficult to spit), nausea, dyspnea, fullness and oppression in the chest and epigastric region.

> Tongue: red with yellow and greasy coating
> Pulse: slippery and rapid

Application:

Pneumonia, chronic tracheitis.

Modification:

1. With intense heat in the lung, add:

石 膏	Shi Gao (Gypsum)	*Gypsum Fibrosum*
知 母	Zhi Mu (Anemarrhena)	*Rhizoma Anemarrhenae*

2. With dry stool or constipation, add:

大 黄	Da Huang (Rhubarb)	*Radix et Rhizoma Rhei*

Generic Name:

Pinellia Expectorant Pills

Qīng Shī Huà Tán Tāng 清濕化痰湯
(Ching-shih-hua-tan-tang)
(Decoction to eliminate Phlegm and Dampness)

Constituents:

天南星	Tian Nan Xing (Arisaema)	6-9 gm.	*Rhizoma Arisaematis*
半 夏	Ban Xia (Pinellia tuber)	6-9 gm.	*Rhizoma Pinelliae*
茯 苓	Fu Ling (Poria)	6-9 gm.	*Poria*
陳 皮	Chen Pi (Citrus peel)	3-6 gm.	*Pericarpium Citri Reticulatae*
白芥子	Bai Jie Zi (Brassica)	6-9 gm.	*Semen Sinapis Albae*
蒼 术	Cang Zhu (Atractylodes)	6-9 gm.	*Rhizoma Atractylodis*
羌 活	Qing Huo (Notopterygium)	6-9 gm.	*Radix Notopterygii*
白 芷	Bai Zhi (Angelica)	6-9 gm.	*Radix Angelicae Dahuricae*
黃 芩	Huang Qin (Scutellaria)	6-9 gm.	*Radix Scutellariae*
竹 瀝	Zhu Li (Bamboo sap)	6-9 gm.	*Saccus Bambusae*
生 薑	Sheng Jiang (Ginger)	3-6 gm.	*Rhizoma Zingiberis Recens*
甘 草	Gan Cao (Licorice)	3-6 gm.	*Radix Glycyrrhizae*

Action:

To resolve phlegm and dampness

Indication:

For a person with migratory pain all over the body, and also lumps in the neck or shoulder. The symptoms are: migratory pain over the whole body and the four limbs, chills and fever, cough and asthma, fullness in the chest, lumps in the neck and shoulder, may have cold sensation in certain areas.

> Tongue: with thin frothy coating
> Pulse: deep and slippery

Application:

Arthralgia, intercostal neuralgia, lymphatic glandula, stiffness of the shoulder with cold sensation.

Generic Name:

Pinellia and Arisaema Combination

Qīng Shǔ Yì Qì Tāng (I) 清暑益氣湯 《溫熱經緯》

(Ching-Shu-I-Chi-Tang) (I)
(Decoction to Clear Summer-heat and Replenish *Qi*) (I)

Constituents:

西瓜翠衣	Xi Gua Cui Yi (Watermelon peel)	20-30 gm.	*Exocarpium Citrulli*
西洋參	Xi Yang Shen (American ginseng)	3-6 gm.	*Radix Panacis Quinquefolii*
荷　梗	He Geng (Lotus stem)	6-9 gm.	*Rhizoma Nelumbinis*
石　斛	Shi Hu (Dendrobium)	6-9 gm.	*Herba Dendrobii*
麥門冬	Mai Men Dong (Ophiopogon)	9-12 gm.	*Radix Ophiopogonis*
黃　連	Huang Lian (Coptis)	1-3 gm.	*Rhizoma Coptidis*
知　母	Zhi Mu (Anemarrhena)	3-6 gm.	*Rhizoma Anemarrhenae*
竹　葉	Zhu Ye (Bamboo leaf)	3-6 gm.	*Folium Bambusae*
甘　草	Gan Cao (Licorice)	1-3 gm.	*Radix Glycyrrhizae*
粳　米	Jing Mi (Oryza)	10-15 gm.	*Semen Oryzae*

Action:

1. To clear the summer heat and replenish the *Qi*
2. To nourish the *Yin* (vital essence) and promote the secretion of body fluids.

Indication:

For a person with affection of summer heat and deficiency of *Yin* (vital essence). The symptoms are: high fever, with profuse perspiration, thirst, fatigue, fidgetiness.

> Tongue: pale or red
> Pulse: feeble and rapid

Application:

Common cold in the summer, summer fever in children, heat-stroke, thermoplegia, sun-stroke.

Contraindication:

For a person with affection of summer-heat and dampness.

Modification:

For prolonged fever in children, add:

白　薇	Bai Wei (Swallowwort)	*Radix Cynanchi Atrati*
地骨皮	Di Gu Pi (Lycium bark)	*Cortex Lycii Radicis*

and eliminate:

黃　連	Huang Lian (Coptis)	*Rhizoma Coptidis*

Qīng Shǔ Yì Qì Tāng (II) 清暑益氣湯 〈脾胃論〉
(Ching-Shu-I-Chi-Tang) (II)
(Decoction to Clear Summer-heat and Replenish *Qi*) (II)

Constituents:

黄 芪	Huang Qi (Astragalus)	9-12 gm.	*Radix Astragali*
人 參	Ren Shen (Ginseng)	1-3 gm.	*Radix Ginseng*
白 术	Bai Zhu (White atractylodes)	3-6 gm.	*Rhizoma Atractylodis Macrocephalae*
蒼 术	Cang Zhu (Atractylodes)	3-6 gm.	*Rhizoma Atractylodis*
神 曲	Shen Qu (Medicated leaven)	6-9 gm.	*Massa Fermentata Medicinalis*
澤 瀉	Ze Xie (Alisma)	6-9 gm.	*Rhizoma Alismatis*
陳 皮	Chen Pi (Citrus peel)	1-3 gm.	*Pericarpium Citri Reticulatae*
青 皮	Qing Pi (Green tangerine peel)	3-6 gm.	*Pericarpium Citri Reticulatae Viridae*
麥門冬	Mai Men Dong (Ophiopogon)	6-9 gm.	*Radix Ophiopogonis*
五味子	Wu Wei Zi (Schisandra)	3-6 gm.	*Fructus Schisandrae*
當歸身	Dang Gui (Chinese angelica)	6-9 gm.	*Radix Angelicae Sinensis*
黄 柏	Huang Bai (Phellodendron)	3-6 gm.	*Cortex Phellodendri*
葛 根	Ge Gen (Pueraria)	6-9 gm.	*Radix Puerariae*
升 麻	Sheng Ma (Cimicifuga)	3-6 gm.	*Rhizoma Cimicifugae*
炙甘草	Zhi Gan Cao (Baked licorice)	1-3 gm.	*Radix Glycyrrhizae Praeparatae*

Action:

1. To clear the summer-heat and replenish *Qi*
2. To promote the secretion of body fluids
3. To dispel dampness

Indication:

For a person with *Qi* (vital energy) deficiency and affection of summer-heat and dampness. The symptoms are: fever, headache, thirst, spontaneous perspiration, lassitude of the four limbs, loss of appetite, fullness sensation in the chest, heaviness sensation of the body, loose stool, urine color amber and scanty.

Tongue: with greasy coating
Pulse: feeble and rapid

Application:

Common cold in the summer, summer fever in children, heat-stroke, sun-stroke, thermoplegia.

Generic Name:

Astragalus and Atractylodes Combination

180

Qīng Wēn Bài Dú Yǐn 清瘟敗毒飲
(Ching-Wen-Pai-Tu-Yin)
(Antiphlogistic Decoction for Epidemic Diseases)

Constituents:

石　膏	Shi Gao (Gypsum)	20-30 gm.	*Gypsum Fibrosum*
犀　角	Xi Jiao (rhinoceros horn)	3-6 gm.	*Cornu Rhinoceri*
生地黃	Sheng Di Huang (Rehmannia)	20-30 gm.	*Radix Rehmanniae*
黃　連	Huang Lian (Coptis)	9-12 gm.	*Rhizoma Coptidis*
黃　芩	Huang Qin (Scutellaria)	9-12 gm.	*Radix Scutellariae*
梔　子	Zhi Zi (Gardenia)	3-6 gm.	*Fructus Gardeniae*
知　母	Zhi Mu (Anemarrhena)	9-12 gm.	*Rhizoma Anemarrhenae*
玄　參	Xuan Shen (Scrophularia)	6-9 gm.	*Radix Scrophulariae*
連　翹	Lian Qiao (Forsythia)	6-9 gm.	*Fructus Forsythiae*
桔　梗	Jie Geng (Platycodon)	6-9 gm.	*Radix Platycodi*
赤芍藥	Chi Shao Yao (Red peony)	10-15 gm.	*Radix Paeoniae Rubra*
牡丹皮	Mu Dan Pi (Moutan bark)	9-12 gm.	*Cortex Moutan Radicis*
鮮竹葉	Zhu Ye (Bamboo leaf)	9-12 gm.	*Folium Bambusae*
甘　草	Gan Cao (Licorice)	3-6 gm.	*Radix Glycyrrhizae*

Action:

    1. To eliminate heat and toxin
    2. To purge the fire and cool the blood

Indication:

For a person with intense heat in both the *Qi* (Secondary defensive) system and Xue (Blood) system of the body. The symptoms are: high body temperature, intensive thirst, chapped lips, headache, restlessness, spitting blood, nose-bleeding, macula on the skin, mania, spasms or convulsions.

    Tongue: dark red, dry or prickly
    Pulse: floating, gigantic, rapid/ or deep, thready, rapid

Application:

Encephalitis B, epidemic meningitis, septicemia, acute leukemia, uremia.

Modification:

    1. With blood stasis, add:

大青葉	Da Qing Ye (Isatis leaf)	*Folium Isatidis*
紫　草	Zi Cao (Lithospermum)	*Radix Lithospermi*

    2. With convulsions, add:

蟬　蛻	Chan Tui (Ciccada slough)	*Periostracum Cicadae*
僵　蠶	Jiang Can (White-stiff silkworm)	*Bombyx Batryticatus*

Qīng Yí Tāng　　清胰湯
(Ching-I-Tang)
(Decoction for Acute Pancreatitis)

Constituents:

柴　胡	Chai Hu (Bupleurum)	12-15 gm.	Radix Bupleuri
白芍藥	Bai Shao Yao (White peony)	6-9 gm.	Radix Paeoniae Alba
黄　芩	Huang Qin (Scutellaria)	6-9 gm.	Radix Scutellariae
胡黃連	Hu Huang Lian (Picrorhiza)	6-9 gm.	Radix Picrorrhizae
木　香	Mu Xiang (Saussurea)	6-9 gm.	Radix Saussureae
延胡索	Yan Hu Suo (Corydalis)	6-9 gm.	Rhizoma Corydalis
大　黃	Da Huang (Rhubarb)	12-15 gm.	Radix et Rhizoma Rhei
芒　硝	Mang Xiao (Mirabilitum)	6-9 gm.	Natrii Sulfas

Action:

1. To soothe the liver and invigorate the circulation of *Qi* (vital energy)
2. To purge the intense heat and fire
3. Purgative

Indication:

For a person with acute pancreatitis due to stagnation of *Qi* (vital energy) in the liver, and intense heat in the spleen and stomach. The symptoms are: fullness and pain in the chest and abdomen (refused to be pressed), thirst, constipation, amber colored urine.

> Tongue: with thin white or yellow coating
> Pulse: wiry/taut and rapid

Application:

Acute pancreatitis

Modification:

If complicated with biliary ascariasis, add:

使君子	Shi Jun Zi (Quisqualis fruit)	Fructus Quisqualis
苦楝皮	Ku Lian Pi (Melia bark)	Cortex Meliae
檳　榔	Bing Lang (Areca seed)	Semen Arecae

Qīng Yíng Tāng　　清營湯

(Ching-Ying-Tang)
(Decoction to Dispel Pathogenic Heat from *Ying* System)

Constituents:

犀　角 Xi Jiao (Rhinoceros horn)	6-9 gm.	*Cornus Rhinoceri*
生地黃 Sheng Di Huang (Rehmannia)	10-15 gm.	*Radix Rehmanniae*
玄　參 Xuan Shen (Scrophularia)	6-9 gm.	*Radix Scrophulariae*
麥門冬 Mai Men Dong (Ophiopogon)	6-9 gm.	*Radix Ophiopogonis*
竹　葉 Zhu Ye (Bamboo leaf)	3-6 gm.	*Folium Bambusae*
黃　連 Huang Lian (Coptis)	1-3 gm.	*Rhizoma Coptidis*
金銀花 Jin Yin Hua (Lonicera flower)	6-9 gm.	*Flos Lonicerae*
連　翹 Lian Qiao (Forsythia)	6-9 gm.	*Fructus Forsythiae*
丹　參 Dan Shen (Salvia root)	3-6 gm.	*Radix Salviae Miltiorrhizae*

Action:

1. To dispel pathogenic heat from the *Ying* (nutrient) system
2. To nourish the *Yin* (vital essence)

Indication:

For a person with pathogenic heat penetrated into the *Ying* (nutrient) system. The symptoms are: fever (especially at night), thirst or no thirst, delirium, restlessness, insomnia, skin with macula.

　　　　Tongue: dark red and dry
　　　　Pulse: thready and rapid

Application:

Encephalitis B, epidemic meningitis, septicemia.

Contraindication:

For a person with white and slippery tongue coating, indicating the presence of dampness.

Modification:

1. With convulsions, add:

鈴羊角 Ling Yang Jiao (Antelope horn)	*Cornu Antelopis*
鉤　藤 Gou Teng (Uncaria)	*Ramulus Uncariae cum Uncis*

2. With excessive heat and phlegm, add:

竹　茹 Zhu Ru (Bamboo shavings)	*Caulus Bambusae in Taenis*

Qīng Zào Jiù Fèi Tāng　　清燥救肺湯
(Ching-Tsao-Chiu-Fei-Tang)
(Decoction to eliminate the Dryness in the Lung)

Constituents:

桑　葉	Sang Ye (Mulberry leaf)	6-9 gm.	*Folium Mori*
石　膏	Shi Gao (Gypsum)	10-15 gm.	*Gypsum Fibrosum*
阿　膠	E Jiao (Donkey-hide gelatin)	6-9 gm.	*Colla Corii Asini*
麥門冬	Mai Men Dong (Ophiopogon)	6-9 gm.	*Radix Ophiopogonis*
胡麻仁	Hu Ma Ren (Flax)	3-6 gm.	*Semen Lini*
人　參	Ren Shen (Ginseng)	3-6 gm.	*Radix Ginseng*
杏　仁	Xing Ren (Apricot seed)	3-6 gm.	*Semen Armeniacae Amarum*
枇杷葉	Pi Pa Ye (Loquat leaf)	6-9 gm.	*Folium Eriobotryae*
甘　草	Gan Cao (Licorice)	3-6 gm.	*Radix Glycyrrhizae*

Action:

To eliminate drought/dryness and moisten the lung.

Indication:

For a person with depletion of *Qi* (vital energy) and *Yin* (vital essence) due to the warmth and dryness in the lung. The symptoms are: fever, headache, dry cough with no sputum, hiccup with dyspnea, dry throat and nostrils.

> Tongue: red and dry with thin white coating
> Pulse: weak, thready or rapid

Application:

Flu with cough, asthma, upper respiratory tract infection, hemoptysis.

Modification:

1. Cough with blood, add:

側柏葉	Ce Bai Ye (Biota tops)	*Cacumen Biotae*
仙鶴草	Xian He Cao (Agrimony herb)	*Herba Agrimoniae*

2. With profuse sputum, add:

川貝母	Chuan Bei Mu (Tendrilled fritillary)	*Bulbus Fritillariae Cirrhosae*
瓜　蔞	Gua Lou (Trichosanthes)	*Semen Trichosanthis*

3. Dehydration or dryness in blood, add:

生地黃	Sheng Di Huang (Rehmannia)	*Radix Rehmanniae*

4. With extreme heat, add:

犀　角	Xi Jiao (Rhinoceros horn)	*Cornus Rhinoceri*
鈴羊角	Ling Yang Jiao (Antelope horn)	*Cornu Antelopis*
牛　黃	Niu Huang (Ox gallstone)	*Calculus Bovis*

Generic Name:

Eriobotrya and Ophiopogon Combination

Rén Shēn Bài Dú Sàn 人參敗毒散
(Jen-Sheng-Pai-Tu-San)
(Antiphlogistic Powder of Ginseng)

Constituents:

羌 活	Qiang Huo (Notopterygium)	6-9 gm.	*Radix Notopterygii*
獨 活	Du Huo (Pubescent angelica)	6-9 gm.	*Radix Angelicae Pubescentis*
川 芎	Chuan Xiong (Ligusticum)	6-9 gm.	*Rhizoma Ligustici Chuanxiong*
柴 胡	Chai Hu (Bupleurum)	6-9 gm.	*Radix Bupleuri*
薄 荷	Bo He (Mentha)	3-6 gm.	*Herba Menthae*
枳 殼	Zhi Ke (Bitter orange)	6-9 gm.	*Fructus Aurantii*
桔 梗	Jie Geng (Platycodon)	6-9 gm.	*Radix Platycodi*
前 胡	Qian Hu (Peucedanum)	6-9 gm.	*Radix Peucedani*
茯 苓	Fu Ling (Poria)	6-9 gm.	*Poria*
人 參	Ren Shen (Ginseng)	3-6 gm.	*Radix Ginseng*
生 薑	Sheng Jiang (Fresh ginger)	3-6 gm.	*Rhizoma Zingiberis Recens*
甘 草	Gan Cao (Licorice)	3-6 gm.	*Radix Glycyrrhizae*

Action:

1. To dispel external wind, cold and dampness (Diaphoretic)
2. To replenish *Qi* (vital energy)

Indication:

For a person of weak constitution with deficeincy of *Qi* (vital energy) and affection of wind, cold and dampness. The symptoms are: high fever, aversion to cold, no perspiration, headache, neck pain, muscle-ache, stuffy nose, cough with sputum, fullness sensation in the chest and epigastric region.

> Tongue: with white and greasy coating
> Pulse: floating, feeble (perceptible on firm pressure)

Application:

Common cold, influenza, malaria, dysentery, suppurative infections

Contraindication:

For a person with strong constitution.

Modification:

For a person with malaria, add:

草 果	Cao Guo (Tsaoko)	*Fructus Tsaoko*
檳 榔	Bing Lang (Betel nut)	*Semen Arecae*

Generic Name:

Ginseng and Mentha Formula

Rén Shēn Hú Táo Tāng 人參胡桃湯
(Jen-Sheng-Hu-Tao-Tang)
(Decoction of Ginseng and Walnut)

Constituents:

人　參 Ren Shen (Ginseng)	6-9 gm.	*Radix Ginseng*
胡桃仁 Hu Tao (Walnut)	10-15 gm.	*Semen Juglandis Regiae*
生　薑 Sheng Jiang (Fresh ginger)	3-6 gm.	*Rhizoma Zingiberis Recens*

Action:

1. To tonify the lung and kidney
2. Antitussive and anti-asthmatic

Indication:

For a person with deficiency of kidney *Qi* (vital energy), therefore cannot aid the lung to control the process of respiration. The symptoms are: dyspnea, asthma, shortness of breath, soft voice, cough with perspiration, low back pain, hands and feet not warm, edema in the face, fullness in the chest.

Tongue: pale
Pulse: feeble

Application:

Cough, asthma, bronchial asthma, chronic bronchitis, pulmonary emphysema.

Rén Shēn Yǎng Yíng Tāng　人參養營湯
(Jen-Shen-Yang-Ying-Tang)
(Nutrient System Nourishing Decoction with Ginseng)

Constituents:

人 參	Ren Shen (Ginseng)	6-9 gm.	*Radix Ginseng*
熟地黃	Shu Di Huang (Prep. rehmannia)	9-12 gm.	*Radix Rehmanniae Praeparatae*
白 术	Bai Zhu (White atractylodes)	9-12 gm.	*Rhizoma Atractylodis Macrocephalae*
當 歸	Dang Gui (Chinese angelicae)	9-12 gm.	*Radix Angelicae Sinensis*
白 芍	Bai Shao Yao (White peony)	6-9 gm.	*Radix Paeoniae Alba*
茯 苓	Fu Ling (Poria)	9-12 gm.	*Poria*
黃 芪	Huang Qi (Astragalus)	9-12 gm.	*Radix Astragali*
肉 桂	Rou Gui (Cinnamon bark)	1-3 gm.	*Cortex Cinnamomi*
五味子	Wu Wei Zi (Schisandra)	6-9 gm.	*Fructus Schisandrae*
遠 志	Yuan Zhi (Polygala)	6-9 gm.	*Radix Polygalae*
陳 皮	Chen Pi (Citrus peel)	3-6 gm.	*Pericarpium Citri Reticulatae*
炙甘草	Zhi Gan Cao (Baked licorice)	3-6 gm.	*Radix Glycyrrhizae Praeparatae*
生 薑	Sheng Jiang (Fresh ginger)	1-3 gm.	*Rhizoma Zingiberis Recens*
大 棗	Da Zao (Jujube)	3-5 pc.	*Fructus Ziziphus Jujubae*

Action:

1. To replenish *Qi* (vital energy) and blood
2. Sedative and tranquilizing

Indication:

For a person with deficiency of *Qi* (vital energy), blood and *Yang* (vital function). The symptoms are: emaciation, pale face, loss of appetite, insomnia, palpitation, forgetfulness, irregular menstruation.

> Tongue: pale
> Pulse: thready and weak

Application:

Anemia, irregular menstruation, uterine bleeding, insomnia.

Generic Name:

Ren Shen Yang Ying Wan;
Ginseng Nutritive Combination

Rùn Cháng Wán   潤腸丸

(Jun-Chang-Wan)
(The Emollient Pills)

Constituents:

當 歸 Dang Gui (Chinese angelica)	6-9 gm.	*Radix Angelicae Sinensis*
生地黃 Sheng Di Huang (Rehmannia)	6-9 gm.	*Radix Rehmanniae*
桃 仁 Tao Ren (Persica seed)	6-9 gm.	*Semen Persicae*
麻子仁 Ma Zi Ren (Cannabis seed)	10-15 gm.	*Fructus Cannabis*
杏 仁 Xing Ren (Apricot seed)	6-9 gm.	*Semen Armeniacae Amarum*
枳 殼 Zhi Ke (Mature bitter orange)	6-9 gm.	*Fructus Aurantii*

Action:

Emollient

Indication:

For a person with constipation caused by deficiency of blood. The symptoms are: constipation, face pale, dizziness, vertigo, palpitation.

Tongue: pale
Pulse: thready

Application:

Constipation of the anemic or elderly person

Contraindication:

For a pregnant woman.

Modification:

If there is internal heat caused by deficiency of blood and depletion of fluid, dry mouth, add:

玄 參 Xuan Shen (Scrophularia)	*Radix Scrophulariae*
何首烏 He Shou Wu (Polygonum)	*Radix Polygoni Multiflori*
知 母 Zhi Mu (Anemarrhena)	*Rhizoma Anemarrhenae*

Generic Name:

Run Chang Wan (Peach Kernel Pills)

Sān Huáng Sì Wù Tāng　三黄四物湯

(San-Huang-Szu-Wu-Tang)
(Decoction of the Four Ingredients and Three Yellow Colored Herbs)

Constituents:

熟地黄	Shu Di Huang (Prep. rehmannia)	12-15 gm.	*Radix Rehmanniae Praeparatae*
當　歸	Dang Gui (Chinese angelica)	6-9 gm.	*Radix Angelicae Sinensis*
川　芎	Chuan Xiong (Ligusticum)	6-9 gm.	*Rhizoma Ligustici Chuanxiong*
赤芍藥	Chi Shao Yao (Red peony)	6-9 gm.	*Radix Paeoniae Rubra*
大　黄	Da Huang (Rhubarb)	3-6 gm.	*Radix et Rhizoma Rhei*
黄　連	Huang Lian (Coptis)	1-3 gm.	*Rhizoma Coptidis*
黄　芩	Huang Qin (Scutellaria)	6-9 gm.	*Radix Scutellariae*

Action:

1. To replenish blood
2. To purge the fire in the heart channel

Indication:

For a person with excessive fire in the heart channel. The symptoms are: fidgetiness, insomnia, constipation, urination amber in color and with burning sensation, amenorrhea.

> Tongue: dark red, red in the tip, with thin coating
> Pulse: thready and rapid

Application:

Anemia, amenorrhea, constipation.

Sān Jiǎ Fù Mài Tāng 三甲復脈湯
(San-Chia-Fu-Mai-Tang)
(Decoction of Three Shells to Recover the Pulse)

Constituents:

牡蠣	Mu Li (Oyster shell)	20-30 gm.	*Concha Ostreae*
鱉甲	Bie Jia (Tortoise shell)	15-30 gm.	*Carapax Trionycis*
龜版	Gui Ban (Tortoise plastron)	15-30 gm.	*Plastrum Testudinis*
炙甘草	Zhi Gan Cao (Baked licorice)	9-12 gm.	*Radix Glycyrrhizae*
生地黃	Sheng Di Huang (Rehmannia)	15-30 gm.	*Radix Rehmanniae*
白芍藥	Bai Shao Yao (White peony)	9-15 gm.	*Radix Paeoniae Alba*
麥門冬	Mai Men Dong (Ophiopogon)	9-15 gm.	*Radix Ophiopogonis*
火麻仁	Huo Ma Ren (Cannabis seed)	9-12 gm.	*Fructus Cannabis*
阿膠	E Jiao (Donkey-hide gelatin)	12-15 gm.	*Colla Corii Asini*

Action:

1. To subdue the exuberance of *Yang* (vital function) and nourish the *Yin* (Vital essence)
2. To subdue the endogenous wind and nourish blood

Indication:

1. For a person with endogenous wind due to deficiency of blood in the later stage of the febrile disease. The symptoms are: spasms of the hands and feet, clonic convulsions, severe palpitation, fatigue, heat sensation in the palms of the hands and feet.

> Tongue: dark red and dry
> Pulse: thready, rapid and weak

2. For a person with exuberance of *Yang* (vital function) due to deficiency of *Yin* (vital essence). The symptoms are: bleeding, palpitation, dizziness, vertigo, tinnitus, throat dry.

> Tongue: dry with sudden disappearance of the fur on the tongue
> Pulse: thready and wiry/taut

Application:

Convulsions, hypocalcemia, anemia, tinnitus, vertigo.

Modification:

In prostration, add:
五味子 Wu Wei Zi (Schisandra fruit)   *Fructus Schisandrae*
雞子黃 Ji Zi Huang (Egg yolk)
This formula is called Da Ding Feng Zhu (大定風珠)

Sān Jīn Tāng　　三金湯
(San-Chin-Tang)
(Decoction of Three Golds)

Constituents:

金錢草	Jin Qian Cao (Lysimachia)	30-60 gm.	*Herba Lysimachiae*
海金沙	Hai Jin Sha (Lygodium spores)	20-30 gm.	*Spora Lygodii*
冬葵子	Dong Kui Zi (Abutilon seed)	10-15 gm.	*Semen Abutili*
石　葦	Shi Wei (Pyrrosia leaf)	6-9 gm.	*Folium Pyrrosiae*
瞿　麥	Qu Mai (Dianthus)	10-15 gm.	*Herba Dianthi*
雞內金	Ji Nei Jin (Chicken's gizzard skin)	6-9 gm.	*Endothelium Corneum Gigeriae*

Action:

1. To eliminate heat and dampness
2. To invigorate the circulation of vital energy

Indication:

For a person with calculi in the urinary tract. The symptoms are: severe pain around the waist, nausea, vomiting, fever, frequent and painful urination, bloody urine.

Tongue: with thin yellow or white coating
Pulse: slippery and rapid, or taut/wiry and rapid

Application:

Urolithiasis

Modification:

1. With severe pain, add:

蒲　黃	Pu Huang (Bulrush pollen)	*Pollen Typhae*
五靈脂	Wu Ling Zhi (Pteropus excrement)	*Faeces Trogopterorum*

2. With hematuria, add:

槐　花	Huai Hua (Sophora flower)	*Flos Sophorae*
藕　節	Ou Jie (Lotus node)	*Nodus Nelumbinis Rhizomatis*
仙鶴草	Xian He Cao (Agrimony herb)	*Herba Agrimoniae*
小　薊	Xiao Ji (Small thistle)	*Herba Cephalanoploris*

Sān Niù Tāng   三拗湯

(San-Niu-Tang)
(The Stubborn Decoction with Three Ingredients)

Constituents:

麻 黄	Ma Huang (Ephedra)	6-9 gm.	*Herba Ephedrae*
杏 仁	Xing Ren (Apricot seed)	6-9 gm.	*Semen Ameniaceae Amarum*
甘 草	Gan Cao (Licorice)	3-6 gm.	*Radix Glycyrrhizae*

Action:

1. Antitussive
2. Anti-asthmatic

Indication:

For a person with common cold and cough. The symptoms are: fever, headache, dizziness, dyspnea, cough with profuse sputum, asthma, fullness sensation of the chest, general aching of the body.

Tongue: with thin white coating
Pulse: floating and tight

Application:

Common cold, cough, asthma

192

Sān Rén Tāng   三仁湯

(San-Jen-Tang)
(Decoction of Three Kinds of Seeds)

Constituents:

杏　仁	Xing Ren (Apricot seed)	9-12 gm.	*Semen Armeniacae Amarum*
白蔻仁	Bai Kou Ren (Cluster)	3-6 gm.	*Semen Cardamomi Rotundi*
薏苡仁	Yi Yi Ren (Coix)	10-15 gm.	*Semen Coicis*
半　夏	Ban Xia (Pinellia)	6-9 gm.	*Rhizoma Pinelliae*
厚　朴	Hou Po (Magnolia bark)	3-6 gm.	*Cortex Magnoliae Officinalis*
滑　石	Hua Shi (Talc)	10-15 gm.	*Talcum*
通　草	Tong Cao (Ricepaper pith)	3-6 gm.	*Medulla Tetrapanacis*
竹　葉	Zhu Ye (Bamboo leaf)	3-6 gm.	*Folium Bambusae*

Action:

1. To increase the functional activity of vital energy
2. To eliminate heat and dampness

Indication:

For a person with heat and dampness in the body. The symptoms are: headache, intolerance of cold, afternoon fever, face sallow, heaviness sensation in the head and body, chest and abdominal fullness, loss of appetite, nausea, thirsty but do not want to drink water.

     Tongue: with white and greasy coating
     Pulse: soft

Application:

Typhoid fever, gastroenteritis, pyelonephritis, brucellosis (undulant fever).

Modification:

1. With high fever, intolerance of cold, add:

藿　香	Huo Xiang (Agastache)	*Herba Agastachis*
香　薷	Xiang Ru (Elsholtzia)	*Herba Elsholtziae*

2. With intermittent fever, add:

草　果	Cao Guo (Tsao-ko)	*Fructus Tsao-ko*
青　蒿	Qing Hao (Sweet wormwood)	*Herba Artemisiae Chinghao*

3. With amber colored urine, add:

金銀花	Jin Yin Hua (Lonicera flower)	*Flos Lonicerae*
連　翹	Lian Qiao (Forsythia fruit)	*Fructus Forsythiae*
蒲公英	Pu Gong Ying (Dandelion)	*Herba Taraxaci*

Sān Wù Bèi Jí Wán　三物備急丸
(San-Wu-Pei-Chi-Wan)
(Pills of Three Ingredients for Sudden Syncope)

Constituents:

大 黃 Da Huang (Rhubarb)	30 gm.	*Radix et Rhizoma Rhei*
巴 豆 Ba Dou (Croton seed)	30 gm.	*Semen Crotonis*
乾 薑 Gan Jiang (Dry ginger)	30 gm.	*Rhizoma Zingiberis*

Grind the above ingredients into powder. Take 0.3-1.5 gm. each time with luke warm water.

Action:

To purge the stagnation of cold

Indication:

For a person with stagnation of cold in the body in sudden syncope. The symptoms are: acute sharp pain in the abdomen, fullness and distention of the abdomen, face pale, dyspnea, lock-jaw, coma, constipation.

Application:

Food poisoning, intestinal obstruction, lock-jaw.

Contraindication:

For a person of weak or Xu (deficiency) syndrome; for coma caused by summer heat; for an elderly person; for a pregnant woman.

Administer this formula with caution.

Generic Name:

Rhubarb, Ginger and Croton Formula

Sān Zǐ Yǎng Qìng Tāng　三子養親湯
(San-Tzu-Yang-Ching-Tang)
(Decoction of Three Seeds Nursing the Parents)

Constituents:

紫蘇子	Zi Su Zi (Perilla seed)	6-9 gm.	*Fructus Perillae*
白芥子	Bai Jie Zi (Brassica seed)	6-9 gm.	*Semen Sinapis Albae*
萊菔子	Lai Fu Zi (Radish seed)	6-9 gm.	*Semen Raphani*

Action:

1. To descend the upward flow of stomach *Qi* (vital energy)
2. To improve digestion
3. To resolve stagnation of phlegm caused by food

Indication:

For an elderly person with weak spleen and stomach, and stagnation of phlegm due to undigested food. The symptoms are: cough with sputum, hiccup, indigestion, chest distention.

Tongue: with greasy coating
Pulse: slippery

Application:

Chronic bronchitis, pulmonary emphysema

Modification:

1. With constipation or hard formed stool, add:

蜂　蜜　Feng Mi (Honey)

2. With cold sensation, add:

生　薑　Sheng Jiang (Fresh ginger)　　　*Rhizoma Zingiberis Recens*

3. For asthma and cough with profuse sputum, add:

半　夏	Ban Xia (Pinellia)	*Rhizoma Pinelliae*
陳　皮	Chen Pi (Citrus peel)	*Pericarpium Citri Reticulatae*
茯　苓	Fu Ling (Poria)	*Poria*
甘　草	Gan Cao (Licorice)	*Radix Glycyrrhizae*

The name of this formula is called Er Chen Tang （二陳湯）

or add:

麻　黃	Ma Huang (Ephedra)	*Herba Ephedrae*
杏　仁	Xing Ren (Apricot seed)	*Semen Armeniacae Amarum*
甘　草	Gan Cao (Licorice)	*Radix Glycyrrhizae*

The name of this formula is called San Niu Tang （三拗湯）

Sāng Jú Yīn　桑菊飲
(Sang-Chu-Yin)
(Decoction of Morus Leaf and Chrysanthemum)

Constituents:

桑 葉	Sang Ye (Morus leaf)	6-9 gm.	*Folium Mori*
菊 花	Ju Hua (Chrysanthemum)	3-6 gm.	*Flos Chrysanthemi*
薄 荷	Bo He (Mentha)	3-6 gm.	*Herba Menthae*
杏 仁	Xing Ren (Apricot seed)	6-9 gm.	*Semen Armeniacae Amarum*
桔 梗	Jie Geng (Platycodon)	6-9 gm.	*Radix Platycodi*
連 翹	Lian Qiao (Forsythia)	6-9 gm.	*Fructus Forsythiae*
蘆 根	Lu Gen (Phragmites)	6-9 gm.	*Rhizoma Phragmitis*
甘 草	Gan Cao (Licorice)	3-6 gm.	*Radix Glycyrrhizae*

Action:

1. Diaphoretic
2. To dispel wind and heat
3. Antitussive

Indication:

For a person with common cold due to exterior affection of wind and heat (initial stage). The symptoms are: cough, fever, with slight thirst.

Tongue: with thin white coating
Pulse: floating and rapid

Application:

Common cold, influenza, acute bronchitis, acute tonsillitis, epidemic conjunctivitis.

Modification:

1. With cough and profuse sputum, add:

瓜蔞皮	Gua Lou Pi (Trichosanthes peel)	*Pericarpium Trichosanthis*
浙貝母	Zhe Bei Mu (Thunberg fritillary bulb)	*Bulbus Fritillariae Thunbergii*

2. With bloody sputum, add:

白茅根	Bai Mao Gen (Imperata)	*Rhizoma Imperatae*
藕 節	*Ou Jie (Lotus node)*	*Nodus Nelumbinis Rhizomatis*

3. For conjunctivitis, add:

草決明	Cao Jue Ming (Cassia)	*Semen Cassiae Torae*
夏枯草	Xia Ku Cao (Prunella spike)	*Spica Prunellae*

Generic Name:

Sang Chu Yin Pien;
Morus and Chrysanthemum Combination

Sāng Piāo Xiāo Sàn　桑螵蛸散

(Sang-Piao-Hsiao-San)
(Manthis Egg-case Powder)

Constituents:

桑螵蛸	Sang Piao Xiao (Manthis egg-case)	9-12 gm.	*Ootheca Mantidis*
龍骨	Long Gu (Dragon bone)	10-20 gm.	*Os Draconis*
人參	Ren Shen (Ginseng)	6-9 gm.	*Radix Ginseng*
茯神	Fu Shen (Poria)	6-9 gm.	*Poria*
石菖蒲	Shi Chang Pu (Acorus)	6-9 gm.	*Rhizoma Acori Graminei*
遠志	Yuan Zhi (Polygala)	3-6 gm.	*Radix Polygalae*
當歸	Dang Gui (Chinese angelica)	6-9 gm.	*Radix Angelicae Sinensis*
龜板	Gui Ban (Tortoise plastron)	10-15 gm.	*Plastrum Testudinis*

Action:

1. To regulate the heart and kidney
2. To consolidate the essence of life

Indication:

For a person with both heart and kidney asthenia. The symptoms are: frequent urination or enuresis, involuntary seminal discharge, absentmindedness, forgetfulness.

Tongue: light red with white coating
Pulse: deep and weak

Application:

Enuresis, spermatorrhea, diabetes mellitus, neurasthenia.

Contraindication:

For a person with frequent urination with burning sensation, urine color amber, which is due to excess fire in the lower burner.

Modification:

1. For spermatorrhea, add:
山茱萸　Shan Zhu Yu (Cornus fruit)　　*Fructus Corni*
沙苑蒺藜　Sha Yuan Ji Li (Chinese milk vetch)　*Semen Astragali*
2. For enuresis, add:
覆盆子　Fu Pen Zi (Raspberry fruit)　　*Fructus Rubi*
益智仁　Yi Zhi Ren (Black cardamon seed)　*Fructus Alpiniae*
3. For neurasthenia with insomnia, forgetfulness and palpitation, add:
五味子　Wu Wei Zi (Schisandra fruit)　　*Fructus Schisandrae*
酸棗仁　Suan Zao Ren (Wild jujube seed)　*Semen Ziziphi Spinosae*

Generic Name:

Manthis Formula

Sāng Xìng Tāng 桑杏湯

(San-Hsing-Tang)
(Decoction of Morus and Apricot Seed)

Constituents:

桑 葉	Sang Ye (Mulberry leaf)	6-9 gm.	*Folium Mori*
杏 仁	Xing Ren (Apricot seed)	6-9 gm.	*Semen Armeniacae Amarum*
淡豆豉	Dan Dou Chi (Prepared soybean)	6-9 gm.	*Semen Sojae Praepartatum*
北沙參	Bei Sha Shen (Glehnia root)	9-12 gm.	*Radix Glehniae*
梨 皮	Li Pi (Pear peel)	3-6 gm.	*Fructus Pyri*
梔 子	Zhi Zi (Gardenia fruit)	6-9 gm.	*Fructus Gardeniae*
浙貝母	Zhe Bei Mu (Thunberg fritillary bulb)	3-6 gm.	*Bulbus Fritillarieae Thunbergii*

Action:

1. Disperse wind and external heat and dryness
2. To moisten the lung

Indication:

For a person with cough caused by external wind, heat and dryness. The symptoms are: fever, headache, dry throat with thirst, dry cough with or without sputum.

Tongue: red with thin white coating, but dry
Pulse: Floating and rapid

Application:

Flu with dry cough, upper respiratory tract infection, measles.

Contraindication:

For a person with cough caused by wind and cold.

Modification:

1. If throat is dry and painful, add:
牛蒡子 Niu Bang Zi (Arctium fruit)   *Fructus Arctii*
2. With nose bleeding, add:
白茅根 Bai Mao Gen (Imperata rhizome)   *Rhizoma Imperatae*
3. Cough with yellow and thick sputum, add:
馬兜鈴 Ma Dou Ling (Aristolochia)   *Fructus Aristolochiae*
瓜蔞皮 Gua Lou Pi (Trichosanthes peel)   *Pericarpium Trichosanthis*
4. Last stage of measles, fever with thirst, dry skin, dry throat & nose, and cough with no sputum, add:
蘆 根 Lu Gen (Phragmites rhizome)   *Rhizoma Phragmitis*
天花粉 Tian Hua Fen (Trichosanthes root)   *Radix Trichosanthis*

Shā Shēn Mài Mén Dōng Tāng　　沙參麥門冬湯
(Sha-Sheng-Mai-Men-Tung-Tang)
(Decoction of Glehnia/Adenophora and Ophiopogon)

Constituents:

沙 參	Sha Shen (Adenophora root)	6-9 gm.	*Radix Adenophorae*
麥門冬	Mai Men Dong (Ophiopogon)	6-9 gm.	*Radix Ophiopogonis*
玉 竹	Yu Zhu (Polygonatum rhizome)	6-9 gm.	*Rhizoma Polygonati Odorati*
天花粉	Tian Hua Fen (Trichosanthes root)	9-12 gm.	*Radix Trichosanthis*
扁 豆	Bian Dou (Dolichos seed)	10-15 gm.	*Semen Dolichi*
桑 葉	Sang Ye (Mulberry leaf)	6-9 gm.	*Folium Mori*
甘 草	Gan Cao (Licorice)	3-6 gm.	*Radix Glycyrrhizae*

Action:

To nourish the lung and stomach and promote the secretion of body fluids.

Indication:

For a person with deficient body fluids in the lung and stomach due to dryness. The symptoms are: dry throat, thirst, dry cough with little or no sputum.

> Tongue: red
> Pulse: weak and rapid

Application:

Cough, bronchitis.

Generic Name:

Adenophora and Ophiopogon Combination

Shāo Fù Zhú Yū Tāng　少腹逐瘀湯
(Shao-Fu-Chu-Yu-Tang)
(Decoction for Removing Blood Stasis in the Lateral Abdomen)

Constituents:

當　歸	Dang Gui (Chinese angelica)	6-9 gm.	*Radix Angelicae Sinensis*
川　芎	Chuan Xiong (Ligusticum)	3-6 gm.	*Rhizoma Ligustici Chuanxiong*
赤芍藥	Chi Shao Yao (Red peony)	6-9 gm.	*Radix Paeoniae Rubra*
小茴香	Xiao Hui Xiang (Fennel)	3-6 gm.	*Fructus Foeniculi*
延胡索	Yan Hu Suo (Corydalis)	3-6 gm.	*Rhizoma Corydalis*
五靈脂	Wu Ling Zhi (Trogopterus dung)	3-6 gm.	*Faeces Trogopterorum*
沒　藥	Mo Yao (Myrrh)	3-6 gm.	*Resina Myrrhae*
肉　桂	Rou Gui (Cinnamon bark)	3-6 gm.	*Cortex Cinnamomi*
乾　薑	Gan Jiang (Dry ginger)	3-6 gm.	*Rhizoma Zingiberis*
蒲　黃	Pu Huang (Bulrush pollen)	6-9 gm.	*Pollen Typhae*

Action:

1. To invigorate blood circulation and remove stasis
2. To relieve pain by warming the channels

Indication:

For a person with blood stasis in the lateral abdomen. The symptoms are: abdominal pain with no lumps, or with lumps but no pain, abdominal distention, irregular menstruation, lumbago during menstruation, blood color purplish black and with clots, or uterine bleeding with abdominal pain.

Application:

Dysmenorrhea, amenorrhea, irregular menstruation, uterine bleeding.

Modification:

1. Chronic abdominal pain (continuous and mild), add:

黨　參	Dang Shen (Codonopsis)	*Radix Codonopsis Pilosulae*
阿　膠	E Jiao (Donkey-hide gelatin)	*Colla Corii Asini*

2. Abdominal pain during menstruation, refused to be pressed, increased blood volume, use fresh ginger instead of dry ginger, and add:

熟地黃	Shu Di Huang (Prep. rehmannia)	*Radix Rehmanniae Praeparatae*
肉　桂	Rou Gui (Cinnamon bark)	*Cortex Cinnamomi*

3. With severe pain during menstruation, add:

木　香	Mu Xiang (Saussurea root)	*Radix Saussureae*
白芍藥	Bai Shao Yao (White peony)	*Radix Paeoniae Alba*

Sháo Yào Tāng   芍藥湯

(Shao-Yao-Tang)
(Decoction of Paeonia)

Constituents:

白芍藥	Bai Shao (White peony)	10-15 gm.	*Radix Paeoniae Alba*
黃 連	Huang Lian (Coptis)	6-9 gm.	*Rhizoma Coptidis*
黃 芩	Huang Qin (Scutellaria)	6-9 gm.	*Radix Scutellariae*
大 黃	Da Huang (Rhubarb)	6-9 gm.	*Radix et Rhizoma Rhei*
當 歸	Dang Gui (Chinese angelica)	6-9 gm.	*Radix Angelicae Sinensis*
肉 桂	Rou Gui (Cinnamon bark)	3-6 gm.	*Cortex Cinnamomi*
木 香	Mu Xiang (Saussurea)	3-6 gm.	*Radix Saussureae*
檳 榔	Bing Lang (Areca)	3-6 gm.	*Semen Arecae*
甘 草	Gan Cao (Licorice)	3-6 gm.	*Radix Glycyrrhizae*

Action:

1. To eliminate heat and toxin
2. To relieve pain by regulating the circulation of *Qi* and blood.

Indication:

For a person with inflammation of the intestines caused by heat, dampness or bacterial toxin. The symptoms are: abdominal pain, bloody stool with red and white mucous, tenesmus, burning sensation of the anus, urination short and dark in color, diarrhea.

Tongue: with thick yellow and greasy coat
Pulse: superficial

Contraindication:

For a person with flu or exterior syndrome.

Application:

Bacterial dysentery, amoebic dysentery, allergic colitis, acute enteritis.

Modification:

1. If the tongue is dry and yellow, with depletion of fluid, subtract:
肉 桂 Rou Gui (cinnamon bark)   *Cortex Cinnamomi*
2, If the stool color is dark purple, with increased heat and toxin, add:
黃 柏 Huang Bai (Phellodendron)   *Cortex Phellodendri*
3. With indigestion, caused by stagnation of food, add:
山 楂 Shan Zha (Crataegus fruit)   *Fructus Crataegi*

Generic Name:

Peony Combination

Shé Chuáng Zǐ Chōng Xǐ Jì　蛇床子沖洗劑

(She-Chuang-Chi-Chung-Hsi-Chi)
(Decoction of Cnidium Fruit for Vaginitis)

Constituents:

蛇床子	She Chuang Zi (Cinidium fruit)	20-30 gm.	*Fructus Cnidii*
苦 参	Ku Shen (Sophora root)	6-9 gm.	*Radix Sophorae Flavescentis*
川楝子	Chuan Lian Zi (Sichuan chinaberry)	3-6 gm.	*Frcutus Meliae Toosendan*
黄 柏	Huang Bai (Phellodendron)	6-9 gm.	*Cortex Phellodendri*
枸杞梗	Gou Qi Gen (Lycium root)	12-15 gm.	*Radix Lycii*
枯 礬	Ku Fan (Alum)	12-15 gm.	*Alumen*

Action:

1. To eliminate dampness
2. Parasiticide

Indication:

For a person with trichomonas vaginalis, with symptoms of foul vaginal
discharges.

Application:

Trichomonas vaginalis.

Comment:

The formula is used for external wash only. Perform twice daily.

Shè Gān Má Huáng Tāng   射干麻黄湯

(She-Kan-Ma-Huang-Tang)
(Decoction of Belamcanda and Ephedra)

Constituents:

射 干	She Gan (Belamcanda)	6-9 gm.	*Rhizoma Belamcandae*
麻 黄	Ma Huang (Ephedra)	6-9 gm.	*Herba Ephedrae*
細 辛	Xi Xin (Asarum)	3-6 gm.	*Herba Asari*
紫 菀	Zi Wan (Aster root)	6-9 gm.	*Radix Asteris*
款冬花	Kuan Dong Hua (Tussilago)	6-9 gm.	*Flos Farfarae*
半 夏	Ban Xia (Pinellia)	6-9 gm.	*Rhizoma Pinelliae*
五味子	Wu Wei Zi (Schisandra)	6-9 gm.	*Fructus Schisandrae*
生 薑	Sheng Jiang (Fresh ginger)	3-6 gm.	*Rhizoma Zingiberis Recens*
大 棗	Da Zao (Jujube)	3-5 pc.	*Fructus Ziziphus Jujubae*

Action:

1. To warm the lung and dispel cold
2. Antitussive, expectorant, anti-asthmatic

Indication:

For a person with cough and asthma due to cold. The symptoms are: cough, dyspnea, wheezing, sputum clear and scanty, color white and frothy, stuffiness sensation in the chest and epigastric region, face color pale or cyanotic, no thirst, or feel thirsty but like to drink hot water, aversion to cold, headache, body-ache.

Tongue: with white and slippery coating
Pulse: wiry and slippery, or floating and tight

Application:

Cough, asthma, asthmatic bronchitis, pulmonary emphysema.

Shēn Fù Tāng 參附湯

(Sheng-Fu-Tang)
(Decoction of Ginseng and Aconite)

Constituents:

人 參 Ren Shen (Ginseng)	12-15 gm.	*Radix Ginseng*
炮附子 Pao Fu Zi (Baked aconite)	9-12 gm.	*Radix Aconiti Praeparatae*

Action:

1. To restore the *Yang* (vital function) from collapse and shock with cold limbs
2. To replenish the *Qi* (vital energy).

Indication:

1. For depletion of *Yang* (vital function) and *Qi* (vital energy), with symptoms of cold hands and feet, perspiration, weakness in breathing, intolerance of cold, pulse fainting.

2. For deficiency in the vital energy of the *Yang* channels with coldness. The symptoms are: cold hands and feet, spontaneous perspiration, intolerance of cold, abdominal pain and cold, loose stools, upset stomach.

Application:

Prostration, cardiac failure, post-surgical bleeding, uterine bleeding.

Comment:

In this prescription, the ginseng cannot be replaced by:

黨 參 Dang Shen (Codonopsis)	*Radix Codonopsis Pilosulae*
西洋參 Xi Yang Shen (American ginseng)	*Radix Panax Americana*

Shēn Jiè Sàn 參蚧散

(Sheng-Chieh-San)
(Powder of Ginseng and Gecko)

Constituents:

人 參	Ren Shen (Ginseng)	9 gm.	*Radix Ginseng*
蛤 蚧	Ge Jie (Gecko)	1 pair	*Gecko*

Grind the above ingredients into powder. Take 1-1.5 gm. each time, 2 to 3 times daily.

Action:

1. To reinforce the lung and kidney
2. Antitussive and anti-asthmatic

Indication:

For a person with chronic cough due to asthenia of both lung and kidney. The symptoms are: cough with asthma, dyspnea, voice low and weak, fatigue.

> Tongue: pale
> Pulse: slow and weak

Application:

Chronic cough, pulmonary emphysema, pulmonary cardiac diseases.

Shēn Líng Bái Zhú Sàn   參苓白术散
(Sheng-Ling-Pai-Chu-San)
(Powder of Ginseng, Poria and White Atractylodes)

Constituents:

人 參	Ren Shen (Ginseng)	9-12 gm.	*Radix Ginseng*
蓮子肉	Lian Zi Rou (Lotus seed)	15-20 gm.	*Semen Nelumbinis*
山 藥	Shao Yao (Dioscorea)	10-15 gm.	*Rhizoma Dioscoreae*
白 术	Bai Zhu (White atractylodes)	9-12 gm.	*Rhizoma Atractylodis Macrocephalae*
茯 苓	Fu Ling (Poria)	10-15 gm.	*Poria*
白扁豆	Bai Bian Dou (Dolichos)	15-20 gm.	*Semen Dolichi*
薏苡仁	Yi Yi Ren (Coix)	20-30 gm.	*Semen Coicis*
砂 仁	Sha Ren (Cardamon)	3-6 gm.	*Fructus Amomi*
桔 梗	Jie Geng (Platycodon)	6-9 gm.	*Radix Platycodi*
炙甘草	Zhi Gan Cao (Baked licorice)	3-6 gm.	*Radix Glycyrrhizae Praeparatae*

Action:

1. To replenish the *Qi* (vital energy)
2. To reinforce the spleen and stomach
3. To resolve dampness due to spleen deficiency

Indication:

For a person with dampness due to spleen and stomach *Qi* (vital energy) deficiency. The symptoms are: weak muscle strength of the arms and legs, abdominal distention, indigestion, vomiting and diarrhea, face pale.

> Tongue: white and greasy
> Pulse: feeble and moderate

Application:

Chronic gastro-enteritis, edema, anemia, pulmonary tuberculosis, chronic nephritis, infantile diarrhea.

Contraindication:

For a person with Shi (excessive) syndromes.

Modification:

With stagnant flow of Qi, add:
陳 皮 Chen Pi (Citrus peel)   *Pericarpium Citri Reticulatae*

Generic Name:

Shen Ling Baizhu Pien;
Ginseng and Atractylodes Formula

Shēn Sū Yǐn 參蘇飲
(Sheng-Su-Yin)
(Decoction of Ginseng and Perilla Leaf)

Constituents:

人 參	Ren Shen (Ginseng)	3-6 gm.	Radix Ginseng
紫蘇葉	Zi Su Ye (Perilla Leaf)	6-9 gm.	Folium Perillae
陳 皮	Chen Pi (Citrus peel)	3-6 gm.	Pericarpium Citri Reticulatae
葛 根	Ge Gen (Pueraria root)	6-9 gm.	Radix Puerariae
前 胡	Qian Hu (Peucedanum root)	6-9 gm.	Radix Peucedani
半 夏	Ban Xia (Pinellia)	6-9 gm.	Rhizoma Pinelliae
茯 苓	Fu Ling (Poria)	6-9 gm.	Poria
枳 殼	Zhi Ke (Bitter Orange)	6-9 gm.	Fructus Aurantii
桔 梗	Jie Geng (Platycodon)	6-9 gm.	Radix Platycodi
木 香	Mu Xiang (Saussurea)	3-6 gm.	Radix Saussureae
甘 草	Gan Cao (Licorice)	3-6 gm.	Radix Glycyrrhizae

Action:

1. Diaphoretic
2. Expectorant
3. To replenish *Qi* (vital energy)
4. To regulate the activity of the stomach

Indication:

For a person of weak constitution with exterior affection of wind and cold and interior retention of phlegm. The symptoms are: fever, aversion to cold, headache, stuffy nose, cough with profuse sputum, chest fullness.

Tongue: with white coating
Pulse: weak

Application:

Common cold.

Generic Name:

Ginseng and Perilla Combination

Shēn Tòng Zhú Yū Tāng　身痛逐瘀湯
(Shen-Tong-Chu-Yu-Tang)
(Decoction to Relieve Muscle-ache)

Constituents:

桃　仁	Tao Ren (Persica seed)	6-9 gm.	*Semen Persicae*
紅　花	Hong Hua (Carthamus)	6-9 gm.	*Flos Carthami*
當　歸	Dang Gui (Chinese angelica)	6-9 gm.	*Radix Angelicae Sinensis*
川　芎	Chuan Xiong (Ligusticum)	3-6 gm.	*Rhizoma Ligustici Chuanxiong*
羌　活	Qiang Huo (Notopterygium)	3-6 gm.	*Radix Notopterygii*
秦　艽	Qin Jiao (Large leaf gentian)	3-6 gm.	*Radix Gentianae*
地　龍	Di Long (Earthworm)	3-6 gm.	*Lumbricus*
沒　藥	Mo Yao (Myrrh)	3-6 gm.	*Resina Myrrhae*
五靈脂	Wu Ling Zhi (Trogopterus dung)	3-6 gm.	*Faeces Trogopterorum*
香　附	Xiang Fu (Cyperus tuber)	1-3 gm.	*Rhizoma Cyperi*
川牛膝	Chuan Niu Xi (Cyathula)	6-9 gm.	*Radix Cyathulae*
甘　草	Gan Cao (Licorice)	3-6 gm.	*Radix Glycyrrhizae*

Action:

1. To invigorate the circulation of *Qi* (vital energy) and blood, and remove blood stasis in the channels
2. To relieve pain and arthralgia

Indication:

For a person with muscle-ache of the neck, back, legs, shoulder or whole body due to obstruction of the flow of *Qi* and blood in the channels.

> Tongue: with red purplish spots
> Pulse: wiry/taut and hesitant

Application:

Muscle-ache of the whole body, arthralgia, rheumatoid arthritis, lumbago.

Modification:

1. With increased body temperature, add:
蒼　术 Cang Zhu (Atractylodes)　　　*Rhizoma Atractylodis*
黃　柏 Huang Bai (Phellodendron)　　*Cortex Phellodendri*
2. With fatigue and weakness, add:
黃　芪 Huang Qi (Astragalus)　　　　*Radix Astragali*
3. With lumbago, add:
杜　仲 Du Zhong (Eucommia bark)　　*Cortex Eucommiae*
巴戟天 Ba Ji Tian (Morinda root)　　*Radix Morindae Officinalis*

Shēng Huà Tāng 生化湯

(Sheng-Hua-Tang)
(Decoction for Removing Stagnant Blood and Promoting Hemogenesis)

Constituents:

當 歸	Dang Gui (Chinese angelica)	15-20 gm.	*Radix Angelicae Sinensis*
川 芎	Chuan Xiong (Ligusticum)	6-9 gm.	*Rhizoma Ligustici Chuanxiong*
桃 仁	Tao Ren (Persica seed)	6-9 gm.	*Semen Persicae*
炮 薑	Pao Jiang (Stir-baked ginger)	1-3 gm.	*Rhizoma Zingiberis*
炙甘草	Zhi Gan Cao (Baked licorice)	1-3 gm.	*Radix Glycyrrhizae Praeparatae*

Action:

1. To remove stagnant blood and promote hemogenesis
2. To relieve pain by warming the channels and collaterals

Indication:

For a person with retention of lochia, and pain in the lower abdomen after childbirth. The symptoms are: color of blood dark purplish, lower abdomen hard and cold and painful, refused to be pressed.

Tongue: with purple spots
Pulse: deep and hesitant

Application:

Retention of lochia, postpartum care.

Modification:

1. With severe coldness, add:

附 子	Fu Zi (Aconite)	*Radix Aconiti Praeparatae*
肉 桂	Rou Gui (Cinnamon bark)	*Cortex Cinnamomi*

2. With severe abdominal pain, add:

五靈脂	Wu Ling Zhi (Trogopterus dung)	*Faeces Trogopterorum*
蒲 黃	Pu Huang (Bulrush pollen)	*Pollen Typhae*
延胡索	Yan Hu Suo (Corydalis)	*Rhizoma Corydalis*

3. With no symptoms of lochia retention, eliminate:

桃 仁	Tao Ren (Persica seed)	*Semen Persicae*

Generic Name:

Tang-kuei and Ginger Combination

Shēng Jiāng Xiè Xīn Tāng   生薑瀉心湯
(Sheng-Chiang-Hsieh-Hsin-Tang)
(The Stomach Purging Decoction with Fresh Ginger)

Constituents:

半 夏	Ban Xia (Pinellia)	9-12 gm.	*Rhizoma Pinelliae*
黃 連	Huang Lian (Coptis)	3-6 gm.	*Rhizoma Coptidis*
黃 芩	Huang Qin (Scutellaria)	6-9 gm.	*Radix Scutellariae*
生 薑	Sheng Jiang (Fresh ginger)	9-12 gm.	*Rhizoma Zingiberis Recens*
人 參	Ren Shen (Ginseng)	6-9 gm.	*Radix Ginseng*
炙甘草	Zhi Gan Cao (Baked licorice)	3-6 gm.	*Radix Glycyrrhizae Praeparatae*
大 棗	Da Zao (Jujube)	3-5 pc.	*Fructus Ziziphus Jujubae*

Action:

1. To eliminate heat and water accumulation in the stomach
2. To relieve fullness and oppression sensation in the stomach

Indication:

For a person with abdominal fullness and oppression due to accumulation of heat and water in the stomach. The symptoms are: stomach upset, fullness and oppression sensation in the chest and abdomen, retch, percussion of fluid in the hypochondriac region, borborygmus, diarrhea.

Tongue: with thin yellow and greasy coating
Pulse: wiry/taut and rapid

Application:

Acute gastroenteritis

Generic Name:

Pinellia and Ginger Combination

Shēng Má Gé Gēn Tāng   升麻葛根湯
(Sheng-Ma-Ko-Ken-Tang)
(Decoction of Cimicifuga and Pueraria)

Constituents:

升 麻	Sheng Ma (Cimicifuga)	3-6 gm.	*Rhizoma Cimicifugae*
葛 根	Ge Gen (Pueraria root)	9-12 gm.	*Radix Puerariae*
赤芍藥	Chi Shao Yao (Red peony)	6-9 gm.	*Radix Paeoniae Rubra*
炙甘草	Zhi Gan Cao (Baked licorice)	3-6 gm.	*Radix Glycyrrhizae Praeparatae*

Action:

1. To dispel exterior wind and heat factors (Diaphoretic)
2. To promote the eruption of measles

Indication:

For a person with measles. The symptoms are: fever, intolerance of wind, headache, cough, blood-shot eyes, thirst.

        Tongue: red with dry coating
        Pulse: floating and rapid

Application:

Measles, influenza.

Modification:

1. To promote the eruption of measles, add:

薄 荷	Bo He (Mentha)	*Herba Menthae*
牛蒡子	Niu Bang Zi (Arctium)	*Fructus Arctii*
蟬 蛻	Chan Tui (Ciccada slough)	*Periostracum Cicadae*
金銀花	Jin Yin Hua (Lonicera flower)	*Flos Lonicerae*
荊 芥	Jing Jie (Schizonepeta)	*Herba Schizonepetae*

2. With painful and swollen throat, add:

桔 梗	Jie Geng (Platycodon)	*Radix Platycodi*
馬 勃	Ma Bo (Lasiophaera)	*Fructificatio Lasiosphaerae*
玄 參	Xuan Shen (Scrophularia)	*Radix Scrophulariae*

Generic Name:

Cimicifuga and Pueraria Combination

Shēng Mài Sàn 生脈散

(Sheng-Mai-San)
(Powder to Activate the Vascular System)

Constituents:

人 參	Ren Shen (Ginseng)	6-9 gm.	*Radix Ginseng*
麥門冬	Mai Men Dong (Ophiopogon)	6-9 gm.	*Radix Ophiopogonis*
五味子	Wu Wei Zi (Schizandra)	6-9 gm.	*Fructus Schizandrae*

Action:

1. To replenish the *Qi* (vital energy) and *Yin* (vital essence)
2. To promote the secretion of body fluids
3. Anhidrotic

Indication:

1. For a person with deficiency of *Qi* (vital energy) and *Yin* (vital essence) due to extreme summer heat. The symptoms are: fatigue, shortness of breath, thirst, profuse perspiration.

> Tongue: red with dry coating
> Pulse: feeble and weak

2. For a person with lung asthenia and chronic cough, thin sputum, shortness of breath, spontaneous perspiration, dry mouth.

> Tongue: dry
> Pulse: feeble and weak

Application:

Chronic cough, pulmonary tuberculosis, neurasthenia, coronary heart disease, angina pectoris, arrhythmia, chronic bronchitis, thermoplegia, cor pulmonale, cardiac failure, myocardial infarction, summer stroke.

Contraindication:

For a person with flu in the summer (initial stage) or mild cough.

Shí Huī Sàn 　　十灰散

(Shih-Hui-San)
(Powder of Ten Ingredients in Ash)

Constituents:

大 薊	Da Ji (Japanese thistle)	10 gm.	Radix Cirsii Japonici
小 薊	Xiao Ji (Small thistle)	10 gm.	Herba Cephalanoploris
荷 葉	He Ye (Lotus leaf)	10 gm.	Folium Nelumbinis
茜草根	Xi Cao Gen (Madder root)	10 gm.	Radix Rubiae
側柏葉	Ce Bai Ye (Biota tops)	10 gm.	Cacumen Biotae
白茅根	Bai Mao Gen (Imperata rhizome)	10 gm.	Rhizoma Imperatae
棕櫚皮	Zong Lu Pi (Trachycarpus stipule fiber)	10 gm.	Fibra Stipulae Trachycarpi
梔 子	Zhi Zi (Gardenia fruit)	10 gm.	Fructus Gardeniae
大 黄	Da Huang (Rhubarb)	10 gm.	Radix et Rhizoma Rhei
牡丹皮	Mu Dan Pi (Moutan bark)	10 gm.	Cortex Moutan Radicis

Burn the above ingredients into ashes. Mix with fresh lotus node or white turnip juice with ink, and make into pills. The above 10 ingredients can also be used in decoction.

Action:

1. Astringent and hemostatic
2. To eliminate heat in the blood by cooling method.

Indication:

For all kinds of bleeding due to excessive fire in the liver and stomach, e.g. epistaxis, hemoptysis, hematemesis, spitting and coughing with blood.

Application:

Epistaxis, hemoptysis, hematemesis, spitting and coughing with blood.

Shí Pí Sàn   實脾散
(Shi-Pi-San)
(Spleen Tonic for Edema)

Constituents:

附 子	Fu Zi (Aconite)	6-9 gm.	*Radix Aconiti Praeparatae*
乾 薑	Gan Jiang (Dry ginger)	6-9 gm.	*Rhizoma Zingiberis*
厚 朴	Hou Po (Magnolia)	6-9 gm.	*Cortex Magnoliae Officinalis*
木 香	Mu Xiang (Saussurea)	6-9 gm.	*Radix Saussureae*
大腹皮	Da Fu Pi (Areca peel)	6-9 gm.	*Pericarpium Arecae*
草 果	Cao Guo (Tsaoko)	6-9 gm.	*Fructus Tsaoko*
白 术	Bai Zhu (White atractylodes)	6-9 gm.	*Rz. Atractylodis Macrocephalae*
茯 苓	Fu Ling (Poria)	6-9 gm.	*Poria*
木 瓜	Mu Gua (Chaenomeles)	6-9 gm.	*Fructus Chaenomelis*
炙甘草	Zhi Gan Cao (Baked licorice)	3 gm.	*Radix Glycyrrhizae Praeparatae*
生 薑	Sheng Jiang (Fresh ginger)	5 pc.	*Rhizoma Zingiberis Recens*
大 棗	Da Zao (Jujube)	1 pc.	*Fructus Ziziphus Jujubae*

Action:

To strengthen the spleen and activate the *Yang Qi* by warming and eliminating water (Diuretic by warming)

Indication:

For a person with edema and deficiency of Spleen *Yang*. The symptoms are: edema in the lower part of the body with heavy sensation, distention in the chest and abdomen, cold hands and feet, no thirst, urination scanty, stools loose.

> Tongue: pale with greasy coat
> Pulse: deep, and slow or thready

Application:

Chronic nephritis, edema caused by cardiac failure.

Modification:

If urination is scanty, add:

澤 瀉	Ze Xie (Alisma)	*Rhizoma Alismatis*
豬 苓	Zhu Ling (Polyporus)	*Polyporus Umbellatus*

Shí Quán Dà Bǔ Tāng　　十全大補湯

(Shih-Chuan-Ta-Pu-Tang)
(The Tonification Decoction with Ten Ingredients)

Constituents:

黄 芪	Huang Qi (Astragalus)	6-9 gm.	Radix Astragali
肉 桂	Rou Gui (Cinnamon bark)	3-6 gm.	Cortex Cinnamomi
人 参	Ren Shen (Ginseng)	6-9 gm.	Radix Panax Ginseng
熟地黄	Shu Di Huang (Prep. rehmannia)	9-12 gm.	Radix Rehmanniae Praeparatae
白 术	Bai Zhu (White atractylodes)	9-12 gm.	Rhizoma Atractylodis Macrocephalae
當 歸	Dang Gui (Chinese angelica)	9-12 gm.	Radix Angelicae Sinensis
白芍藥	Bai Shao Yao (White peony)	6-9 gm.	Radix Paeoniae Alba
川 芎	Chuan Xiong (Ligusticum)	3-6 gm.	Rhizoma Ligustici Chuanxiong
茯 苓	Fu Ling (Poria)	6-9 gm.	Poria
炙甘草	Zhi Gan Cao (Baked licorice)	3-6 gm.	Radix Glycyrrhizae Praeparatae

The following 2 ingredients may be added:

生 薑	Sheng Jiang (Fresh ginger)	1-3 gm.	Rhizoma Zingiberis Recens
大 棗	Da Zao (Jujube)	3-5 pc.	Fructus Ziziphus Jujubae

Action:

1. To replenish *Yang* (Vital function)
2. To replenish *Qi* (vital energy) and blood

Indication:

For a person with deficiency of *Qi* (vital energy), blood, *Yang* (vital function) with cold sensation. The symptoms are; cold hands and feet, face pale or sallow, dizziness, general fatigue, shortness of breath, palpitation, loss of appetite, anemia.

Tongue: pale with thin white coating
Pulse: thready and weak

Application:

Cardiac failure, anemia, uterine bleeding, chronic abscess, postpartum care.

Generic Name:

Ten Flavor Tea;
Ginseng and Tang-kuei Ten Combination

Shí Wěi Sàn　　石葦散

(Shih-Wei-San)
(Powder of Pyrrosia Leaf)

Constituents:

石 葦	Shi Wei (Pyrrosia leaf)	6-9 gm.	*Folium Pyrrosiae*
木 通	Mu Tong (Akebia)	3-6 gm.	*Caulis Akebiae*
車前子	Che Qian Zi (Plantago seed)	6-9 gm.	*Semen Plantaginis*
瞿 麥	Qu Mai (Dianthus; Pink)	3-6 gm.	*Herba Dianthi*
冬葵子	Dong Kui Zi (Abutilon seed)	3-6 gm.	*Semen Abutili*
滑 石	Hua Shi (Talc)	6-9 gm.	*Talcum*
甘 草	Gan Cao (Licorice)	1-3 gm.	*Radix Glycyrrhizae*

Action:

1. Diuretic
2. To eliminate stone in the urinary tract

Indication:

For a person with stones in the urinary tract. The symptoms are: urination with burning pain, urine color yellowish amber and turbid, with small stones, sudden discontinuation of urination, subtle pain in the lower abdomen and lower back.

　　Tongue: with greasy coating
　　Pulse: wiry/taut or rapid

Application:

Urolithiasis, cystitis, urethritis, gallstone, acute nephritis, calculi of all kinds.

Contraindication:

1. For urolithiasis, add:

金錢草 Jin Qian Cao (Lysimachia)	*Herba Lysimachiae*
海金沙 Hai Jin Sha (Lygodium spores)	*Spora Lygodii*
雞內金 Ji Nei Jin (Chicken's gizzard skin)	*Endothelium Corneum Gigeriae*

2. For hematuria, add:

小 薊 Xiao Ji (Small thistle)	*Herba Cephalanoploris*
蒲 黃 Pu Huang (Bulrush pollen)	*Pollen Typhae*
牡丹皮 Mu Dan Pi (Moutan bark)	*Cortex Moutan Radicis*

Shī Xiào Sàn　　失笑散
(Shih-Hsiao-San)
(Losing the Smile Powder)

Constituents:

五靈脂 Wu Ling Zhi (Pteropus excrement)　　10-15 gm.　　*Faeces Trogopterorum*
蒲　黃 Pu Huang (Bulrush pollen)　　10-15 gm.　　*Pollen Typhae*

Grind the above ingredients into powder. Take 6 gm. each time with rice wine or vinegar.

Action:

1. To invigorate the blood circulation and remove stasis
2. To disperse lumps or hardening
3. To relieve pain

Indication:

For a person with blood stasis in the body. The symptoms are: irregular menstruation, lower abdominal pain, dysmenorrhea, retention of lochia.

Tongue: dark red with purple spots
Pulse: hesitant or wiry/taut and tight

Application:

Retention of lochia, dysmenorrhea, angina pectoris, amenorrhea.

Modification:

1. With stagnation of vital energy, add:
川楝子 Chuan Lian Zi (Sichuan chinaberry)　　*Fructus Meliae Toosendan*
香　附 Xiang Fu (Cyperus tuber)　　*Rhizoma Cyperi*
2. With cold sensation, add:
當　歸 Dang Gui (Chinese angelica)　　*Radix Angelicae Sinensis*
艾　葉 Ai Ye (Artemisia)　　*Folium Artemisia Argyi*
3. With pain in the chest and abdomen after child-birth, add:
山　楂 Shan Zha (Crataegus fruit)　　*Fructus Crataegi*

Generic Name:

Pteropus and Bulrush Formula

Shī Xiào Wán (Zhī Shí Xiāo Pǐ Wán) 失笑丸 (枳實消痞丸)
(Shih-Hsiao-Wan) (Chi-Chih-Hsiao-Pi-Wan)
(Losing the Smile Pills) or
(Pills with Immature Bitter Orange for Abdominal Distention)

Constituents:

枳 實	Zhi Shi (Immature bitter orange)	12-15 gm.	*Fructus Aurantii Immaturus*
厚 朴	Hou Po (Magnolia bark)	9-12 gm.	*Cortex Magnoliae Officinalis*
人 參	Ren Shen (Ginseng)	6-9 gm.	*Radix Ginseng*
白 术	Bai Zhu (White atractylodes)	6-9 gm.	*Rhizoma Atractylodis Macrocephalae*
茯 苓	Fu Ling (Poria)	6-9 gm.	*Poria*
黄 連	Huang Lian (Coptis)	12-15 gm.	*Rhizoma Coptidis*
麥 芽	Mai Ya (Malt)	6-9 gm.	*Fructus Hordei Germinatus*
神 曲	Shen Qu (Medicated leaven)	9-12 gm.	*Massa Fermentata Medicinalis*
炙甘草	Zhi Gan Cao (Baked licorice)	3-6 gm.	*Radix Glycyrrhizae Praeparatae*
生 薑	Sheng Jiang (Fresh ginger)	3-6 gm.	*Rhizoma Zingiberis Recens*

Grind the above ingredients into powder and made into pills.
Take 6-9 gm. each time with luke warm water.

Action:

1. To eliminate fullness and oppression of the abdomen
2. To strengthen the spleen and stomach

Indication:

For a person with oppression or distention of the abdomen due to
deficiency or asthenia of spleen and stomach. The symptoms are: loss of
appetite, fatigue, indigestion, constipation, fullness and oppression in the
epigastric region and chest, abdominal distention.

> Tongue: with white and thick coating
> Pulse: wiry/taut

Application:

Chronic gastritis, gastric ulcer, indigestion, chronic cholecystitis.

Shí Zăo Tāng   十棗湯
(Shih-Tsao-Tang)
(Decoction of Ten Jujubes)

Constituents:

大戟 Da Ji (Euphorbia)	20 gm.	*Radix Euphorbiae*
芫花 Yuan Hua (Genkwa)	20 gm.	*Flos Genkwa*
甘遂 Gan Sui (Kansui)	20 gm.	*Radix Euphorbiae Kansui*
大棗 Da Zao (Jujube)	20 gm.	*Fructus Ziziphus Jujubae*

Action:

To dispel the stagnanation of water in the channels and bowels and visceras (Cathartic)

Indication:

For a person with edema or accumulation of water in the chest, hypochondrium or other bowels or visceras. The symptoms are: fluid in the hypochondrium, pain in the chest and hypochondria on coughing, fullness in the epigastric region, dry vomiting, shortness of breath, headache, dizziness.

Tongue: with white coating
Pulse: wiry/taut and deep

Application:

Edema, ascites, pleurisy with effusion, liver cirrhosis, chronic nephritis.

Contraindication:

For a person of weak constitution or a pregnant woman.

Generic Name:

Jujube Combination

Shū Chī Yǐn Zǐ　　疏齒飲子

(Shu-Chih-Yin-Chi)
(Formula for Edema by Irrigation)

Constituents:

商　陸	Shang Lu (Pokeberry root)	6-9 gm.	*Radix Phytolaccae*
茯苓皮	Fu Ling Pi (Poria peel)	20-30 gm.	*Poria*
澤　瀉	Ze Xie (Alisma)	9-12 gm.	*Rhizoma Alismatis*
木　通	Mu Tong (Akebia)	9-12 gm.	*Caulis Akebiae*
赤小豆	Chi Xiao Dou (Adsuki bean)	12-15 gm.	*Semen Phaseoli*
椒　目	Jiao Mu (Zanthoxylum)	6-9 gm.	*Pericarpium Zanthoxyli*
檳　榔	Bing Lang (Areca seed)	6-9 gm.	*Semen Arecae*
大腹皮	Da Fu Pi (Areca peel)	12-15 gm.	*Pericarpium Arecae*
羌　活	Qiang Huo (Notopterygium)	6-9 gm.	*Radix Notopterygii*
秦　艽	Qin Jiao (Gentian root)	6-9 gm.	*Radix Gentianae*
生　薑	Sheng Jiang (Fresh ginger)	3-6 gm.	*Rz. Zingiberis Recens*

Action:

To eliminate edema with purgative and diuretic effect.

Indication:

For a person with edema with shi (excess) syndromes and exterior affection of wind and dampness. The symptoms are: edema all over the body, skin color with bright texture, abdominal fullness, with irritable heat and thirst sensation, urination scanty and with amber color, stools dry.

> Tongue: with yellow and greasy coat
> Pulse: deep and rapid

Application:

Edema (cardiac or nephritic), cor pulmonale, pericarditis, pleuritis.

Shū Gān Wán　　舒肝丸

(Shu-Kan-Wan)
(Liver-soothing Pills)

Constituents:

柴　胡	Chai Hu (Bupleurum)	6-9 gm.	*Radix Bupleuri*
延胡索	Yan Hu Suo (Corydalis)	3-6 gm.	*Rhizoma Corydalis*
白芍藥	Bai Shao Yao (White peony)	6-9 gm.	*Radix Paeoniae Alba*
茯　苓	Fu Ling (Poria)	6-9 gm.	*Poria*
薑　黃	Jiang Huang (Tumeric)	3-6 gm.	*Rhizoma Curcumae Longae*
厚　朴	Hou Po (Magnolia bark)	6-9 gm.	*Cortex Magnoliae Officinalis*
陳　皮	Chen Pi (Citrus peel)	3-6 gm.	*Pericarpium Citri Reticulatae*
枳　殼	Zhi Ke (Bitter orange)	6-9 gm.	*Fructus Aurantii*
沉　香	Chen Xiang (Saussurea)	3-6 gm.	*Lignum Aquilariae Resinatum*
木　香	Mu Xiang (Saussurea)	3-6 gm.	*Radix Saussureae*
川楝子	Chuan Lian Zi (Sichuan chinaberry)	3-6 gm.	*Fructus Meliae Toosendan*
豆蔻仁	Dou Kou Ren (Cluster)	3-6 gm.	*Amomum Cardamomum*
砂　仁	Sha Ren (Cardamon)	3-6 gm.	*Fructus Amomi*

Action:

1. To soothe the liver and regulate the stomach
2. To circulate the flow of liver *Qi*
3. To relieve pain

Indication:

For a person with pain in the costal and epigastric region due to stagnation of *Qi* (vital energy) in the liver and stomach. The symptoms are: depression, pain and fullness over the costal and epigastric region, eructation, indigestion, acid regurgitation, loss of appetite.

> Tongue: with white or yellow greasy coating
> Pulse: wiry/taut

Application:

Hypochondriac pain, hepatitis, irregular menstruation, acid regurgitation.

Generic Name:

Shu Kan Wan

Shū Jīng Huó Xuè Tāng   舒經活血湯
(Shu-Ching-Huo-Hsieh-Tang)
(Decoction for Removing Blood Stasis in the Channels)

Constituents:

當 歸	Dang Gui (Chinese angelica)	6-9 gm.	*Radix Angelicae Sinenss*
川 芎	Chuan Xiong (Ligusticum)	6-9 gm.	*Rhizoma Ligustici Chuanxiong*
地 黃	Di Huang (Rehmannia)	9-12 gm.	*Radix Rehmanniae*
芍 藥	Shao Yao (Paeonia root)	6-9 gm.	*Radix Paeoniae*
桃 仁	Tao Ren (Persica seed)	9-12 gm.	*Semen Persicae*
茯 苓	Fu Ling (Poria)	6-9 gm.	*Poria*
蒼 术	Cang Zhu (Atractylodes)	6-9 gm.	*Rhizoma Atractylodis*
羌 活	Qiang Huo (Notopterygium)	6-9 gm.	*Radix Notopterygii*
白 芷	Bai Zhi (Angelica root)	6-9 gm.	*Radix Angelicae Dahuricae*
陳 皮	Chen Pi (Citrus peel)	3-6 gm.	*Pericarpium Citri Reticulatae*
威靈仙	Wei Ling Xian (Clematis)	6-9 gm.	*Radix Clematidis*
防 己	Fang Ji (Stephania)	6-9 gm.	*Radix Stephaniae Tetrandrae*
防 風	Fang Feng (Ledebouriella)	6-9 gm.	*Radix Ledebouriellae*
龍膽草	Long Dan Cao (Gentiana)	6-9 gm.	*Radix Gentianae*
懷牛膝	Huai Niu Xi (Achyranthes)	6-9 gm.	*Radix Achyranthis Bidentatae*
生 薑	Sheng Jiang (Fresh Ginger)	3-6 gm.	*Rhizoma Zingiberis Recens*
甘 草	Gan Cao (Licorice)	3-6 gm.	*Radix Glycyrrhizae*

Action:

1. To invigorate the circulation of blood in the channels and strengthen the tendons
2. To dispel wind, cold and dampness (Anti-rheumatic)

Indication:

For a person with pain in the abdomen and lower part of the body (below the waist). The symptoms are: muscle-ache, low back pain, sciatica, abdominal fullness, edema, intolerance of wind and cold.

     Tongue: pale or pink with purple spots
     Pulse: hesistant or tight

Application:

Gout, arthritis, lumbago, sciatica, edema, hemiplegia, purpura, postpartum pain.

Generic Name:

Clematis and Stephania Combination

Sì Jūn Zǐ Tāng　　四君子湯
(Szu-Chun-Tzu-Tang)
(The Four Noble Ingredients Decoction)

Constituents:

人 參	Ren Shen (Ginseng)	6-9 gm.	*Radix Ginseng*
白 朮	Bai Zhu (White atactylodes)	6-9 gm.	*Rhizoma Atractylodis Macrocephalae*
茯 苓	Fu Ling (Poria)	6-9 gm.	*Poria*
甘 草	Gan Cao (Licorice)	3-6 gm.	*Radix Glycyrrhizae*

Action:

1. To replenish the vital energy
2. To tonify and strengthen the spleen and stomach

Indication:

For a person with deficiency of *Qi* (vital energy) of the spleen and stomach, with poor transportation of food nutrients. The symptoms are: face pale, voice soft, muscle weakness in the arms and legs, abdominal distention, loss of appetite, vomiting, borborygmus and diarrhea.

Tongue: light color with thin coating
Pulse: weak

Application:

Chronic gastritis, gastric and duodenal ulcer

Modification:

1. With stagnant flow of *Qi* (vital energy), add:

陳 皮 Chen Pi (Citrus peel)　　　　*Pericarpium Citri Reticulatae*
This is named Yi Kung San (異功散)

2. With damp phlegm, add:

陳 皮 Chen Pi (Citrus peel)　　　　*Pericarpium Citri Reticultae*
半 夏 Ban Xia (Pinellia)　　　　*Rhizoma Pinelliae*
This is named Liu Jun Zi Tang (Six Major Herb Combination)
(六君子湯)

3. With deficiency of both *Qi* and blood, use this formula together with Si Wu Tang (Tang-Kuei Four Combination) (四物湯)

This is now named Ba Zhen Tang (Tang-kuei and Ginseng Eight Combination) (八珍湯)

Generic Name:

Four Major Herb Combination

Sì Miào Yǒng Ān Tāng　　四妙勇安湯

(Shih-Miao-Yung-An-Tang)
(Decoction for Thromboangiitis with Four Effective Ingredients)

Constituents:

金銀花	Jin Yin Hua (Lonicera flower)	20-30 gm.	*Flos Lonicerae*
玄 參	Xuan Shen (Scrophularia)	20-30 gm.	*Radix Scrophulariae*
當 歸	Dang Gui (Chinese angelica)	10-15 gm.	*Radix Angelicae Sinensis*
甘 草	Gan Cao (Licorice)	5-10 gm.	*Radix Glycyrrhizae*

Action:

1. To eliminate heat and toxin
2. To invigorate the blood circulation
3. To replenish the *Yin* (vital essence)

Indication:

For a person with gangrene of the extremities, with manifestations of local inflammation, purulent abscess, thirst, annoying heat.

Tongue: red
Pulse: rapid

Application:

Thromboangiitis

Modification:

1. Thromboangiitis of the upper extremities, add:

桂 枝	Gui Zhi (Cinnamon twig)	*Ramulus Cinnamomi*
薑 黃	Jiang Huang (Tumeric rhizome)	*Rhizoma Curcumae Longae*

2. Thromboangiitis of the lower extremities, add:

川牛膝	Chuan Niu Xi (Cyathula root)	*Radix Cyathulae*
黃 柏	Huang Bai (Phellodendron)	*Cortex Phellodendri*

3. With severe pain, add:

乳 香	Ru Xiang (Mastic)	*Resina Olibani*
沒 藥	Mo Yao (Myrrh)	*Resina Myrrhae*

4. With blood clots, add:

桃 仁	Tao Ren (Persica seed)	*Semen Persicae*
紅 花	Hong Hua (Carthamus)	*Flos Carthami*

Sì Nì Sàn   四逆散

(Szu-Ni-San)
(Powder for Relieving Depression with Cold Limbs)

Constituents:

柴 胡 Chai Hu (Bupleurum)	9-12 gm.	*Radix Bupleuri*
枳 實 Zhi Shi (Immature bitter orange)	6-9 gm.	*Fructus Aurantii Immaturus*
白 芍 Bai Shao Yao (White peony)	9-12 gm.	*Radix paeoniae Alba*
甘 草 Gan Cao (Licorice)	3-6 gm.	*Radix Glycyrrhizae*

Action:

1. To regulate the liver and spleen
2. To eliminate the heat in the interior of the body

Indication:

1. For a person with depressed liver in which the flow of vital energy is impeded by pathogenic heat in the interior of the body. The symptoms are: coldness in the extremities, abdominal pain, diarrhea.

> Tongue: pale with white coating
> Pulse: wiry/taut

2. For a person with disharmony between liver and spleen, accompanied with costal or abdominal pain, and menstrual complaints.

Application:

Syncope (due to heat), chronic hepatitis, gastric neuralgia, intercostal neuralgia, biliary ascariasis, hernia, pancreatitis, acute appendicitis.

Modification:

1. With hypochondriac pain, add:

延胡索 Yan Hu Suo (Corydalis tuber)	*Rhizoma Corydalis*
郁 金 Yu Jin (Curcuma root)	*Radix Curcumae*

2. With jaundice, add:

茵陳蒿 Yin Chen Hao (Capillaris)	*Herba Artemisiae Capillaris*
郁 金 Yu Jin (Curcuma root)	*Radix Curcumae*

3. With pain caused by blood stasis, add:

丹 參 Dan Shen (Salvia root)	*Radix Salviae Miltiorrhizae*
五靈脂 Wu Ling Zhi (Trogopterus dung)	*Faeces Trogopterorum*

Generic Name:

Bupleurum and Chih-shih Formula

Sì Nì Tāng　四逆湯

(Szu-Ni-Tang)
(Decoction for Treating Vital Prostration with Cold Limbs)

Constituents:

附 子 Fu Zi (Aconite)	10-15 gm.	*Radix Aconiti Praeparatae*
乾 薑 Gan Jiang (Dry ginger)	6-9 gm.	*Rhizoma Zingiberis*
炙甘草 Zhi Gan Can (Baked licorice)	10-15 gm.	*Radix Glycyrrhizae Praeparatae*

Action:

To restore the *Yang* (vital function) from collapse and shock.

Indication:

1. For depletion of *Yang* (vital function) in the Shao-yin channel. The symptoms are: cold hands and feet, intolerance of cold, like to sleep with the body curled up, fatigue, watery diarrhea with undigested food in the stool, vomiting, abdominal pain, no thirst.

> Tongue: pale or dark purple
> Pulse: deep and faint

2. For depletion of *Yang* (vital function) due to profuse perspiration, or intake of diaphoretics by mistake.

Application:

Prostration, cardiac failure

Modification:

1. For chronic rheumatoid arthritis caused by cold, add:

桂 枝 Gui Zhi (Cinnamon twig)	*Ramulus Cinnamomi*
白 芍 Bai Shao (White peony)	*Radix Paeoniae Alba*

2. For edema caused by deficiency and coldness of the spleen and stomach, add:

黨 參 Dang Shen (Codonopsis)	*Radix Codonopsis Pilosulae*
茯 苓 Fu Ling (Poria)	*Poria*
澤 瀉 Ze Xie (Alisma)	*Rhizoma Alismatis*

3. If diarrhea stopped suddenly, add:

人 參 Ren Shen (Ginseng)	*Radix Ginseng*

This formula is called Si Ni Jia Ren Shen Tang（四逆加人參湯）

Comment:

If the person's face is red and look irritable, he should take this decoction cold.

Generic Name:

Aconite and G. L. Combination

Sì Shén Wán   四神丸

(Szu-Shen-Wan)
(Pills of Four Miraculous Drugs)

Constituents:

補骨脂 Bu Gui Zi (Psoralea)	9-12 gm.	*Fructus Psoraleae*
吳茱萸 Wu Zhu Yu (Evodia)	6-9 gm.	*Fructus Evodiae*
肉豆蔻 Rou Dou Kou (Nutmeg)	6-9 gm.	*Semen Myristicae*
五味子 Wu Wei Zi (Schisandra)	6-9 gm.	*Fructus Schisandrae*
生　薑 Sheng Jiang (Fresh ginger)	1-3 gm.	*Rhizoma Zingiberis Recens*
大　棗 Da Zao (Jujube)	3-5 pc.	*Fructus Ziziphus Jujubae*

Action:

1. To warm the kidney and spleen
2. Anti-diarrhetic

Indication:

For a person with diarrhea due to spleen and kidney deficiency and coldness. The symptoms are: diarrhea in the early morning, loss of appetite, indigestion, abdominal pain, low back pain, hands and feet cold, fatigue, weakness.

> Tongue: light color
> Pulse: deep and slow

Application:

Chronic or habitual diarrhea before dawn in chronic colitis, chronic dysentery, intestinal tuberculosis.

Modification:

1. With prolapse of rectum, add:

黄　芪 Huang Qi (Astragalus)	*Radix Astragali*
升　麻 Sheng Ma (Cimicifuga)	*Rhizoma Cimicifugae*

2. For cold hands and feet, add:

附　子 Fu Zi (Aconite)	*Radix Aconiti Praeparatae*
肉　桂 Rou Gui (Cinnamon bark)	*Cortex Cinnamomi*

3. With lower abdominal pain, add:

茴　香 Hui Xiang (Fennel fruit)	*Fructus Foeniculi*
木　香 Mu Xiang (Saussurea root)	*Radix Saussureae*

and eliminate:

五味子 Wu Wei Zi (Schisandra)	*Fructus Schisandrae*
吳茱萸 Wu Zhu Yu (Evodia)	*Fructus Evodiae*

Sì Shēng Wán　　四生丸

(Shih-Sheng-Wan)
(Pills of Four Fresh Ingredients)

Constituents:

生 荷 葉	Sheng He Ye (Lotus leaf)	20 gm.	*Folium Nelumbinis*
生 艾 葉	Sheng Ai Ye (Artemisia)	15 gm.	*Folium Artemisiae Argyi*
生側柏葉	Sheng Ce Bai Ye (Biota tops)	15 gm.	*Cacumen Biotae*
生 地 黃	Sheng Di Huang (Fresh rehmannia)	20 gm.	*Radix Rehmanniae*

Grind the above fresh ingredients into powder, make into pills.
Or boil the above fresh ingredients into decoction.

Action:

To stop bleeding by cooling the heat in the blood.

Indication:

For all kinds of bleeding pertaining to the upper part of the body. The symptoms are: spitting blood, nose bleeding, color fresh red, mouth and throat dry.

Tongue: red or dark red
Pulse: wiry, rapid and forceful

Application:

Spitting blood, epistaxis, tuberculosis, bronchiectasis, ulcer.

Modification:

1. If bleeding is excessive, add:

白茅根	Bai Mao Gen (Imperata)	*Rhizoma Imperatae*
小 薊	Xiao Ji (Small thistle)	*Herba Cephalanoploris*
藕 節	Ou Jie (Lotus node)	*Nodus Nelumbinis Rhizomatis*
仙鶴草	Xian He Cao (Agrimony)	*Herba Agrimoniae*

2. To eliminate blood clots, add:

茜草根	Xi Cao Gen (Madder root)	*Radix Rubiae*
牡丹皮	Mu Dan Pi (Moutan bark)	*Cortex Moutan Radicis*

Sì Wù Tāng　　四物湯

(Szu-Wu-Tang)
(The Four Ingrediets Decoction)

Constituents:

熟地黃	Shu Di Huang (Prep. rehmannia)	10-15 gm.	*Radix Rehmanniae*
當　歸	Dang Gui (Chinese angelica)	9-12 gm.	*Radix Angelicae Sinensis*
川　芎	Chuan Xiong (Ligusticum)	6-9 gm.	*Rhizoma Ligustici Chuanxiong*
白芍藥	Bai Shao Yao (White peony)	9-12 gm.	*Radix Paeoniae Alba*

Action:

1. To nourish and replenish blood
2. To regualte the flow of blood circulation

Indication:

For a person with anemia and stagnant blood circulation. The symptoms are: face sallow, lips and finger nails pale, dizziness, vertigo, tinnitis, irregular menstruation, decreased flow of blood, abdominal pain or amennorhea.

Tongue: light color
Pulse: thready and weak, or thready and hesitant

Application:

Anemia, irregular menstruation, threatened abortion, post-partum anemia.

Contraindication:

For a person with anemia and diarrhea due to spleen deficiency; excessive loss of blood, or dehydration.

Modification:

1. With blood stasis, add:

桃　仁	Tao Ren (Persica seed)	*Semen Persicae*
紅　花	Hong Hua (Carthamus)	*Flos Carthami*

This is named Tao Hong Sì Wù Tang (桃紅四物湯)

2. For post-partum and uterine bleeding, add:

阿　膠	E Jiao (Donkey-hide gelatin)	*Colla Corii Asini*
艾　葉	Ai Ye (Artemisia)	*Folium Artemisiae Argyi*

This is named Jiao Ai Tang (膠艾湯)

3. Dysmennorhea caused by anemia and blood stasis, add:

益母草	Yi Mu Cao (Leonurus)	*Herba Leonuri*
香　附	Xiang Fu (Cyperus tuber)	*Rhizoma Cyperi*
延胡索	Yan Hu Suo (Corydalis tuber)	*Rhizoma Corydalis*

Generic Name:

Tang-kuei Four Combination

Sū Hé Xiāng Wán   蘇合香丸
(Su-Ho-Hsiang-Wan)
(Styrax Pills)

Constituents:

蘇合香	Su He Xiang (Styrax)	6-9 gm.	*Styrax Liquidus*
青木香	Qing Mu Xiang (Birthwort)	6-9 gm.	*Radix Aristolochiae*
香 附	Xiang Fu (Cyperus)	6-9 gm.	*Rhizoma Cyperi*
檀 香	Tan Xiang (Sandalwood)	3-6 gm.	*Lignum Santali Albi*
安息香	An Xi Xiang (Benzoin)	3-6 gm.	*Benzoinum*
沉 香	Chen Xiang (Aquilaria)	1-3 gm.	*Lignum Aquilariae Resinatum*
麝 香	She Xiang (Musk)	.2-.5 gm.	*Moschus*
丁 香	Ding Xiang (Cloves)	1-2 gm.	*Flos Caryophylli*
乳 香	Ru Xiang (Mastic)	3-6 gm.	*Resina Olibani*
冰 片	Bing Pian (Borneol)	.5-1 gm.	*Borneolum*
犀 角	Xi Jiao (Rhinoceros horn)	.5-1 gm.	*Cornus Rhinoceri*
白 术	Bai Zhu (White atractylodes)	6-9 gm.	*Rhizoma Atractylodis Macrocephalae*
硃 砂	Zhu Sha (Cinnabar)	.5-1 gm.	*Cinnabaris*
蓽 拔	Bi Ba (Long pepper)	3-6 gm.	*Fructus Piperis Longi*
訶 子	He Zi (Terminalia)	6-9 gm.	*Fructus Chebulae*

Action:

1. Warming
2. Resuscitating

Indication:

For a person with coma due to apoplexy, stroke, or cholera. The symptoms are: lock-jaws, coma, loss of consciousness, abdominal pain, face pale and white, oral and nasal breath cold, hands and feet cold.

> Tongue: white and slippery
> Pulse: deep, slow and forceful; or wiry, tight and forceful

Application:

Stroke, apoplexy, cholera, coronary heart disease, angina pectoris.

Contraindication:

For a pregnant woman.

Generic Name:

Kuan Hsin Su Ho Wan;
Su He Xiang Pills;
Styrax Formula

Sū Zǐ Jiàng Qì Tāng   蘇子降氣湯

(Su-Tzu-Chiang-Chi-Tang)
(Decoction of Perilla Seed to Descend the Flow of *Qi*)

Constituents:

蘇　子	Su Zi (Perilla seed)	6-9 gm.	*Fructus Perillae*
半　夏	Ban Xia (Pinellia tuber)	6-9 gm.	*Rhizoma Pinelliae*
厚　朴	Hou Po (Magnolia bark)	6-9 gm.	*Cortex Magnoliae Officinalis*
前　胡	Qian Hu (Peucedanum root)	6-9 gm.	*Radix Peucedani*
肉　桂	Rou Gui (Cinnamon bark)	3-6 gm.	*Cortex Cinnamomi*
當　歸	Dang Gui (Chinese angelica)	6-9 gm.	*Radix Angelicae Sinensis*
炙甘草	Zhi Gan Cao (Baked licorice)	3-6 gm.	*Radix Glycyrrhizae Praeparatae*
陳　皮	Chen Pi (Citrus peel)	3-6 gm.	*Pericarpium Citri Reticulatae*

The following may be added:

紫蘇葉	Zi Su Ye (Perilla leaf)	6-9 gm.	*Folium Perillae*
生　薑	Sheng Jiang (Fresh ginger)	1-3 gm.	*Rhizoma Zingiberis Recens*
大　棗	Da Zao (Jujube)	3-5 pc.	*Fructus Ziziphus Jujubae*

Action:

1. To descend the upward flow of *Qi* and relieve asthma
2. To resolve phlegm due to coldness

Indication:

For a person with asthma due to cold phlegm in the lung and with deficiency in the kidney. The symptoms are: cough with dyspnea, shortness of breath, asthma and profuse saliva and sputum, epigastric fullness, dizziness, vertigo, lumbar pain, weakness in the body and feet, edema.

Tongue: white, slippery or greasy
Pulse: tight and slippery

Application:

Bronchial asthma, chronic bronchitis, pulmonary emphysema

Contraindication:

For a person with asthma caused by:
1. Deficiency of lung and kidney
2. Accumulation of heat and phlegm in the lung

Modification:

1. With aversion to wind and chills, add:

麻　黄	Ma Huang (Ephedra)	*Herba Ephedrae*
杏　仁	Xing Ren (Apricot seed)	*Semen Armeniacae Amarum*

2. With deficiency of vital energy, add:

黨　參	Dang Shen (Codonopsis)	*Radix Codonopsis Pilosulae*
五味子	Wu Wei Zi (Schisandra fruit)	*Fructus Schisandrae*

Generic Name: Perilla Fruit Combination

Suān Zǎo Rén Tāng　　酸棗仁湯

(Suan-Tsao-Jen-Tang)
(Decoction of Wild Jujube Seed)

Constituents:

酸棗仁 Suan Zao Ren (Wild jujube)	10-15 gm.	*Semen Ziziphi Spinosae*
茯　苓 Fu Ling (Poria)	9-12 gm.	*Poria*
川　芎 Chuan Xiong (Ligusticum)	6-9 gm.	*Rhizoma Ligustici Chuanxiong*
知　母 Zhi Mu (Anemarrhena)	6-9 gm.	*Rhizoma Anemarrhenae*
甘　草 Gan Cao (Licorice)	3-6 gm.	*Radix Glycyrrhizae*

Action:

1. Sedative
2. To nourish the blood in liver
3. To clear the heat in liver

Indication:

For a person with deficiency of blood in the liver. The symptoms are: fidgetiness, insomnia, excessive dreams, palpitation, dizziness, dry mouth and throat

> Tongue: red
> Pulse: wiry, thready and rapid

Application:

Insomnia, neurasthenia

Modification:

1. With heart and spleen asthenia, add:

黨　參 Dang Shen (Codonopsis)	*Radix Codonopsis Pilosulae*
龍　齒 Long Chi (Dragon's teeth)	*Dens Draconis*

2. With night perspiration, add:

柏子仁 Bai Zi Ren (Biota seed)	*Semen Biotae*
五味子 Wu Wei Zi (Schisandra fruit)	*Fructus Schisandrae*

3. For neurasthenia with fidgetiness and insomnia, add:

旱蓮草 Han Lian Cao (Eclipta)	*Herba Ecliptae*
女貞子 Nu Zhen Zi (Ligustrum fruit)	*Fructus Ligustri Lucidi*

4. With palpitation, add:

龍　齒 Long Chi (Dragon's teeth)	*Dens Draconis*
牡　蠣 Mu Li (Oyster shell)	*Concha Ostreae*

Generic Name:

Tabellae Suan Zao Ren Tang;
Zizyphus Combination

Suō Quán Wán　　縮泉丸

(Suo-Chuan-Wan)
(Pills for Enuresis)

Constituents:

益智仁	Yi Zhi Ren (Black cardamon)	9-12 gm.	*Fructus Alpiniae*
烏　藥	Wu Yao (Lindera)	9-12 gm.	*Radix Linderae*
山　藥	Shan Yao (Dioscorea)	9-12 gm.	*Rhizoma Dioscoreae*

Action:

1. To warm the spleen and kidney
2. To relieve enuresis

Indication:

For a person with urination difficulty due to deficiency of spleen and kidney. The symptoms are: lumbago, urination (frequent, clear, and prolonged), or bed-wetting, spermatorrhea, leukorrhea.

   Tongue: pale with white coating
   Pulse: deep and weak

Application:

Enuresis, spermatorrhea, leukorrhea, lumbago.

Tài Shān Pán Shí Sàn　泰山盤石散
(Tai-Shan-Pan-Shih-San)
(Powder for Threatened Abortion)

Constituents:

人 參	Ren Shen (Ginseng)	6-9 gm.	*Radix Ginseng*
黄 芪	Huang Qi (Astragalus)	6-9 gm.	*Radix Astragali*
當 歸	Dang Gui (Chinese angelica)	6-9 gm.	*Radix Angelicae Sinensis*
川續斷	Chuan Xu Duan (Dipsacus)	6-9 gm.	*Radix Dipsaci*
黄 芩	Huang Qin (Scutellaria)	3-6 gm.	*Radix Scutellariae*
川 芎	Chuan Xiong (Ligusticum)	6-9 gm.	*Rhizoma Ligustici Chuanxiong*
白芍藥	Bai Shao Yao (White peony)	6-9 gm.	*Radix Paeoniae Alba*
熟地黄	Shu Di Huang (Prep. rehmannia)	9-12 gm.	*Radix Rehmanniae Praeparatae*
白 术	Bai Zhu (White atractylodes)	6-9 gm.	*Rhizoma Atractylodis Macrocephalae*
砂 仁	Sha Ren (Cardamon)	3-6 gm.	*Fructus Amomi*
炙甘草	Zhi Gan Cao (Baked licorice)	3-6 gm.	*Radix Glycyrrhizae Praeparatae*
糯 米	Nuo Mi (Glutinous rice)	20-30 gm.	*Semen Oryzae Glutinosae*

Action:

1. To replenish *Qi* (vital energy) and blood
2. To prevent miscarriage

Indication:

For a person with deficiency of *Qi* (vital energy) & blood, and has threatened abortion. The symptoms are: malaise, lack of appetite, miscarriage, color of blood is light red, ptosis of visceras, lower abdomen pain (constant), face sallow, palpitation, insomnia.

Tongue: pale with thin coating
Pulse: slippery and weak

Application:

Threatened abortion.

Modification:

1. With low back pain, add:
杜 仲 Du Zhong (Eucommia bark)　　*Cortex Eucommiae*
桑寄生 Sang Ji Sheng (Mulberry mistletoe)　*Ramulus Loranthi*
2. With excessive bleeding, add:
阿 膠 E Jiao (Donkey-hide gelatin)　*Colla Asini*
仙鶴草 Xian He Cao (Agrimony)　　*Herba Agrimoniae*
3. With ptosis of visceras, add:
升 麻 Sheng Ma (Cimicifuga)　　*Rhizoma Cimicifugae*

Táo Hé Chéng Qì Tāng 桃核承氣湯
(Tao-Ho-Cheng-Chi-Tang)
(Purgative Decoction of Persica Seed)

Constituents:

桃 仁	Tao Ren (Persica seed)	6-9 gm.	*Semen Persicae*
桂 枝	Gui Zhi (Cinnamon)	3-6 gm.	*Ramulus Cinnamomi*
大 黃	Da Huang (Rhubarb)	6-9 gm.	*Radix et Rhizoma Rhei*
芒 硝	Mang Xiao (Mirabilitum)	3-6 gm.	*Natrii Sulfas*
炙甘草	Zhi Gan Cao (Baked licorice)	3-6 gm.	*Radix Glycyrrhizae Praeparatae*

Action:

To eliminate heat and blood stasis.

Indication:

For a person with heat and blood stasis in the lower part of the body (lower burner). The symptoms are: acute abdominal pain, neurosis, delirium, thirst, stool hard/firm, no difficulty in urination, increased body temperature at night.

> Tongue: red and dry
> Pulse: deep and forceful, or hesistant

Application:

Irregular menstruation, dysmenorrhea, amenorrhea, acute pelvic inflammation, retention of lochia, intestinal obstruction.

Modification:

1. With severe blood stasis, add:

當 歸	Dang Gui (Chinese angelica)	*Radix Angelicae Sinensis*
紅 花	Hong Hua (Carthamus)	*Flos Carthami*

2. With *Qi* (vital energy) stagnation, add:

香 附	Xiang Fu (Cyperus tuber)	*Rhizoma Cyperi*
青 皮	Qing Pi (Green tangerine peel)	*Pericarpium Citri Reticulatae Viridae*

3. With retention of lochia, add:

五靈脂	Wu Ling Zhi (Trogopterus dung)	*Faeces Trogopterorum*
蒲 黃	Pu Huang (Bulrush pollen)	*Pollen Typhae*

Generic Name:

Persica and Rhubarb Combination

Táo Huā Tāng   桃花湯
(Tao-Hua-Tang)
(Decoction of Peach Flower)

Constituents:

赤石脂	Chi Shi Zhi (Red halloysite)	20-25 gm.	*Halloysitum rubrum*
乾 薑	Gan Jiang (Dry ginger)	6-9 gm.	*Rhizoma Zingiberis*
粳 米	Jing Mi (Rice)	20-30 gm.	*Semen Oryzae*

Action:

Relieving diarrhea with astringents

Indication:

For a person with chronic diarrhea, stools bloody and purulent, red or dull red, abdominal pain with preference to heat and pressure.

Tongue: pale with white coating
Pulse: slow and weak

Application:

Chronic diarrhea with bloody and purulent stools.

Modification:

1. With deficiency of spleen and kidney with interior cold symptoms, add:
附 子 Fu Zi (Aconite)   *Radix Aconiti Praeparatae*
2. With severe abdominal pain, add:
白芍藥 Bai Shao Yao (White peony)   *Radix Paeoniae Alba*
桂 枝 Gui Zhi (Cinnamon)   *Ramulus Cinnamomi*
3. With prolapse, add:
黨 參 Dang Shen (Codonopsis)   *Radix Codonopsis Pilosulae*
肉豆蔻 Rou Dou Kou (Nutmeg)   *Semen Myristicae*

Comment:

The dissection color of red halloysite is like a peach flower, therefore this formula is named the "Decoction of Peach Flower."

Tiān Má Gōu Téng Yǐn   天麻鉤藤飲
(Tien-Ma-Kou-Teng-Yin)
(Decoction of Gastrodia and Uncaria)

Constituents:

天 麻	Tian Ma (Gastrodia tuber)	6-9 gm.	*Rhizoma Gastrodiae*
鉤 藤	Gou Teng (Uncaria)	6-9 gm.	*Ramulus Uncariae Uncis*
石決明	Shi Jue Ming (Sea-ear shell)	3-6 gm.	*Concha Haliotidis*
桑寄生	Sang Ji Sheng (Mulberry mistletoe)	6-9 gm.	*Ramulus Loranthi*
杜 仲	Du Zhong (Eucommia bark)	6-9 gm.	*Cortex Eucommiae*
川牛膝	Chuan Niu Xi (Cyathula root)	6-9 gm.	*Radix Cyathulae*
梔 子	Zhi Zi (Gardenia fruit)	3-6 gm.	*Fructus Gardeniae*
黃 芩	Huang Qin (Scutellaria)	6-9 gm.	*Radix Scutellariae*
益母草	Yi Mu Cao (Leonurus)	6-9 gm.	*Herba Leonuri*
夜交藤	Ye Jiao Teng (Fleeceflower)	6-9 gm.	*Caulis Polygoni Multiflori*
茯 神	Fu Shen (Poria)	3-6 gm.	*Poria*

Action:

To subdue the endogenous wind in the liver channel (Antihypertensive)

Indication:

For a person with endogenous wind in the liver channel due to excessive liver *Yang* (vital function). The symptoms are: headache, vertigo, paralysis or convulsions, trembling movement of the tongue, insomnia, coma, deviation of the mouth and eyes, hemiplegia.

> Tongue: red
> Pulse: wiry/taut and rapid

Application:

Hypertension, puerperal eclampsia, hemiplegia, trigeminal neuralgia.

Tiān Tāi Wū Yào Sàn　　天台烏藥散

(Tien-Tai-Wu-Yao-San)
(The Lindera Root Powder)

Constituents:

烏　藥 Wu Yao (Lindera)	10-15 gm.	*Radix Linderae*
茴　香 Hui Xiang (Fennel fruit)	10-15 gm.	*Fructus Foeniculi*
高良姜 Gao Liang Jiang (Galanga)	10-15 gm.	*Rhizoma Galangae*
青　皮 Qing Pi (Green tangerine peel)	10-15 gm.	*Pericarpium Citri Reticulatae Viridae*
木　香 Mu Xiang (Saussurea)	10-15 gm.	*Radix Saussureae*
檳　榔 Bing Lang (Areca seed)	10-15 gm.	*Semen Arecae*
川楝子 Chuan Lian Zi (Sichuan chinaberry)	10-15 gm.	*Fructus Meliae Toosendan*
巴　豆 Ba Dou (Croton seed)	10-15 gm.	*Semen Crotonis*

Grind the above ingredients into powder, and take 3 gm. each time.

Action:

1. To invigorate the circulation of *Qi* (vital energy) in liver
2. To dispel cold and relieve pain

Indication:

For a person with hernia caused by stagnation of cold and vital energy, with manifestation of pain in the lower lateral abdomen, radiating to the genital region.

> Tongue: pale with white coating
> Pulse: deep, slow or wiry/taut

Application:

Hernia, inguinal hernia, scrotal hernia, hernia of the vagina or testis, hypochondriac pain.

Modification:

1. For hernia, add:

橘　核 Ju He (Tangerine seed)	*Semen Citri Reticulatae*
荔枝核 Li Zhi He (Lychee seed)	*Semen Litchi*

2. With cold, add:

吳茱萸 Wu Zhu Yu (Evodia fruit)	*Fructus Evodiae*
肉　桂 Rou Gui (Cinnamon bark)	*Cortex Cinnamomi*

Tiān Wáng Bǔ Xīn Dān 天王補心丹
(Tien-Wang-Pu-Hsin-Tan)
(The King's Mind-easing Tonic Pills)

Constituents:

生地黃	Sheng Di Huang (Fresh rehmannia)	10-15 gm.	*Radix Rehmanniae*
玄　參	Xuan Shen (Scrophularia)	9-12 gm.	*Radix Scrophulariae*
麥門冬	Mai Men Dong (Ophiopogon)	9-12 gm.	*Radix Ophiopogonis*
天門冬	Tian Men Dong (Asparagus)	9-12 gm.	*Radix Asparagi*
丹　參	Dan Shen (Salvia)	9-12 gm.	*Radix Salviae Miltiorrhizae*
當　歸	Dang Gui (Chinese angelica)	6-9 gm.	*Radix Angelicae Sinensis*
茯　苓	Fu Ling (Poria)	9-12 gm.	*Poria*
柏子仁	Bai Zi Ren (Biota seed)	9-12 gm.	*Semen Biotae*
遠　志	Yuan Zhi (Polygala root)	6-9 gm.	*Radix Polygalae*
五味子	Wu Wei Zi (Schisandra)	9-12 gm.	*Fructus Schisandrae*
酸棗仁	Suan Zao Ren (Wild jujube)	9-12 gm.	*Semen Ziziphi Spinosae*
桔　梗	Jie Geng (Platycodon)	6-9 gm.	*Radix Platycodi*
硃　砂	Zhu Sha (Cinnabar)	1-3 gm.	*Cinnabaris*
人　參	Ren Shen (Ginseng)	6-9 gm.	*Radix Ginseng*

Action:

1. To nourish the *Yin* (vital essence) of heart and kidney
2. Febrifugal
3. Sedative

Indication:

For a person with deficiency of blood and vital essence of heart and kidney. The symptoms are: forgetfulness, insomnia, restlessness, fatigue, nocturnal emission, dry stool, oral suppurative infection.

> Tongue: red with thin coating
> Pulse: thready and rapid

Application:

Neurasthenia, insomnia, hypertension, hyperthyroidism.

Contraindication:

For a person with spleen and stomach asthenia with loose stools, or stagnancy of phlegm and dampness.

Generic Name:

Tien Wang Bu Xin Wan;
Emperor's Tea;
Ginseng and Zizyphus Formula

Tiáo Gān Tāng 調肝湯

(Tiao-Kan-Tang)
(Regulating the Liver Decoction)

Constituents:

山藥	Shao Yao (Dioscorea)	9-12 gm.	*Rhizoma Dioscoreae*
阿膠	E Jiao (Donkey-hide gelatin)	9-12 gm.	*Colla Corii Asini*
當歸	Dang Gui (Chinese angelica)	6-9 gm.	*Radix Angelicae Sinensis*
白芍藥	Bai Shao Yao (White peony)	6-9 gm.	*Radix Paeoniae Alba*
山茱萸	Shan Zhu Yu (Cornus)	6-9 gm.	*Fructus Corni*
巴戟天	Ba Ji Tian (Morinda)	6-9 gm.	*Radix Morindae Officinalis*
澤蘭	Ze Lan (Bugleweed)	9-12 gm.	*Herba Lycopi*
丹參	Dan Shen (Salvia)	6-9 gm.	*Radix Salviae Miltiorrhizae*
甘草	Gan Cao (Licorice)	3-6 gm.	*Radix Glycyrrhizae*

Action:

1. To replenish the *Yin* (vital essence) of liver and kidney
2. To regulate menstruation flow

Indication:

For a person with amenorrhea due to asthenia of liver and kidney. The symptoms are: delayed menstruation, amenorrhea, retarded growth or maturity in puberty, face sallow, chest flat, breast underdeveloped, cold sensation in the lower abdomen, dizziness or vertigo, vaginal discharges clear and scanty.

> Tongue: pale with thin coating
> Pulse: thready and weak

Application:

Amenorrhea, irregular menstruation, retarded maturity.

Tiáo Wèi Chéng Qì Tāng 調味承氣湯

(Tiao-Wei-Cheng-Chi-Tang)
(The Stomach Regulating Purgative Decoction)

Constituents:

大 黃 Da Huang (Rhubarb)	10-20 gm.	*Radix et Rhizoma Rhei*
芒 硝 Mang Xiao (Mirabilitum)	10-20 gm.	*Natrii Sulfas*
炙甘草 Zhi Gan Cao (Baked licorice)	3-6 gm.	*Radix Glycyrrhizae Praeparatae*

Add Mang Xiao (Mirabilitum) last in the cooking process.

Action:

To eliminate heat and dryness (Slow purgative)

Indication:

For a person with heat and dryness in the Yang-ming visceras (stomach and intestines). The symptoms are: tidal fever, sweating from the hands and feet, constipation, delirium, no abdominal fullness or distention, no oppression or fullness in the chest or epigastric region.

> Tongue: with yellow coating
> Pulse: deep and forceful

Application:

Acute simple intestinal obstruction, acute cholecystitis, acute appendicitis, constipation.

Generic Name:

Rhubarb and Mirabilitum Combination

Tíng Lì Dà Zǎo Xiè Fèi Tāng   葶藶大棗瀉肺湯
(Ting-Li-Ta-Tsao-Hsieh-Fei-Tang)
(Decoction to Purge the Lung with Lepidium and Jujube)

Constituents:

葶藶子 Ting Li Zi (Lepidium)	10-15 gm.	*Semen Lepidii*
大　棗 Da Zao (Jujube)	12-15 pc.	*Fructus Ziziphus Jujubae*

Action:

1. To eliminate water and phlegm in the lung
2. To relieve cough and asthma

Indication:

For a person with asthma and edema of the face and eyes. The symptoms are: cough with profuse sputum, asthma, chest distention, edema of the face and eyes, dysuria, cannot sleep.

> Tongue: with white and greasy coating
> Pulse: slippery

Application:

Cardiac edema and asthma, chronic bronchitis, asthmatic bronchitis.

Generic Name:

Lepidium and Jujube Combination

Tōng Mài Sì Nì Tāng 通脈四逆湯
(Tung-Mọ-Tzu-Ni-Tang)
(Decoction for Treating Vital Prostration with Cold Limbs by Invigorating the Vascular System)

Constituents:

附 子	Fu Zi (Aconite)	10-15 gm.	*Radix Aconiti Praeparatae*
乾 薑	Gan Jiang (Dry ginger)	12-18 gm.	*Rhizoma Zingiberis*
炙甘草	Zhi Gan Cao (Baked licorice)	10-15 gm.	*Radix Glycyrrhizae Praeparatae*

Action:

1. To restore the *Yang* (vital function) from collapse and shock with cold limbs
2. To invigorate the vascular system (blood circulation)

Indication:

For a person with depletion of *Yang* (vital function) in the Shao-yin channel. The symptoms are: diarrhea with undigested food in the stool, vomiting, face red, cold hands and feet, body is cold on the exterior but hot in the interior, no symptoms of aversion to cold.

> Tongue: pale or dark purple
> Pulse: deep and faint

Application:

Prostration, cardiac failure

Comment:

This formula is very similar to Si Ni Tang (四逆湯)
(Aconite and G. L. Combination.)

The only difference is the amount of dry ginger (乾薑) is doubled in this formula.

Generic Name:

Licorice, Aconite and Ginger Pulse Combination

Tōng Qiào Huó Xuè Tāng　　通竅活血湯

(Tong-Chiao-Huo-Hsieh-Tang)
(Decoction to Invigorate Blood Circulation and Open the Orifices)

Constituents:

麝 香	She Xiang (Musk)	.1-.2 gm.	*Moschus*
桃 仁	Tao Ren (Persica seed)	6-9 gm.	*Semen Persicae*
紅 花	Hong Hua (Carthamus)	6-9 gm.	*Flos Carthami*
川 芎	Chuan Xiong (Ligusticum)	3-6 gm.	*Rhizoma Ligustici Chuanxiong*
赤芍藥	Chi Shao Yao (Red peony)	3-6 gm.	*Radix Paeoniae Rubra*
老 葱	Cong (Old spring onion)	3 pc.	*Herba Allii Fistulosi*
生 薑	Sheng Jiang (Fresh ginger)	3-6 gm.	*Rhizoma Zingiberis Recens*
大 棗	Da Zao (Jujube)	3-5 pc.	*Fructus Ziziphus Jujubae*
黃 酒	Rice Wine		

Action:

To invigorate blood circulation and open the orifices

Indication:

For a person with blood stasis in the head and face. The symptoms are: headache, dizziness, deafness, loss of hair, face pale with cyanosis, phthisis, weakness of the muscles.

Application:

Cerebral concussion, post-concussion syndromes, phthisis, infantile malnutrition.

Tòng Xiè Yào Fāng (Bái Zhú Sháo Yào Sàn)

痛瀉要方 (白术芍藥散)

(Tung-Hsieh-Yao-Fang) (Pai-Chu-Shao-Yao-San)

(Powder of White Atractylodes and White Peony for Diarrhea with Abdominal Pain)

Constituents:

白 术	Bai Zhu (White atractylodes)	6-9 gm.	*Rhizoma Atractylodis acrocephalae*
白芍藥	Bai Shao Yao (White peony)	6-9 gm.	*Radix Paeoniae Alba*
陳 皮	Chen Pi (Citrus peel)	3-6 gm.	*Pericarpium Citri Reticulatae*
防 風	Fang Feng (Ledebouriella)	6-9 gm.	*Radix Ledebouriellae*

Action:

1. To soothe the liver and relieve pain
2. To strengthen the spleen and stop diarrhea

Indication:

For a person with diarrhea and abdominal pain. The symptoms are: abdominal pain, borborygmus, diarrhea, pain is not relieved after diarrhea.

Tongue: with thin white coating
Pulse: wiry/taut and slow

Application:

Allergic colitis, enteritis.

Modification:

With watery diarrhea, add:
升 麻 Sheng Ma (Cimicifuga)   *Rhizoma Cimicifugae*

Tōng Yū Jiān 通瘀煎
(Tong-Yu-Chian)
(Decoction for Blood Stasis)

Constituents:

當歸尾	Dang Gui Wei (Chinese angelica)	12-15 gm.	*Radix Angelicae Sinensis*
紅 花	Hong Hua (Safflower)	6-9 gm.	*Flos Carthami*
山 楂	Shan Zha (Crataegus)	9-12 gm.	*Fructus Crataegi*
烏 藥	Wu Yao (Lindera)	6-9 gm.	*Radix Linderae*
木 香	Mu Xiang (Saussurea)	6-9 gm.	*Radix Saussureae*
香 附	Xiang Fu (Cyperus)	6-9 gm.	*Rhizoma Cyperi*
青 皮	Qing Pi (Green tangerine peel)	3-6 gm.	*Pericarpium Citri Reticulatae Viridae*
澤 瀉	Ze Xie (Alisma)	6-9 gm.	*Rhizoma Alismatis*

Action:

To invigorate blood circulation and remove stasis

Indication:

For a person with coma due to blood stasis, lockjaw, face red, lips cyanotic.

Tongue: red
Pulse: deep and wiry

Modification:

1. With anger, irritability, disturbance of sleep and increased nightmares, add:

鉤 藤	Gou Teng (Uncaria stem with hooks)	*Ramulus Uncariae cum Uncis*
石決明	Shi Jue Ming (Abalone shell)	*Concha Haliotidis*
龍膽草	Long Dan Cao (Gentiana)	*Radix Gentianae*
牡丹皮	Mu Dan Pi (Moutan bark)	*Cortex Moutan Radicis*

2. With headache, dizziness and disturbance of liver Yang, add:

菊 花	Ju Hua (Chrysanthemum flower)	*Flos Chrysanthemi*
枸杞子	Gou Qi Zi (Lycium fruit)	*Fructus Lycii*
珍珠母	Zhen Zhu Mu (Mother-of-pearl)	*Concha Margaritifera Usta*

246

Tòu Nóng Sàn 透膿散

(Tou-Nung-San)
(The Anti-purulent Powder)

Constituents:

穿山甲	Chuan Shan Jia (Ageater scales)	3-9 gm.	*Squama Manitis*
皂角刺	Zao Jiao Ci (Gleditsia spine)	9-15 gm.	*Spina Gleditsiae*
黄 芪	Huang Qi (Astragalus)	9-15 gm.	*Radix Astragali*
當 歸	Dang Gui (Chinese angelica)	6-9 gm.	*Radix Angelicae Sinensis*
川 芎	Chuan Xiong (Ligusticum)	6-9 gm.	*Rhizoma Ligustici Chuanxiong*

Action:

1. To speed up the process of pus formation
2. To replenish *Qi* (vital energy) and blood

Indication:

For a person with purulent deep-rooted boils and carbuncles

Modification:

To eliminate heat and toxin, add:

白 芷	Bai Zhi (Angelica)	*Radix Angelicae Dahuricae*
金銀花	Jin Yin Hua (Lonicera flower)	*Flos Lonicerae*
牛蒡子	Niu Bang Zi (Arctium fruit)	*Fructus Arctii*

This formula is also called Tou Nung San (透膿散)

Wán Dài Tāng　完帶湯
(Wan-Tai Tang)
(Decoction for Morbid Leukorrhea)

Constituents:

人 參	Ren Shen (Ginseng)	6-9 gm.	*Radix Ginseng*
白 术	Bai Zhu (White atractylodes)	20-30 gm.	*Rhizoma Atractylodis Macrocephalae*
山 藥	Shan Yao (Dioscorea)	20-30 gm.	*Radix Dioscoreae*
蒼 术	Cang Zhu (Atractylodes)	6-9 gm.	*Rhizoma Atractylodis*
陳 皮	Chen Pi (Citrus peel)	2-3 gm.	*Pericarpium Citri Reticulatae*
車前子	Che Qian Zi (Plantago seed)	6-9 gm.	*Semen Plantaginis*
白芍藥	Bai Shao Yao (White peony)	12-15 gm.	*Radix Paeoniae Alba*
柴 胡	Chai Hu (Bupleurum)	2-3 gm.	*Radix Bupleuri*
荊芥穗	Jing Jie Sui (Schizonepeta)	2-3 gm.	*Spica Schizonepetae*
甘 草	Gan Cao (Licorice)	2-3 gm.	*Radix Glycyrrhizae*

Action:

1. To strength the spleen and stomach
2. To eliminate dampness and leukorrhea

Indication:

For a person with hypofunction of the spleen, leukorrhea, color white or pale yellow, clear, odorless, face pale, malaise, stool loose.

Tongue: pale pink with white coat
Pulse: slow, soft or weak

Application:

Leukorrhea

Modification:

1. With severe low back pain, add:

菟絲子 Tu Si Zi (Dodder seed)　　　*Semen Cuscutae*
杜　仲 Du Zhong (Eucommia bark)　　*Cortex Eucommiae*

2. With Abdominal pain, add:

烏　药 Wu Yao (Lindera root)　　　*Radix Linderae*
茴　香 Hui Xiang (Fennel)　　　Fructus Foeniculi

Wěi Jīng Tāng　　葦莖湯
(Wei-Ching-Tang)
(Decoction of Phragmites Stem)

Constituents:

葦 莖 Wei Jing (Phragmites stem)	10-20 gm.	*Ramus Phragmitis*
薏苡仁 Yi Yi Ren (Coix)	10-20 gm.	*Semen Coicis*
冬瓜仁 Dong Gua Ren (Benincasa)	10-20 gm.	*Semen Benincasae*
桃 仁 Tao Ren (Persica seed)	5-10 gm.	*Semen Persicae*

Action:

1. To eliminate heat and phlegm in the lung
2. Anti-purulent

Indication:

For a person with lung abscess. The symptoms are: fever, cough with yellow and foul odor sputum, spitting blood, dull pain in the chest (especially while coughing), skin dry and squamous.

    Tongue: red with yellow and greasy coating
    Pulse: slippery and rapid

Application:

Lung abscess, measles, bronchitis, pneumonia, whooping cough.

Modification:

1. Before pustulation, add:
金銀花 Jin Yin Hua (Lonicera flower)　　*Flos Lonicerae*
魚腥草 Yu Xing Cao (Houttuynia)　　*Herba Houttuyniae*
2. After pustulation, add:
桔 梗 Jie Geng (Platycodon)　　*Radix Platycodi*
浙貝母 Zhe Bei Mu (Thunberg fritillary)　　*Bulbus Fritillariae Thunbergii*
甘 草 Gan Cao (Licorice)　　*Radix Glycyrrhizae*
3. For cough with profuse sputum, add:
浙貝母 Zhe Bei Mu (Thunberg fritillary)　　*Bulbus Fritillariae Thunbergii*
瓜蔞皮 Gua Lou Pi (Trichosanthes peel)　　*Pericarpium Trichosanthis*

Wèi Líng Tāng 胃苓湯

(Wei-Ling-Tang)

(Decoction to Dispel Dampness in the Spleen and Stomach)

Constituents:

澤	瀉	Ze Xie (Alisma)	9-12 gm.	*Rhizoma Alismatis*
茯	苓	Fu Ling (Poria)	6-9 gm.	*Poria*
豬	苓	Zhu Ling (Polyporus)	6-9 gm.	*Polyporus Umbellatus*
桂	枝	Gui Zhi (Cinnamon twig)	3-6 gm.	*Ramulus Cinnamomi*
白	术	Bai Zhu (White atractylodes)	6-9 gm.	*Rhizoma Atractylodis Macrocephalae*
蒼	术	Cang Zhu (Atractylodes)	6-9 gm.	*Rhizoma Atractylodis*
厚	朴	Hou Po (Magnolia bark)	6-9 gm.	*Cortex Magnoliae Officinalis*
陳	皮	Chen Pi (Citrus peel)	3-6 gm.	*Pericarpium Citri Recticulatae*
甘	草	Gan Cao (Licorice)	1-3 gm.	*Radix Glycyrrhizae*
生	薑	Sheng Jiang (Fresh ginger)	1-3 gm.	*Rhizoma Zingiberis Recens*
大	棗	Da Zao (Jujube)	3-5 pc.	*Fructus Ziziphus Jujubae*

Action:

1. To dispel the dampness in the spleen
2. To regulate the flow of vital energy in spleen and stomach (Carminative)

Indication:

For a person with dampness accumulated in the spleen and stomach. The symptoms are: abdominal fullness, loss of appetite, sensation of heaviness in the head and body, edema in face and the eyes, watery diarrhea, urination scanty.

> Tongue: with white and greasy coating
> Pulse: soft and thready

Application:

Chronic gastritis, gastric neurosis, ascites, nephritic and cardiac edema, enteritis, urinary retention, scrotal hydrocele.

Wēn Dǎn Tāng 溫胆湯

(Wen-Tan-Tang)
(The Gallbladder Warming Decoction)

Constituents:

半 夏	Ban Xia (Pinellia)	6-9 gm.	Rhizoma Pinelliae
陳 皮	Chen Pi (Citrus peel)	6-9 gm.	Pericarpium Citri Reticulatae
茯 苓	Fu Ling (Poria)	9-12 gm.	Poria
枳 實	Zhi Shi (Immature bitter orange)	6-9 gm.	Fructus Aurantii Immaturus
竹 茹	Zhu Ru (Bamboo shavings)	6-9 gm.	Caulus Bambusae in Taenis
甘 草	Gan Cao (Licorice)	1-3 gm.	Radix Glycyrrhizae
大 棗	Da Zao (Jujube)	3-5 pc.	Fructus Ziziphus Jujubae

Action:

1. Expectorant
2. Sedative

Indication:

For a person with profuse phlegm and timidity due to disharmony between liver and stomach. The symptoms are: profuse sputum of white color, foamy, nausea and vomiting, dizziness, palpitation, insomnia, restlessness, timidity.

> Tongue: white with greasy coating
> Pulse: slippery

Application:

Chronic tracheitis, bronchitis, pulmonary emphysema, insomnia, timidity.

Modification:

1. With biter mouth, vexation, add:
黄 連 Huang Lian (Coptis)　　　　Rhizoma Coptidis
This formula is called Huang Lian Wen Dan Tang (黃連溫胆湯)

2. With headache, dizziness, vertigo, nausea and vomiting, add:
藿 香 Huo Xiang (Agastache)　　Herba Agastachis
石菖蒲 Shi Chang Pu (Acorus)　　Rhizoma Acori Graminei

3. With summer heat and dampness, add:
青 蒿 Qing Hao (Sweet wormwood)　Herba Artemisiae Chinghao
黄 芩 Huang Qin (Scutellaria)　　Radix Scutellariae

Generic Name:

Bamboo and Hoelen Combination

Wēn Jīng Tāng   溫經湯
(Wen-Ching-Tang)
(The Collateral Warming Decoction)

Constituents:

吳茱萸	Wu Zhu Yu (Evodia fruit)	3-6 gm.	*Fructus Evodiae*
桂　枝	Gui Zhi (Cinnamon)	3-6 gm.	*Ramulus Cinnamomi*
當　歸	Dang Gui (Chinese angelica)	6-9 gm.	*Radix Angelicae Sinensis*
川　芎	Chuan Xiong (Ligusticum)	6-9 gm.	*Rhizoma Ligustici Chuanxiong*
白芍藥	Bai Shao Yao (White peony)	6-9 gm.	*Radix Paeoniae Alba*
阿　膠	E Jiao (Donkey-hide gelatin)	6-9 gm.	*Colla Corii Asini*
麥門冬	Mai Men Dong (Ophiopogon)	6-9 gm.	*Radix Ophiopogonis*
牡丹皮	Mu Dan Pi (Moutan bark)	6-9 gm.	*Cortex Moutan Radicis*
人　參	Ren Shen (Ginseng)	3-6 gm.	*Radix Ginseng*
半　夏	Ban Xia (Pinellia)	6-9 gm.	*Rhizoma Pinelliae*
生　薑	Sheng Jiang (Fresh ginger)	6-9 gm.	*Rhizoma Zingiberis Recens*
甘　草	Gan Cao (Licorice)	3-6 gm.	*Radix Glycyrrhizae*

Action:

1. To warm the channels and collaterals and dispel cold
2. To nourish blood and remove blood stasis

Indication:

For a person with irregular menstruation due to deficiency and coldness in the Chong (Vital) and Ren (Conception) channels. The symptoms are: irregular menstrual flow (early or delayed), increased body temperature in the evening, heat sensation in the palms and soles, mouth and throat dry, abdominal pain with coldness, incapability to conceive.

Application:

Irregular menstruation, dysmenorrhea, uterine bleeding, infertility, chronic pelvic inflammation.

Modification:

1. Severe abdominal pain and coldness, add:

艾　葉	Ai Ye (Artemisia)	*Folium Artemisiae Argyi*
肉　桂	Rou Gui (Cinnamon bark)	*Cortex Cinnamomi*

and eliminate: Dan Pi (丹皮) (Moutan bark), Mai Men Dong (麥門冬) (Ophiopogon) and Gui Zhi (桂枝) (Cinnamon twig).

2. Uterine bleeding, increased blood flow, color light, add:

艾　葉	Ai Ye (Artemisia)	*Folium Artemisiae Argyi*
熱地黃	Shu Di Huang (Prep. rehmannia)	*Radix Rehmanniae Praeparatae*

Generic Name:

Tang-kuei and Evodia Combination

Wēn Pí Tāng 溫脾湯
(Wen-Pi-Tang)
(The Spleen Warming Decoction)

Constituents:

大 黃 Da Huang (Rhubarb)	6-9 gm.	*Radix et Rhizoma Rhei*
附 子 Fu Zi (Aconite)	6-9 gm.	*Radix Aconiti Praeparatae*
人 參 Ren Shen (Ginseng)	3-6 gm.	*Radix Ginseng*
乾 薑 Gan Jiang (Dry ginger)	3-6 gm.	*Rhizoma Zingiberis*
甘 草 Gan Cao (Licorice)	3-6 gm.	*Radix Glycyrrhizae*

Action:

1. Cathartic
2. To replenish the spleen *Yang* (vital function)

Indication:

For a person with chronic diarrhea or constipation due to deficiency of spleen *Yang* (vital function). The symptoms are: constipation, or dysentery with blood and mucus, abdominal pain, hands and feet cold.

Tongue: pale with white coating
Pulse: deep and wiry/taut

Application:

Constipation, chronic bacterial dysentery, irritable colon, intestinal tuberculosis.

Modification:

1. With severe abdominal pain, add:

肉 桂 Rou Gui (Cinnamon bark)   *Cortex Cinnamomi*
木 香 Mu Xiang (Saussurea)   *Radix Saussureae*

2. With vomiting, add:

制半夏 Ban Xia (Pinellia)   *Rhizoma Pinelliae Praeparatae*
砂 仁 Sha Ren (Cardamon)   *Fructus Amomi*

Wǔ Líng Sàn　　五苓散

(Wu-Ling-San)
(Powder of Five Drugs with Poria)

Constituents:

澤　瀉	Ze Xie (Alisma)	9-12 gm.	*Rhizoma Alismatis*
茯　苓	Fu Ling (Poria)	6-9 gm.	*Poria*
豬　苓	Zhu Ling (Polyporus)	6-9 gm.	*Polyporus Umbellatus*
桂　枝	Gui Zhi (Cinnamon twig)	3-6 gm.	*Ramulus Cinnamomi*
白　术	Bai Zhu (White atractylodes)	6-9 gm.	*Radix Atractylodis Macrocephalae*

Action:

1. Diuretic
2. Diaphoretic
3. To strengthen the spleen

Indication:

1. For a person with interior accumulation of water and exterior symptom-complex. The symptoms are: fever, thirst, headache, edema, diarrhea, vomiting immediately after the intake of water, difficulty in urination.

> Tongue: white and slippery
> Pulse: floating and rapid

2. For a person with stagnation of water and dampness in the body, resulting in edema, diarrhea, dysuria, cholera, vomiting.

3. For a person with retention of fluid in the body, with manifestation of dizziness, spitting saliva, shortness of breath, cough, palpitation below the umbilicus.

Application:

Chronic nephritic edema, acute gastritis, cardiac edema, gastrectasis, ascites due to liver cirrhosis, urinary retention, scrotal hydrocele, acute enteritis, with diarrhea.

Modification:

1. With indigestion and dampness, resulting in diarrhea and decreased urination, eliminate:
桂　枝 Gui Zhi (Cinnamon twig)　　　*Ramulus Cinnamomi*
This formula is called Si Ling San (四苓散)

2. With jaundice and dysuria, add:
茵陳蒿 Yin Chen Hao (Capillaris)　　　*Herba Artemisiae Capillaris*
This formula is called Yin Chen Wu Ling San (茵陳五苓散)

Generic Name:

Hoelen Five Herbs Formula

Wū Méi Wán　　烏梅丸
(Wu-Mei-Wan)
(Pills of Mume/Black Plums)

Constituents:

烏 梅	Wu Mei (Mume; Black plum)	10-15 gm.	*Fructus Mume*
細 辛	Xi Xin (Asarum)	1-3 gm.	*Herba Asari*
乾 薑	Gan Jiang (Dry ginger)	6-9 gm.	*Rhizoma Zingiberis*
蜀 椒	Shu Jiao (Zanthoxylum)	1-3 gm.	*Pericarpium Zanthoxyli*
桂 枝	Gui Zhi (Cinnamon twig)	6-9 gm.	*Ramulus Cinnamomi*
附 子	Fu Zi (Aconite)	6-9 gm.	*Radix Aconiti Praeparatae*
黃 連	Huang Lian (Coptis)	3-6 gm.	*Rhizoma Coptidis*
黃 柏	Huang Bai (Phellodendron)	6-9 gm.	*Cortex Phellodendri*
人 參	Ren Shen (Ginseng)	6-9 gm.	*Radix Ginseng*
當 歸	Dang Gui (Chinese angelica)	6-9 gm.	*Radix Angelicae Sinensis*

Action:

1. To warm the internal visceras
2. To replenish the vital energy of the body
3. To dispel the parasites (Anthelmintic)

Indication:

For a person with coldness in the extremities due to ascaris infestation. The symptoms are: recurrent abdominal pain, vomiting (sometimes with ascaris), hands and feet cold, chronic diarrhea.

Tongue: map-like shedding
Pulse: hidden, or wiry and tight

Application:

Ascariasis, biliary ascariasis, chronic dysentery, chronic gastritis.

Modification:

1. To increase the anthelmintic effect, add:

使 君 子	Shi Jun Zi (quisqualis fruit)	*Fructus Quisqualis*
檳 榔	Bing Lang (Areca seed; Betel nut)	*Semen Arecae*
苦楝根皮	Ku Lian Gen Pi (Melia root-bark)	*Cortex Meliae Azedarachis*
榧 子	Fei Zi (Torreya nut)	*Semen Torreyae*

2. To excrete the parasite through stools, add:

大 黃	Da Huang (Rhubarb)	*Radix et Rhizoma Rhei*

3. If the hands and feet are not cold, subtract:

桂 枝	Gui Zi (Cinnamon twig)	*Ramulus Cinnamomi*
附 子	Fu Zi (Aconite)	*Radix Aconiti Praeparatae*

Generic Name:

Mume Formula

Wǔ Mó Yǐn Zǐ   五磨飲子

(Wu-Mo-Yin-Chih)
(Aromatic Formula with Five Herbs)

Constituents:

烏 藥	Wu Yao (Lindera root)	6-9 gm.	*Radix Linderae*
沉 香	Chen Xiang (Aquilaria wood)	6-9 gm.	*Lignum Aquilariae Resinatum*
木 香	Mu Xiang (Saussurea)	6-9 gm.	*Radix Saussureae*
檳 榔	Bing Lang (Areca seed)	6-9 gm.	*Semen Arecae*
枳 實	Zhi Shi (Immature bitter orange)	3-6 gm.	*Fructus Aurantii Immaturus*

Action:

To relieve the stagnant liver *Qi* in the lung and chest

Indication:

For a person with chest pain caused by stagnation of liver *Qi*. The symptoms are asthma, chest pain, irritability in the throat, insomnia, heart palpitation. The person may have coma with lockjaw and closed fist, and cold extremities.

> Tongue: with thin coat
> Pulse: wiry

Application:

Chest pain with phlegm and asthma, coma.

Modification:

1. With insomnia and palpitation, add:

酸棗仁	Suan Zao Ren (Wild jujube)	*Semen Ziziphi Spinosae*
遠 志	Yuan Zhi (Polygala root)	*Radix Polygalae*
茯 神	Fu Shen (Poria)	*Poria*
夜交藤	Ye Jiao Teng (Fleeceflower stem)	*Caulis Polygoni Multiflori*

2. With high blood pressure and dizziness, add:

鉤 藤	Gou Teng (Uncaria stem with hooks)	*Ramulus Uncariae cum Uncis*
石決明	Shi Jue Ming (Abalone shell)	*Concha Haliotidis*
磁 石	Ci Shi (Magnetite)	*Magnetitum*

3. With increased obstruction of phlegm, add:

胆南星	Dan Nan Xing (Processed arisaema)	*Rhizoma Arisaematis*
浙貝母	Zhe Bei Mu (Fritillary bulb)	*Bulbus Fritillariae Thunbergii*
橘 紅	Ju Hong (Tangerine peel)	*Pericarpium Citri Reticulatae*
竹 瀝	Zhu Li (Bamboo sap)	*Saccus Bambusae*

Wǔ Pí Yǐn (Wǔ Pí Sàn) 五皮飲 (五皮散)

(Wu-Pi-Yin, Wu-Pi-San)
(Decoction or Powder with Five Kinds of Peels)

Constituents:

茯苓皮 Fu Ling Pi (Poria peel)	9-12 gm.	*Poria*
桑白皮 Sang Bai Pi (Mulberry bark)	9-12 gm.	*Cortex Mori Radicis*
生薑皮 Sheng Jiang Pi (Ginger peel)	6-9 gm.	*Rhizoma Zingiberis Recens*
大腹皮 Da Fu Pi (Areca peel)	9-12 gm.	*Pericarpium Arecae*
陳　皮 Chen Pi (Citrus peel)	6-9 gm.	*Pericarpium Citri Reticulatae*

Actions:

1. Diuretic, to reduce edema
2. To strengthen the spleen and regulate *Qi* circulation

Indications:

For a person with edema due to retention of water in the skin caused by deficiency of spleen *Qi*. The symptoms are: edema over the whole body, heaviness sensation of the body, distention in the chest and abdomen, rapid breathing, dysuria.

Tongue: white and slippery
Pulse: thready, moderate, or slippery

Application:

Cardiac and nephritic edema, edema during pregnancy, generalized edema in the summer.

Modification:

1. Subtract Sang Bai Pi (Mulberry Bark) *Cortex Mori Radicis* and add:
五加皮 Wu Jia Pi (Acanthopanax Root Bark) *Cortex Acanthopanacis Radicis*
This formula is also called Wu Pi Yin (五皮飲)

2. Subtract Sang Bai Pi (Mulberry Bark) *Cortex Mori Radicis* and add:
白　术 Bai Zhu (White Atractylodes)　*Rhizoma Atractylodis Macrocephalae*
This formula is used for edema during pregnancy and is called Bai Zhu San (白术散)

3. For edema of the upper part of the body, add:
防　風 Fang Feng (Ledebouriella)　*Radix Ledebouriellae*
羌　活 Qiang Huo (Notopterygium)　*Rz. seu Rx. Notopterygii*

4. For edema of the lower part of the body, add:
防　己 Fang Ji (Stephania root)　*Radix Stephaniae Tetrandrae*
澤　瀉 Ze Xie (Alisma tuber)　*Rhizoma Alismatis*

Generic Name:

Hoelen and Areca Combination

Wū Tóu Tāng   烏頭湯 （乌头汤）
(Wu-Tou-Tang)
(Decoction of Sichuan Aconite)

Constituents:

川烏頭	Chuan Wu Tou (Sichuan aconite)	9-15 gm.	*Radix Aconiti*
麻 黃	Ma Huang (Ephedra)	6-9 gm.	*Herba Ephedrae*
黃 芪	Huang Qi (Astragalus)	6-15 gm.	*Radix Astragali*
白芍藥	Bai Shao Yao (White peony)	6-9 gm.	*Radix Paeoniae Alba*
炙甘草	Zhi Gan Cao (Baked licorice)	6-9 gm.	*Radix Glycyrrhizae Praeparatae*
蜂 蜜	Feng Mi (Honey)	60 gm.	

Action:

1. To dispel cold and reinforce the *Yang* (vital function)
2. To replenish *Qi* and blood
3. Analgesic

Indication:

For a person with arthritis due to cold. The symptoms ar: arthritic pain all over the body, difficulty in flexion and extension, severe pain, hands and feet cold.

Tongue: white and greasy coating
Pulse: deep and thready

Application:

Arthritis (due to cold), arthralgia.

Wǔ Wèi Xiāo Dú Yǐn   五味消毒飲

(Wu-Wei-Hsiao-Tu-Yin)
(The Antiseptic Decoction with Five Ingredients)

Constituents:

金銀花	Jin Yin Hua (Lonicera flower)	12-15 gm.	*Flos Lonicerae*
野菊花	Ye Ju Hua (Wild chrysanthemum)	9-12 gm.	*Flos Chrysanthemi*
紫花地丁	Zi Hua Di Ding (Viola)	12-15 gm.	*Herba Violae*
蒲公英	Pu Gong *Ying* (Dandelion)	12-15 gm.	*Herba Taraxaci*
天葵子	Tian Kui Zi (Semiaquilgia seed)	6-9 gm.	*Semen Semiaquilegiae*

Action:

1. To eliminate heat and toxin
2. Anti-inflammatory

Indication:

For a person with all kinds of boils and carbuncles with inflammations. The symptoms are: local inflammation with pus, deep-rooted boils, very firm/hard and painful.

Tongue: with yellow and greasy coating
Pulse: rapid

Application:

Deep-rooted boils, acne, carbuncles and furnacles.

Modification:

1. With severe heat, add:

黃連	Huang Lian (Coptis)	*Rhizoma Coptidis*
半枝蓮	Ban Zhi Lian (Barbat skullcap)	*Herba Scutellariae Barbatae*

2. With inflammation, add:

防風	Fang Feng (Ledebouriella)	*Radix Ledebouriellae*
蟬蛻	Chan Tui (Ciccada slough)	*Periostracum Cicadae*

3. With heat and toxin in blood (septicemia), add:

赤芍藥	Chi Shao Yao (Red peony)	*Radix Paeoniae Rubra*
牡丹皮	Mu Dan Pi (Moutan bark)	*Cortex Moutan Radicis*
生地黃	Sheng Di Huang (Fresh rehmannia)	*Radix Rehmanniae*

4. For abscess in the breasts, add:

瓜蔞皮	Gua Lou Pi (Trichosanthes peel)	*Pericarpium Trichosanthis*
浙貝母	Zhe Bei Mu (Fritillary bulb)	*Bulbus Fritillariae Thunbergii*
牡丹皮	Mu Dan Pi (Moutan bark)	*Cortex Moutan Radicis*

Wū Yào Shùn Qì Sàn   烏藥順氣散

(Wu-Yao-Shun-Chi-San)
(The Lindera Powder for Regulating Qi)

Constituents:

烏 藥	Wu Yao (Lindera)	10-15 gm.	*Radix Linderae*
僵 蠶	Jiang Can (Stiff silkworm)	3-6 gm.	*Bombyx Batryticatus*
川 芎	Chuan Xiong (Ligusticum)	6-9 gm.	*Rhizoma Ligustici Chuanxiong*
白 芷	Bai Zhi (Angelica root)	6-9 gm.	*Radix Angelicae Dahuricae*
麻 黃	Ma Huang (Ephedra)	6-9 gm.	*Herba Ephedrae*
桔 梗	Jie Geng (Platycodon)	6-9 gm.	*Radix Platycodi*
枳 殼	Zhi Ke (Mature bitter orange)	3-6 gm.	*Fructus Aurantii*
陳 皮	Chen Pi (Citrus peel)	3-6 gm.	*Pericarpium Citri Reticulatae*
乾 薑	Gan Jiang (Ginger)	3-6 gm.	*Rhizoma Zingiberis*
甘 草	Gan Cao (Licorice)	3-6 gm.	*Radix Glycyrrhizae*

Action:

1. To dispel wind by regulating the flow of *Qi* (external and internal)
2. To resolve the stagnation of phlegm

Indication:

For a person with stroke or cerebral hemorrhage. The symptoms are: muscle-ache, paralysis, hemiplegia, trigeminal neuralgia or Bell's palsy, difficulty of speech, deviation of the eyes and mouth, dyspnea.

> Tongue: with frothy or greasy coating
> Pulse: full/firm

Application:

Syncope, stroke, cerebral hemorrhage, hemiplegia, trigeminal neuralgia, Bell's palsy.

Generic Name:

Lindera Formula

Wú Zhū Yú Tāng　　吳茱萸湯

(Wu-Chu-Yu-Tang)
(Decoction of Evodia)

Constituents:

吳茱萸	Wu Zhu Yu (Evodia)	9-12 gm.	*Fructus Evodiae*
人　參	Ren Shen (Ginseng)	9-12 gm.	*Radix Ginseng*
生　薑	Sheng Jiang (Fresh ginger)	18-21 gm.	*Rhizoma Zingiberis Recens*
大　棗	Da Zao (Jujube)	4-6 pc.	*Fructus Ziziphus Jujubae*

Action:

1. To warm the liver and stomach
2. Anti-emetic

Indication:

For a person with deficiency and coldness of the liver and stomach. The symptoms are: headache, retch or vomit with saliva/mucus immediately after intake of food, acid regurgitation, abdominal pain, fullness in the epigastric region.

Tongue: pale with white and slippery coating
Pulse: slow and weak

Application:

Acute and chronic gastritis, morning sickness, neurotic headache, Meniere's disease.

Modification:

1. With increased vomiting, add:

半　夏	Ban Xia (Pinellia)	*Rhizoma Pinelliae*
陳　皮	Chen Pi (Citrus peel)	*Pericarpium Citri Reticulatae*
砂　仁	Sha Ren (Amomum fruit)	*Fructus Amomi*

2. With severe headache, add:

藁　本	Gao Ben (Straw seed)	*Rz. et Radix Ligustici Sinensis*
白　芷	Bai Zhi (Angelica)	*Radix Angelicae Dahuricae*
川　芎	Chuan Xiong (Chuanxiong)	*Rhizoma Ligustici Chuanxiong*
當　歸	Dang Gui (Chinese angelica)	*Radix Angelicae Sinensis*

Caution:

This decoction may induce further vomiting. It may be taken cold, or divided into smaller dosages.

Generic Name:

Evodia Combination

Xī Jiǎo Dì Huáng Tāng　　犀角地黄湯

(Hsi-Chiao-Ti-Huang-Tang)
(Decoction of Rhinoceros Horn and Rehmannia)

Constituents:

犀　角 Xi Jiao (Rhinoceros horn)	3-6 gm.	*Cornus Rhinoceri*
生地黄 Di Huang (Fresh rehmannia)	20-30 gm.	*Radix Rehmanniae*
赤芍藥 Chi Shao Yao (Red peony)	10-15 gm.	*Radix Paeoniae Rubra*
牡丹皮 Mu Dan Pi (Moutan bark)	9-12 gm.	*Cortex Moutan Radicis*

Action:

1. To dispel pathogenic heat from the *Xue* (Blood) system
2. To remove blood stasis by cooling effect.

Indication:

1. For a person with epidemic febrile diseases with pathogenic heat in the *Xue* (Blood) system. The symptoms are: high fever, delirium. Tongue dark red with prickly coating. Pulse thready and rapid.

2. For a person with excessive heat and random flow of blood, manifested by spitting blood, epistaxis, bloody stool, hematuria, macula colored purplish black. Tongue dark red with prickly fur.

3. For a person with syndromes of accumulated pathogenic heat and blood stasis, with black stools.

Application:

Acute leukemia, acute icteric hepatotrophy, uremia, hepatic coma, septicemia, boils, local inflammations.

Modification:

1. For spitting blood and epistasis, add:
白茅根 Bai Mao Gen (Imperata rhizome)　　*Rhizoma Imperatae*
側柏葉 Ce Bai Ye (Biota tops)　　*Cacumen Biotae*

2. For bloody stool, add:
槐　花 Huai Hua (Sophora flower)　　*Flos Sophorae*
紫　草 Zi Cao (Lithospermum)　　*Radix Lithospermi*

3. With mania, add:
黄　芩 Huang Qin (Scutellaria)　　*Radix Scutellariae*
大　黄 Da Huang (Rhubarb)　　*Radix et Rhizoma Rhei*

Generic Name:

Rhinoceros and Rehmannia Combination

Xiāng Rú Sàn   香薷散

(Hsiang-Ju-San)
(Decoction of Elsholtzia)

Constituents:

香 薷	Xiang Ru (Elsholtzia)	9-12 gm.	*Herba Elsholtziae*
白扁豆	Bai Bian Dou (Dolichos)	6-9 gm.	*Semen Dolichi*
厚 朴	Hou Po (Magnolia bark)	6-9 gm.	*Cortex Magnoliae Officinalis*

Action:

1. Diaphoretic
2. To dispel cold and dampness
3. To regulate the spleen and stomach

Indication:

For a person with exterior affection of cold, and interior dampness. The symptoms are: fever, intolerance of cold, headache, heavy sensation of the head, no perspiration, fullness sensation in the chest, fatigue, abdominal pain, vomiting, diarrhea.

Tongue: with white greasy coating
Pulse: floating

Application:

Common cold, heat-stroke, gastroenteritis, bacterial dysentery.

Contraindication:

For a person with common cold in the winter time.

Modification:

To clear the summer heat, add:
金銀花 Jin Yin Hua (Lonicera flower)   *Flos Lonicerae*
連 翹 Lian Qiao (Forsythia)   *Fructus Forsythiae*
This prescription is called Xin Jia Xiang Ru Yin (新加香薷飲)

Generic Name:

Elsholtzia Combination

Xiāng Shā Liù Jūn Zǐ Tāng   香砂六君子湯
(Hsiang-Sha-Liu-Chun Tzu-Tang)
(Saussurea, Cardamon and the Six Noble Ingredients Decoction)

Constituents:

木 香	Mu Xiang (Saussurea)	3-6 gm.	*Radix Saussureae*
砂 仁	Sha Ren (Cardamon)	3-6 gm.	*Fructus Amomi*
人 參	Ren Shen (Ginseng)	6-9 gm.	*Radix Ginseng*
白 术	Bai Zhu (White atractylodes)	6-9 gm.	*Rhizoma Atractylodis Macrocephalae*
茯 苓	Fu Ling (Poria)	6-9 gm.	*Poria*
陳 皮	Chen Pi (Citrus peel)	3-6 gm.	*Pericarpium Citri Reticulatae*
半 夏	Ban Xia (Pinellia)	6-9 gm.	*Rhizoma Pinelliae*
炙甘草	Zhi Gan Cao (Baked licorice)	3-6 gm.	*Radix Glycyrrhizae Praeparatae*

Action:

1. To replenish the vital energy of spleen and stomach
2. To relieve abdominal distention due to cold and dampness
3. To relieve morning-sickness

Indication:

For a person with weakness and asthenia of spleen and stomach. The symptoms are: abdominal pain (subtle), chest fullness, belching, nausea, vomiting, diarrhea, loss of appetite, emaciation.

> Tongue: pale with thin white coating
> Pulse: feeble and weak

Application:

Morning sickness, chronic gastritis, gastric and duodenal ulcer.

Modification:

1. For morning sickness, with cold tendency, add:
乾 薑 Gan Jiang (Dry ginger)   *Rhizoma Zingiberis*
2. For morning sickness, with heat tendency, add:
竹 茹 Zhu Ru (Bamboo shavings)   *Caulus Bambusae in Taenis*

Generic Name:

Aplotaxis-Amomum Pills;
Saussurea and Cardamon Combination

Xiāng Sū Sàn　香蘇散

(Hsiang-Su-San)

(Decoction of Cyperus and Perilla Leaf)

Constituents:

香　附	Xiang Fu (Cyperus)	6-9 gm.	*Rhizoma Cyperi*
紫蘇葉	Zi Su Ye (Perilla leaf)	6-9 gm.	*Folium Perillae*
陳　皮	Chen Pi (Citrus peel)	3-6 gm.	*Pericarpium Citri Reticulate*
炙甘草	Zhi Gan Cao (Baked licorice)	3-6 gm.	*Radix Glycyrrhizae Praeparatae*

Action:

1. Diaphoretic
2. Carminative

Indication:

For a person with exterior affection of wind and cold, and interior stagnation of vital energy. The symptoms are: fever, headache, belching, loss of appetite, fullness and oppression in the chest and abdomen.

Tongue: with thin white coating
Pulse: floating

Application:

Common cold (G-I type).

Modification:

1. To increase the diaphoretic effect, add:

葱　白	Cong Bai (Allium bulb)	*Bulbus Allii Fistulosumi*
淡豆豉	Dan Dou Chi (Prepared soybean)	*Semen Sojae Praepartatum*

This formula is called Xiang Su Cong Chi Tang (香蘇葱豉湯)

2. With hiccough, cough with white sputum, add:

紫蘇子	Zi Su Zi (Perilla seed)	*Fructus Perillae*
半　夏	Ban Xia (Pinellia)	*Rhizoma Pinelliae*

3. With abdominal fullness, add:

枳　殼	Zhi Ke (Bitter orange)	*Fructus Aurantii*
厚　朴	Hou Po (Magnolia bark)	*Cortex Magnoliae Officinalis*

4. With indigestion, add:

麥　芽	Mai Ya (Germinated barley)	*Fructus Hordei Germinatus*
神　曲	Shen Qu (Medicated leaven)	*Massa Fermentata Medicinalis*

Generic Name:

Cyperus and Perilla Formula

Xiǎo Chái Hú Tāng   小柴胡湯

(Hsiao-Chai-Hu-Tang)
(Minor Bupleurum Decoction)

Constituents:

柴 胡	Chai Hu (Bupleurum)	12-15 gm.	*Radix Bupleuri*
黄 芩	Huang Qin (Scutellaria)	9-12 gm.	*Radix Scutellariae*
半 夏	Ban Xia (Pinellia)	9-12 gm.	*Rhizoma Pinelliae*
生 薑	Sheng Jiang (Fresh ginger)	3-6 gm.	*Rhizoma Zingiberis Recens*
人 參	Ren Shen (Ginseng)	6-9 gm.	*Radix Ginseng*
甘 草	Gan Cao (Licorice)	3-6 gm.	*Radix Glycyrrhizae*
大 棗	Da Zao (Jujube)	3-5 pc.	*Fructus Ziziphus Jujubae*

Action:

To mediate the Shao-yang (Minor Yang) channel and to treat febrile diseases while the pathogenic factors are neither superficial nor deep-entrenched.

Indication:

For a person with syndrome of the Shao-yang channel which runs between the exterior and interior of the body. The symptoms are: alternate fever and chills, fullness and choking feeling in the chest and costal regions, bitterness in the mouth, dry throat, dizziness, loss of appetite, may tend to vomit.

> Tongue: with thin white coating
> Pulse: wiry/taut

Application:

Malaria, cholecystitis, hepatitis, jaundice, amenorrhea.

Modification:

1. For malaria, add:

常 山	Chang Shan (Dichroa root)	*Radix Dichroae*
草 果	Cao Guo (Tsaoko)	*Fructus Tsao-ko*

2. With deficiency of *Yin* (vital essence), add:

鱉 甲	Bie Jia (Tortoise shell)	*Carapax Trionycis*
青 蒿	Qing Hao (Sweet wormwood)	*Herba Artemisiae Chinghao*

3. With abdominal fullness and pain, add:

延胡索	Yan Hu Suo (Corydalis tuber)	*Rhizoma Corydalis*
香 附	Xiang Fu (Cyperus tuber)	*Rhizoma Cyperi*
枳 實	Zhi Shi (Immature bitter orange)	*Fructus Aurantii Immaturus*

Generic Name:

Minor Bupleurum Decoction

Xiǎo Chéng Qì Tāng   小承氣湯

(Hsiao-Cheng-Chi-Tang)
(Less Drastic Purgative Decoction)

Constituents:

大 黃	Da Huang (Rhubarb)	9-12 gm.	*Radix et Rhizoma Rhei*
厚 朴	Hou Po (Magnolia bark)	6-9 gm.	*Cortex Magnoliae Officinalis*
枳 實	Zhi Shi (Immature bitter orange)	6-9 gm.	*Fructus Aurantii Immaturus*

Action:

To eliminate the intense heat in the stomach and the intestines.
(Cold purgative)

Indication:

For a person with intense heat in the visceras related with the Yang-ming
(the stomach and intestines) channel. The symptoms are: tidal fever,
sweating from the hands and feet, fullness in the chest and epigastric
region, constipation, delirium, abdominal distention, tenesmus.

Tongue: with yellow coating
Pulse: slippery and swift

Application:

Acute simple intestinal obstruction, acute cholecystitis, acute
appendicitis, constipation.

Generic Name:

Minor Rhubarb Combination

Xiāo Fēng Sàn 消風散
(Hsiao-Feng-San)
(Formula for Dispersing Pathogenic Wind)

Constituents:

荆 芥	Jing Jie (Schizonepeta)	3-6 gm.	*Herba Schizonepetae*
防 風	Fang Feng (Ledebouriella)	3-6 gm.	*Radix Ledebouriellae*
牛蒡子	Niu Bang Zi (Arctium)	3-6 gm.	*Fructus Arctii*
蟬 蛻	Chan Tui (Cicada slough)	3-6 gm.	*Periostracum Cicadae*
蒼 朮	Cang Zhu (Atractylodes)	3-6 gm.	*Rhizoma Atractylodis*
苦 參	Ku Shen (Sophora root)	3-6 gm.	*Radix Sophorae*
木 通	Mu Tong (Akebia stem)	3-6 gm.	*Caulis Akebiae*
煅石膏	Duan Shi Gao (Calcinized gypsum)	3 gm.	*Gypsum Fibrosum*
知 母	Zhi Mu (Anemarrhena)	3-6 gm.	*Rhizoma Anemarrhenae*
生地黄	Sheng Di Huang (Rehmannia)	3-6 gm.	*Radix Rehmanniae*
當 歸	Dang Gui (Chinese angelica)	3-6 gm.	*Radix Angelicae Sinensis*
胡麻仁	Hu Ma Ren (Cannabis seed)	3-6 gm.	*Fructus Cannabis*
甘 草	Gan Cao (Licorice)	2-3 gm.	*Radix Glycyrrhizae*

Action:

1. Eliminate heat and disperse pathogenic wind
2. Stop itching, eliminate dampness

Indication:

For a person with eczema and urticaria with inflamed papules and itchiness.

Tongue: pink with white or yellow coating
Pulse: floating, rapid and forceful

Application:

Eczema, urticaria, rubella, dermatitis (allergenic, neurogenic, and drug-related), tinea capitis.

Modification:

1. With excessive pathogenic wind, add:

連 翹	Lian Qiao (Forsythia)	*Fructus Forsythiae*
金銀花	Jin Yin Hua (Honeysuckle)	*Fructus Lonicerae*

2. With excessive heat in blood, add:

赤芍藥	Chi Shao Yao (Red peony)	*Radix Paeoniae Rubra*
紫 草	Zi Cao (Lithospermum)	*Radix Lithospermi*

3. With excessive heat and dampness, add:

地膚子	Di Fu Zi (Kochia fruit)	*Fructus Kochiae*
車前子	Che Qian Zi (Plantago seed)	*Semen Plantaginis*

Xiǎo Huó Luò Dān 小活絡丹

(Hsiao-Huo-Luo-Tan)
(Pills for Activating Circulation in Collateral Channels—Minor)

Constituents:

川烏頭	Chuan Wu Tou (Sichuan aconite)	180 gm.	*Radix Aconiti*
草烏頭	Cao Wu Tou (Aconite)	180 gm.	*Radix Aconiti Transsecti*
天南星	Tian Nan Xing (Arisaema)	180 gm.	*Rhizoma Arisaematis*
地 龍	Di Long (Earthworm)	180 gm.	*Lumbricus*
乳 香	Ru Xiang (Mastic)	60 gm.	*Resina Olibani*
沒 藥	Mo Yao (Myrrh)	60 gm.	*Resina Myrrhae*

Grind the above ingredients into powder and made into pills.

Take 1-2 pills each time, twice daily.

Action:

1. To warm the channels and collaterals
2. To dispel wind and dampness
3. To resolve phlegm and stagnant blood

Indication:

1. For a person with stroke, numbness or paralysis of the hands and feet for a long period of time, pain in the arms and legs.

2. For a person with wind, cold and dampness in the channels and collaterals, with difficulty of muscle movements, wandering pain, and muscle spasms.

Application:

Apoplexy, arthritis, cerebral vascular accident.

Contraindication:

For a pregnant woman; a person with low graded fever due to deficiency of *Yin* (vital essence).

Generic Name:

Xiao Huo Luo Dan

Xiǎo Jì Yǐn Zǐ　　小薊飲子

(Hsiao-Chi-Yin-Tzu)
(Decoction of Small Thistle)

Constituents:

生地黄	Sheng Di Huang (Fresh rehmannia)	15-20 gm.	*Radix Rehmanniae*
小 薊	Xiao Ji (Small thistle)	10-15 gm.	*Herba Cephalanoploris*
炒蒲黄	Pu Huang (Bulrush pollen)	6-9 gm.	*Pollen Typhae*
藕 節	Ou Jie (Lotus node)	6-9 gm.	*Nodus Nelumbinis Rhizomatis*
滑 石	Hua Shi (Talc)	10-15 gm.	*Talcum*
木 通	Mu Tong (Akebia)	3-6 gm.	*Caulis Akebiae*
淡竹葉	Dan Zhu Ye (Lophatherum)	6-9 gm.	*Herba Lophatheri*
梔 子	Zhi Zi (Gardenia fruit)	6-9 gm.	*Fructus Gardeniae*
當 歸	Dang Gui (Chinese angelica)	6-9 gm.	*Radix Angelicae Sinensis*
炙甘草	Zhi Gan Cao (Baked licorice)	3-6 gm.	*Radix Glycyrrhizae Praeparatae*

Action:

1. To cool blood and stop bleeding
2. To eliminate heat

Indication:

For a person with hematuria. The symptoms are: urination with burning pain and heat sensation, urine with blood, color purplish red, with blood clots.

  Tongue: red with yellow coating
  Pulse: rapid and forceful

Application:

Hematuria

Xiǎo Jiàn Zhōng Tāng   小建中湯
(Hsiao-Chien-Chung-Tang)
(Minor Decoction for Restoring the Normal Function of the Middle Burner)

Constituents:

飴 糖	Yi Tang (Maltose)	20-30 gm.	*Saccharum Granorum*
桂 枝	Gui Zhi (Cinnamon twig)	6-9 gm.	*Ramulus Cinnamomi*
白芍藥	Bai Shao Yao (White peony)	10-15 gm.	*Radix Paeoniae Alba*
炙甘草	Zhi Gan Cao (Baked licorice)	3-6 gm.	*Radix Glycyrrhizae*
生 薑	Sheng Jiang (Fresh ginger)	3-6 gm.	*Rhizoma Zingiberis Recens*
大 棗	Da Zao (Jujube)	3-5 pc.	*Fructus Ziziphus Jujubae*

Action:

1. To warm and tonify the spleen and stomach
2. To replenish vital energy
3. To relieve spasmodic pain

Indication:

1. For a person with consumptive disease due to asthenia and accumulation of cold in the spleen and stomach. The symptoms are: abdominal pain (relieved by warmth and pressure) and spasms.

2. For a person with consumptive disease due to deficiency of both *Yin* (vital essence) and *Yang* (vital function), with manifestation of palpitation and vexation.

3. For a person with consumptive disease due to febrile diseases with high fever.

Application:

1. For postpartum weakness, with abdominal pain and spasms, add:
當 歸 Dang Gui (Chinese angelica)   *Radix Angelicae Sinensis*
This formula is called Dang Gui Jian Zhong Tang (當歸健中湯)

2. With dyspnea and spontaneous perspiration, add:
黃 芪 Huang Qi (Astragalus)   *Radix Astragali*
This formula is called Huang Qi Jian Zhong Tang (黃芪建中湯)

Generic Name:

Minor Cinnamon and Peony Combination

Xiāo Luǒ Wán   消瘰丸

(Hsiao-Luo-Wan)
(Pills for Goiter)

Constituents:

浙貝母	Zhe Bei Mu (Thunberg fritillary bulb)	10-15 gm.	*Bulbus Fritillariae Thunbergii*
牡 蠣	Mu Li (Oyster shell)	15-20 gm.	*Concha Ostreae*
玄 參	Xuan Shen (Scrophularia)	10-15 gm.	*Radix Scrophulariae*

Action:

1. To eliminate heat and resolve phlegm
2. To soften hardening and disperse lumps

Indication:

For goiter, scrofula, subcutaneous nodule caused by the accumulation of phlegm and fire. The symptoms are: hard lumps or nodules anterior or posterior to the ear, no change in skin color, throat dry, mouth bitter.

Application:

Simple goiter, hyperthyroidism, thyroiditis, acute simple lymphadenitis.

Modification:

1. If the nodule is hard and large, increase the dosage of Mu Li 牡 蠣 (Oyster shell) and add:

昆 布	Kun Bu (Ecklonia)	*Thallus Eckloniae*
海 藻	Hai Zao (Sargassum)	*Sargassum*
夏枯草	Xia Ku Cao (Prunella spike)	*Spica Prunellae*

2. With increased fire and phlegm, add:

知 母	Zhi Mu (Anemarrhena rhizome)	*Rhizoma Anemarrhenae*
牡丹皮	Mu Dan Pi (Moutan bark)	*Cortex Moutan Radicis*

3. With stagnancy of vital energy in liver, add:

柴 胡	Chai Hu (Bupleurum)	*Radix Bupleuri*
香 附	Xiang Fu (Cyperus tuber)	*Rhizoma Cyperi*
青 皮	Qing Pi (Green tangerine peel)	*Pericarpium Citri Reticulatae Viridae*

Xiǎo Qīng Lóng Tāng　　小青龍湯

(Hsiao-Ching-Lung-Tang)
(Minor Decoction of Blue Dragon)

Constituents:

麻 黄	Ma Huang (Ephedra)	6-9 gm.	*Herba Ephedrae*
桂 枝	Gui Zhi (Cinnamon twig)	9-12 gm.	*Ramulus Cinnamomi*
白芍藥	Bai Shao Yao (White peony)	9-12 gm.	*Radix Paeoniae Alba*
乾 薑	Gan Jiang (Dry ginger)	9-12 gm.	*Rhizoma Zingiberis*
細 辛	Xi Xin (Asarum)	6-9 gm.	*Herba Asari*
五味子	Wu Wei Zi (Schisandra)	9-12 gm.	*Fructus Schisandrae*
半 夏	Ban Xia (Pinellia)	9-12 gm.	*Rhizoma Pinelliae*
炙甘草	Zhi Gan Cao (Baked licorice)	3-6 gm.	*Radix Glycyrrhizae Praeparatae*

Action:

1. Diaphoretic
2. To dispel cold and resolve stagnation of water or fluids
3. To warm the lung

Indication:

For a person with exterior affection of wind and cold, and interior stagnation of water or body fluids. The symptoms are: fever, intolerance of cold, cough, dyspnea, shortness of breath, fullness sensation in the chest, edema with heaviness sensation of the body, no perspiration.

> Tongue: white with greasy coating
> Pulse: floating

Application:

Common cold, influenza, chronic asthmatic bronchitis, bronchial asthma, pulmonary emphysema.

Modification:

1. With internal heat and irritability, add:

石 膏 Shi Gao (Gypsum)　　　　　*Gypsum Fibrosum*

This formula called Xiao Qing Long Jia Shi Gao Tang. (小青龍加石膏湯)

2. With cough, add:

杏 仁 Xing Ren (Apricot seed)　　　　*Semen Armeniacae Amarum*

Generic Name:

Minor Blue Dragon Combination

Xiǎo Xiàn Xiōng Tāng　　小陷胸湯
(Hsiao-Hsien-Hsiung-Tang)
(Minor Decoction Sinking into the Chest)

Constituents:

黄 連	Huang Lian (Coptis)	1-3 gm.	*Rhizoma Coptidis*
半 夏	Ban Xia (Pinellia)	3-6 gm.	*Rhizoma Pinelliae*
瓜蔞仁	Gua Lou Ren (Trichosanthes seed)	9-12 gm.	*Semen Trichosanthis*

Action:

To eliminate heat and phlegm in the chest (Cold purgative)

Indication:

For a person with obstruction of heat and phlegm in the chest. The symptoms are: distention and oppression in the chest and epigastric region, painful if pressed, spitting sticky and yellow sputum.

Tongue: with yellow and greasy coating
Pulse: floating and slippery; or slippery and rapid

Application:

Pleurisy with effusion, bronchitis.

Modification:

1. With intermittent fever, hypochondriac pain, add:

柴 胡	Chai Hu (Bupleurum)	*Radix Bupleuri*
黄 芩	Huang Qin (Scutellaria)	*Radix Scutellariae*
枳 實	Zhi Shi (Immature bitter orange)	*Fructus Aurantii Immaturus*
桔 梗	Jie Geng (Platycodon)	*Radix Platycodi*
生 薑	Sheng Jiang (Fresh ginger)	*Rhizoma Zingiberis Recens*

This formula is called Chai Hu Xian Xiong Tang (柴胡陷胸湯)

2. With nausea and vomiting, add:

竹 茹	Zhu Ru (Bamboo shavings)	*Caulus Bambusae in Taenis*
生 薑	Sheng Jiang (Fresh ginger)	*Rhizoma Zingiberis Recens*

3. With thick and sticky sputum, add:

胆南星	Dan Nan Xing (Arisaema tuber)	*Rhizoma Arisaematis*
浙貝母	Zhe Bei Mu (Thunberg fritillary bulb)	*Bulbus Fritillarieae Thunbergii*

Generic Name:

Minor Trichosanthes Combination

Xiāo Yáo Sàn 逍遙散

(Hsiao-Yao-San)
(The Ease Powder)

Constituents:

柴 胡	Chai Hu (Bupleurum)	6-9 gm.	*Radix Bupleuri*
當 歸	Dang Gui (Chinese angelica)	6-9 gm.	*Radix Angelicae Sinensis*
白芍藥	Bai Shao Yao (White peony)	9-12 gm.	*Radix Paeoniae Alba*
白 术	Bai Zhu (White atractylodes)	6-9 gm.	*Rhizoma Atractylodis Macrocephalae*
茯 苓	Fu Ling (Poria)	9-15 gm.	*Poria*
薄 荷	Bo He (Mentha)	1-3 gm.	*Herba Mentha*
生 薑	Sheng Jiang (Fresh ginger)	1-3 gm.	*Rhizoma Zingiberis Recens*
炙甘草	Zhi Gan Cao (Baked licorice)	3-6 gm.	*Radix Glycyrrhizae Praeparatae*

Action:

1. To regulate/coordinate the function of liver and spleen
2. To relieve the stagnation of vital energy in liver
3. To replenish blood

Indication:

For a person with anemia and stagnancy of *Qi* (vital energy) in liver and spleen. The symptoms are: costal pain, headache, dizziness, mouth and throat dry, lassitude, loss of appetite, irregular menstruation, breast distention, alternate chills and fever as in malaria.

> Tongue: pale red
> Pulse: wiry/taut and feeble

Application:

Chronic hepatitis, irregular menstruation, uterine bleeding, leukorrhea, breast distention.

Modification:

Chronic hepatitis, irregular menstruation, uterine bleeding, leukorrhea, breast distention.

Modification:

For chronic hepatitis, add:

茜草根	Xi Cao Gen (Rubia root)	*Radix Rubiae*
海螵蛸	Hai Piao Xiao (Cuttlefish bone)	*Os Sepiae*
黨 參	Dang Shen (Codonopsis)	*Radix Codonopsis Pilosulae*

Generic Name:

Hsiao Yao Wan;
Bupleurum and Tang-kuei Formula

Xiè Bái Sàn (Xiè Fèi Sàn)   瀉白散 （瀉肺散）
(Hsieh-Pai-San) (Hsieh-Fei-San)
(Powder to Purge the Lung Heat)

Constituents:

地骨皮	Di Gu Pi (Lycium bark)	10-20 gm.	*Cortex Lycii Radicis*
桑白皮	Sang Bai Pi (Morus bark)	10-20 gm.	*Cortex Mori Radicis*
炙甘草	Zhi Gan Cao (Baked licorice)	3-6 gm.	*Radix Glycyrrhizae Praeparatae*
粳 米	Jing Mi (Oryza)	15 gm.	*Semen Oryzae*

Action:

1. To purge the hidden heat in the lung (Febrifugal)
2. Antitussive and anti-asthmatic

Indication:

For a person with cough and asthma due to hidden heat in the lung. The symptoms are: cough, asthma, dyspnea, mouth and throat dry, afternoon fever, hemoptysis.

      Tongue: red with yellow coating
      Pulse: thready and rapid

Application:

Asthma, cough, infantile measles, infantile pneumonia, tracheitis.

Modification:

1. With intense heat in lung channel, add:

黃 芩	Huang Qin (Scutellaria)	*Radix Scutellariae*
知 母	Zhi Mu (Anemarrhena)	*Rhizoma Anemarrhenae*

2. With dry heat and cough, add:

瓜蔞皮	Gua Lou Pi (Trichosanthes peel)	*Pericarpium Trichosanthis*
川貝母	Chuan Bei Mu (Tendrilled fritillary)	*Bulbus Fritillariae Cirrhosae*

3. With tidal fever in the afternoon, add:

青 蒿	Qing Hao (Sweet wormwood)	*Herba Artemisiae Chinghao*
鱉 甲	Bie Jia (Tortoise shell)	*Carapax Trionycis*
銀柴胡	Yin Chai Hu (Stellaria root)	*Radix Stellariae*

4. With thirst and irritable fever, add:

天花粉	Tian Hua Fen (Trichosanthes root)	*Radix Trichosanthis*
知 母	Zhi Mu (Anemarrhena)	*Rhizoma Anemarrhenae*

Generic Name:

Morus and Lycium Formula

Xiè Xīn Tāng (Sān Huáng Xiè Xīn Tāng)
瀉心湯 (三黄瀉心湯)
(Hsieh-Hsin-Tang, San-Huang-Hsieh-Hsin-Tang)
(Decoction to Purge Heat from Heart and Stomach)

Constituents:

大	黃	Da Huang (Rhubarb)	10-15 gm.	*Radix et Rhizoma Rhei*
黃	連	Huang Lian (Coptis)	6-9 gm.	*Rhizoma Coptidis*
黃	芩	Huang Qin (Scutellaria)	9-12 gm.	*Radix Scutellariae*

Action:

To dispel noxious heat and toxin from the heart and stomach (Febrifugal)

Indication:

For a person with noxious heat or fire in the heart and stomach. The symptoms are: fever, face red, eyes red, fidgetiness, insomnia, thirsty, urine yellow, suppurative infection on the skin, bleeding.

> Tongue: tip red with yellow greasy coating
> Pulse: rapid

Application:

Febrile disease, spitting blood, epistaxis, erysipelas, septicemia induced by boils and carbuncles, ulceration of the oral cavity, dysentery, hepatitis.

Modification:

1. With profuse perspiration and cold limbs, add:
附 子 Fu Zi (Aconite)   *Radix Aconiti Praeparatae*
This formula is called Fu Zi Xie Xin Tang (附子瀉心湯)

2. With mouth and tongue dry, add:
天花粉 Tian Hua Fen (Trichosanthes root)   *Radix Trichosanthis*
蘆 根 Lu Gen (Phragmites rhizome)   *Rhizoma Phragmitis*

3. With increased heat and dampness, add:
厚 朴 Hou Po (Magnolia bark)   *Cortex Magnoliae Officinalis*
半 夏 Ban Xia (Pinellia)   *Rhizoma Pinelliae*

4. With severe abdominal pain, add:
延胡索 Yan Hu Suo (Corydalis tuber)   *Rhizoma Corydalis*
木 香 Mu Xiang (Saussurea root)   *Radix Saussureae*
川楝子 Chuan Lian Zi (Sichuan chinaberry) *Fructus Meliae Toosendan*
枳 殼 Zhi Ke (Bitter orange)   *Fructus Aurantii*

Generic Name:

Coptis and Rhubarb Combination

Xīn Yí Sàn　　　辛夷散

(Hsin-I-San)
(Powder of Magnolia Flower)

Constituents:

辛	夷	Xin Yi (Magnolia flower)	6-9 gm.	*Flos Magnoliae*
細	辛	Xi Xin (Asarum)	3-6 gm.	*Herba Asari*
藁	本	Gao Ben (Straw seed)	6-9 gm.	*Rhizoma et Radix Ligustici*
防	風	Fang Feng (Ledebouriella)	6-9 gm.	*Radix Ledebouriellae*
白	芷	Bai Zhi (Angelica)	6-9 gm.	*Radix Angelicae Dahuricae*
川	芎	Chuan Xiong (Ligusticum)	6-9 gm.	*Rz. Ligustici Chuanxiong*
升	麻	Sheng Ma (Cimicifuga)	6-9 gm.	*Rhizoma Cimicifugae*
木	通	Mu Tong (Akebia)	6-9 gm.	*Caulis Akebiae*
甘	草	Gan Cao (Licorice)	3-6 gm.	*Radix Glycyrrhizae*

Action:

1. To disperse wind and cold
2. To open the nasal orifices

Indication:

For a person with symptoms of stuffy nose, profuse nasal discharges, loss of smell, difficulty of breathing.

> Tongue: with white coating
> Pulse: floating and tight

Application:

Stuffy nose, nasal sinusitis, chronic rhinitis, allergic rhinitis, accessary nasal sinuses.

Xìng Sū Sàn 杏蘇散
(Hsing-Su-San)
(Powder of Apricot Seed and Perilla)

Constituents:

杏　仁	Xing Ren (Apricot seed)	6-9 gm.	*Semen Armeniacae Amarum*
紫蘇葉	Zi Su Ye (Perilla leaf)	6-9 gm.	*Folium Perillae*
枳　殼	Zhi Ke (Bitter orange)	6-9 gm.	*Fructus Aurantii*
桔　梗	Jie Geng (Platycodon)	6-9 gm.	*Radix Platycodi*
前　胡	Qian Hu (Peucedanum)	6-9 gm.	*Radix Peucedani*
橘　皮	Ju Pi (Citrus peel)	3-6 gm.	*Pericarpium Citri Reticulatae*
半　夏	Ban Xia (Pinellia)	6-9 gm.	*Rhizoma Pinelliae*
茯　苓	Fu Ling (Poria)	9-12 gm.	*Poria*
生　薑	Sheng Jiang (Fresh ginger)	3-6 gm.	*Rhizoma Zingiberis Recens*
甘　草	Gan Cao (Licorice)	3-6 gm.	*Radix Glycyrrhizae*
大　棗	Da Zao (Jujube)	3-5 pc.	*Fructus Ziziphus Jujubae*

Action:

1. Diaphoretic
2. To dispel wind and cold
3. To soothe the lung and relieve cough

Indication:

For a person with exterior affection of wind and cold, and interior stagnation of phlegm and dampness. The symptoms are: headache, no perspiration, intolerance of cold, cough with thin sputum, nasal obstruction, cough.

     Tongue: white coating
     Pulse: wiry/taut

Application:

Common cold, chronic tracheitis, bronchiectasis, pulmonary emphysema.

Modification:

1. With perspiration, pulse wiry and tight, add:
羌　活 Qiang Huo (Notopterygium)   *Rhizoma seu Radix Notopterygii*
2. With diarrhea and abdominal fullness, add:
蒼　术 Cang Zhu (Atractylodes)   *Rhizoma Atractylodis*
厚　朴 Hou Po (Magnolia bark)   *Cortex Magnoliae Officinalis*
3. With supra-orbital headache, add:
白　芷 Bai Zhi (Angelica root)   *Radix Angelicae Dahuricae*
4. With interior heat, add:
黄　芩 Huang Qin (Scutellaria)   *Radix Scutellariae*

Generic Name:

Apricot Seed and Perilla Formula

Xuán Fù Dài Zhĕ Tāng　　旋覆代赭湯
(Hsuan-Fu-Tai-Che-Tang)
(Decoction of Inula Flower and Hematite)

Constituents:

旋覆花	Xuan Fu Hua (Inula flower)	6-9 gm.	*Flos Inulae*
代赭石	Dai Zhe Shi (Hematite)	10-15 gm.	*Haematitum*
人　參	Ren Shen (Ginseng)	3-6 gm.	*Radix Ginseng*
半　夏	Ban Xia (Pinellia tuber)	6-9 gm.	*Rhizoma Pinelliae*
生　薑	Sheng Jiang (Fresh ginger)	9-12 gm.	*Rhizoma Zingiberis Recens*
炙甘草	Zhi Gan Cao (Baked licorice)	3-6 gm.	*Radix Glycyrrhizae Praeparatae*
大　棗	Da Zao (Jujube)	10-12 pc.	*Fructus Ziziphus Jujubae*

Action:

1. To regulate the stomach and the flow of stomach *Qi* (vital energy)
2. Expectorant, anti-hiccup

Indication:

For a person with phlegm obstruction due to deficiency of *Qi* (vital energy) and upward flow of stomach *Qi*. The symptoms are: epigastric obstruction, hiccup, vomiting with saliva and sputum, nausea, belching, abdominal distention.

      Tongue: white and slippery
      Pulse: wiry/taut and feeble

Application:

Nervous regurgitation, gastro-intestinal neurosis, gastrectasis, incomplete pyloric obstruction, gastric or duodenal ulcer

Contraindication:

For nausea and vomiting due to pregnancy.

Modification:

1. With greasy tongue coating due to phlegm and dampness, add:

厚　朴	Hou Po (Magnolia bark)	*Cortex Magnoliae Officinalis*
茯　苓	Fu Ling (Poria)	*Poria*
陳　皮	Chen Pi (Citrus peel)	*Pericarpium Citri Reticulatae*

2. If the stomach *Qi* (vital energy) is not deficient, eliminate:

人　參	Ren Shen (Ginseng)	*Radix Ginseng*
炙甘草	Zhi Gan Cao (Baked licorice)	*Radix Glycyrrhizae Praeparata*
大　棗	Da Zao (Jujube)	*Fructus Ziziphus Jujubae*

3. If the stomach is very cold, use dry ginger (乾薑) instead of fresh ginger. (生薑)

Generic Name:

Inula and Hematite Combination

Xuè Fǔ Zhú Yū Tāng 血府逐瘀湯

(Hsieh-Fu-Chu-Yu-Tang)

(Decoction for Removing Blood Stasis in Chest)

Constituents:

桃 仁	Tao Ren (Persica seed)	9-12 gm.	*Semen Persicae*
紅 花	Hong Hua (Carthamus)	6-9 gm.	*Flos Carthami*
當 歸	Dang Gui (Chinese angelica)	6-9 gm.	*Radix Angelicae Sinensis*
川 芎	Chuan Xiong (Ligusticum)	3-6 gm.	*Rz. Ligustici Chuanxiong*
赤芍藥	Chi Shao Yao (Red peony)	6-9 gm.	*Radix Paeoniae Rubra*
川牛膝	Chuan Niu Xi (Cyathula)	6-9 gm.	*Radix Cyathulae*
柴 胡	Chai Hu (Bupleurum)	3-6 gm.	*Radix Bupleuri*
桔 梗	Jie Geng (Platycodon)	3-6 gm.	*Radix Platycodi*
枳 殼	Zhi Ke (Bitter orange)	6-9 gm.	*Fructus Aurantii*
生地黃	Sheng Di Huang (Raw rehmannia)	6-9 gm.	*Radix Rehmanniae*
甘 草	Gan Cao (Licorice)	3-6 gm.	*Radix Glycyrrhizae*

Action:

1. To invigorate blood circulation and remove stasis
2. To promote the circulation of *Qi* and relieve pain

Indication:

For a person with pain in the head and chest due to blood stasis or poor circulation. The symptoms are: chronic pain in the head and chest (fixed and piercing), chronic hiccup, irritability, insomnia, emotional upset, increased body temperature especially in the afternoon.

Tongue: dark red with purple spots
Pulse: hesitant, or wiry and tight

Application:

Coronary heart disease, angina pectoris, rheumatic heart disease, cartilage costalgia, functional neurosis, post-concussion syndromes, external injury in the chest

Modification:

1. With hard lumps in the chest, add:

郁 金	Yu Jin (Curcuma)	*Radix Curcumae*
丹 參	Dan Shen (Salvia root)	*Radix Salviae Miltiorrhizae*

and eliminate:

桔 梗	Jie Geng (Platycodon)	*Radix Platycodi*

2. For amenorrhea and dysmenorrhea, add:

香 附	Xiang Fu (Cyperus tuber)	*Rhizoma Cyperi*
益母草	Yi Mu Cao (Leonurus herb)	*Herba Leonuri*

and eliminate Jie Geng (桔梗) (Platycodon) and Chai Hu (柴胡) (Bupleurum).

Yáng Hé Tāng 陽和湯 (阳和汤)

(Yang-Ho-Tang)
(Yang Activating Decoction)

Constituents:

熟地黃	Shu Di Huang (Prep. rehmannia)	20-30 gm.	*Radix Rehmanniae Praeparatae*
鹿角膠	Lu Jiao Jiao (Antler gelatin)	6-9 gm.	*Colla Cornus Cervi*
薑　炭	Jiang Tan (Charcoal ginger)	6 gm.	*Rhizoma Zingiberis*
肉　桂	Rou Gui (Cinnamon bark)	2-3 gm.	*Cortex Cinnamoni*
麻　黃	Ma Huang (Ephedra)	2-3 gm.	*Herba Ephedrae*
白芥子	Bai Jie zi (Brassica seed)	6-9 gm.	*Semen Sinapis Albae*
甘　草	Gan Cao (Licorice)	2-3 gm.	*Radix Glycyrrhizae*

Action:

1. To activate the *Yang* and tonify blood
2. To disperse the cold and reinforce the blood circulation

Indication:

For a person with abscesses of the *Yin*-type, such as inguinal cellulitis, phlegmon, multiple abscesses, arthroncus of the knee. The symptoms are local papules or pustules, no heat sensation, no thirst.

Tongue: pale pink with white coating
Pulse: deep, slow or thready

Application:

Tuberculosis of the lung, bone and periotoneum, chronic osteomyelitis, periostitis, chronic lymphonoditis, rheumatoid arthritis, chronic bronchitis, chronic bronchial asthma, menstrual cramps and thromboangiitis obliterans (Buerger's disease).

Modification:

1. With deficiency of *Qi* (vital energy), add:

黨　參	Dang Shen (Codonopsis)	*Radix Codonopsis Pilosulae*
黃　芪	Huang Qi (Astragalus)	*Radix Astragali*

2. With increased cold symptoms, add:

附　子	Fu Zi (Aconite)	*Radix Aconiti Praeparatae*

Yǎng Xīn Tāng   養心湯 (养心汤)
(Yang-Hsin-Tang)
(Decoction to Nourish the Heart)

Constituents:

人 參	Ren Shen (Ginseng)	9-12 gm.	*Radix Ginseng*
黄 芪	Huang Qi (Astragalus)	20-30 gm.	*Radix Astragali*
茯 神	Fu Shen (Poria)	6-9 gm.	*Poria*
當 歸	Dang Gui (Chinese angelica)	6-9 gm.	*Radix Angelicae Sinensis*
川 芎	Chuan Xiong (Ligusticum)	6-9 gm.	*Rz. Ligustici Chuanxiong*
五味子	Wu Wei Zi (Schisandra)	6-9 gm.	*Fructus Schisandrae*
酸棗仁	Suan Zao Ren (Jujube)	6-9 gm.	*Semen Ziziphi Spinosae*
柏子仁	Bai Zi Ren (Biota)	6-9 gm.	*Semen Biotae*
遠 志	Yuan Zhi (Polygala)	6-9 gm.	*Radix Polygalae*
半 夏	Ban Xia (Pinellia)	6-9 gm.	*Rhizoma Pinelliae*
肉 桂	Rou Gui (Cinnamon bark)	3-6 gm.	*Cortex Cinnamomi*
炙甘草	Zhi Gan Cao (Baked licorice)	3-6 gm.	*Radix Glycyrrhizae Praeparatae*

Action:

To nourish the heart and replenish blood

Indication:

For a person with deficiency of blood in the heart. The symptoms are: anemia, face pallor, malaise, insomnia, forgetfulness, absent-mindedness severe palpitation.

> Tongue: Pale with thin coat
> Pulse: Slow and weak pulse with regular or irregular intervals

Application:

Anemia, neurasthenia, arrhythmia, tuberculosis, depressive psychosis.

Yăng Yīn Qīng Fèi Tāng 養陰清肺湯
(Yang-Yin-Ching-Fei-Tang)
(Decoction to Nourish the *Yin* and Cleanse the Lung)

Constituents:

生地黄	Sheng Di Huang (Raw rehmannia)	15-20 gm.	*Radix Rehmanniae*
玄 參	Xuan Shen (Scrophularia)	10-15 gm.	*Radix Scrophulariae*
麥門冬	Mai Men Dong (Ophiopogon)	10-15 gm.	*Radix Ophiopogonis*
白芍藥	Bai Shao Yao (White peony)	6-9 gm.	*Radix Paeoniae Alba*
牡丹皮	Mu Dan Pi (Moutan bark)	6-9 gm.	*Cortex Moutan Radicis*
川貝母	Chuan Bei Mu (Tendrilled fritillary)	6-9 gm.	*Bulbus Fritillariae Cirrhosae*
薄 荷	Bo He (Mentha)	3-6 gm.	*Herba Menthae*
甘 草	Gan Cao (Licorice)	3-6 gm.	*Radix Glycyrrhizae*

Action:

1. To nourish the *Yin* of the lung and kidney
2. Anti-toxin

Indication:

For a person with dipheria. The symptoms are: pain in the throat with white spots and swelling, fever, dryness in the nose and lips, cough or no cough, wheezing.

Tongue: red
Pulse: weak and rapid

Application:

Dipheria, chronic laryngitis, tuberculosis, tonsillitis.

Modification:

1. If heat in severe, add:

金銀花 Jin Yin Hua (Honeysuckle)	*Flos Lonicerae*
連 翹 Lian Qiao (Forsythia)	*Fructus Forsythiae*

2. With dipheria, add:

黄 芩 Huang Qin (Scutellaria)	*Radix Scutellariae*
連 翹 Lian Qiao (Forsythia)	*Fructus Forsythiae*

3. With inflammation and swelling of the throat, add:

板藍根 Ban Lan Gen (Isatis root)	*Radix Isatidis*
蒲公英 Pu Gong Ying (Dandelion)	*Herba Taraxaci*
射 干 She Gan (Belamcanda)	*Rhizoma Belamcandae*
馬 勃 Ma Bo (Puff-ball)	*Lasiosphaera seu Calvatia*
僵 蠶 Jiang Can (White-stiff silkworm)	*Bombyx Batryticatus*
桔 梗 Jie Geng (Platycodon)	*Radix Platycodi*

4. With exterior symptom-complexes, add:

牛蒡子 Niu Bang Zi (Arctium fruit)	*Fructus Arctii*
蟬 蛻 Chan Tui (Ciccada slough)	*Periostracum Cicadae*

Yī Guàn Jiān   一貫煎

(I-Kuan-Chian)
(The Liver Reinforcing Decoction)

Constituents:

生地黃	Sheng Di Huang (Fresh rehmannia)	10-15 gm.	*Radix Rehmanniae*
北沙參	Bei Sha Shen (Glehnia)	6-9 gm.	*Radix Glehniae*
麥門冬	Mai Men Dong (Ophiopogon)	6-9 gm.	*Radix Ophiopogonis*
當 歸	Dang Gui (Chinese angelica)	6-9 gm.	*Radix Angelicae Sinensis*
枸杞子	Gou Qi Zi (Lycium fruit)	6-9 gm.	*Fructus Lycii*
川楝子	Chuan Lian Zi (Chinaberry)	3-6 gm.	*Fructus Meliae Toosendan*

Action:

1. To replenish the *Yin* (vital essence) of liver and kidney
2. To regulate the flow of liver *Qi* (vital energy)

Indication:

For a person with liver and kidney *Yin* (vital essence) deficiency, and stagnant flow of vital energy in the liver. The symptoms are: pain in the chest and hypochondrium, acid regurgitation, throat dry, mouth bitter and dry.

> Tongue: red, dry
> Pulse: thready and wiry

Application:

Chest pain of chronic hepatitis, gastric and duodenal ulcer, GI neurosis, hypochrondric neuralgia.

Contraindication:

For a person with chest pain due to retention of phlegm.

Modification:

1. For bitter and dry mouth, add:
黃 連 Huang Lian (Coptis)   *Rhizoma Coptidis*
2. With constipation, add:
瓜蔞仁 Gua Lou Ren (Trichosanthes fruit)   *Semen Trichosanthis*
3. With profuse perspiration at night, add:
地骨皮 Di Gu Pi (Lycium bark)   *Cortex Lycii Radicis*
4. With increased sputum, add:
貝 母 Bei Mu (Fritillary bulb)   *Bulbus Fritillariae*
5. With hypochrondric pain and hard lumps, add:
鱉 甲 Bie Jia (Tortoise shell)   *Carapax Trionycis*
6. With irritable heat and thirst, add:
知 母 Zhi Mu (Anemarrhena)   *Rhizoma Anemarrhenae*
石 膏 Shi Gao (Gypsum)   *Gypsum Fibrosum*
7. With severe abdominal pain, add:
白芍藥 Bai Shao Yao (White peony)   *Radix Paeoniae Alba*
甘 草 Gan Cao (Licorice)   *Radix Glycyrrhizae*

Yì Wèi Tāng   益胃湯
(Yi-Wei-Tang)
(The Stomach Tonic Decoction)

Constituents:

沙 參	Sha Shen (Glehnia root)	6-9 gm.	*Radix Glenniae*
麥門冬	Mai Men Dong (Ophiopogon)	6-9 gm.	*Radix Ophiopogonis*
生地黃	Sheng Di Huang (Rehmannia)	9-12 gm.	*Radix Rehmanniae*
玉 竹	Yu Zhu (Polygonatum)	6-9 gm.	*Rhizoma Polygonati Odorati*
冰 糖	Bing Tang (Rock sugar)		

Action:

To replenish the lung *Yin* (vital essence)

Indication:

For a person of depleted *Yin* fluid in the stomach caused by fevrile disease or escess liver fire. The symptoms are: mough and lips dry, hungry but no appetite, retch, hiccough, abdominal pain or epigastric upset, stools dry and hard.

Tongue: red, dry and with thin coating
Pulse: thready and rapid

Application:

Febrile disease (Yang-ming channel), flu.

Yīn Chén Hāo Tāng　　茵陳蒿湯

(Yin-Chen-Hao-Tang)
(Decoction of Capillaris)

Constituents:

茵陳蒿 Yin Chen Hao (Capillaris)	9-12 gm.	*Herba Artemisiae Capillaris*
栀 子 Zhi Zi (Gardenia fruit)	3-6 gm.	*Fructus Gardeniae*
大 黃 Da Huang (Rhubarb)	6-9 gm.	*Radix et Rhizoma Rhei*

Action:

To clear heat and dampness interiorly

Indication:

For a person with jaundice caused by accumulation of heat and dampness. The symptoms are: eyes and the skin color icteric, abdominal fullness, thirst, perspiration in the head, urination decreased.

Tongue: with yellow and greasy coating
Pulse: Sinkig and forceful; or slippery and rapid

Application:

Acute infectious hepatitis, cholecystitis, cholelithiasis.

Modification:

1. With intermittent fever, headache, mouth bitter, add:
柴 胡 Chai Hu (Bupleurum)　　　　*Radix Bupleri*
黃 芩 Huang Qin (Scutellaria)　　　*Radix Scutellariae*
2. With hypochondric pain, abdominal fullness, add:
郁 金 Yu Jin (Curcuma)　　　　　*Radix Curcumae*
枳 實 Zhi Shi (Immature bitter orange)　*Fructus Aurantii Immaturus*
3. With nausea and vomiting, indigestion, add:
竹 茹 Zhu Ru (Bamboo shavings)　　*Caulus Bambusae in Taenis*
神 曲 Shen Qu (Medicated leaven)　　*Massa Fermentata Medicinalis*

Generic Name:

Capillaris Combination

Yín Qiáo Bài Dú Sàn 銀翹敗毒散

(Yin-Chiao-Pai-Tu-San)
(Antiphlogistic Powder of Lonicera Flower and Forsythia)

Constituents:

金銀花 Jin Yin Hua (lonicera flower)	6-9 gm.	*Flos Lonicerae*
連 翹 Lian Qiao (Forsythia)	6-9 gm.	*Fructus Forsythiae*
羌 活 Qiang Huo (Notopterygium)	6-9 gm.	*Rhizoma Notopterygii*
獨 活 Du Huo (Pubescent angelica)	6-9 gm.	*Radix Angelicae Pubescentis*
川 芎 Chuan Xiong (Ligusticum)	6-9 gm.	*Rz. Ligustici Chuanxiong*
柴 胡 Chai Hu (Bupleurum)	6-9 gm.	*Radix Bupleuri*
薄 荷 Bo He (Mentha)	3-6 gm.	*Herba Menthae*
枳 殼 Zhi Ke (Bitter orange)	6-9 gm.	*Fructus Aurantii*
桔 梗 Jie Geng (Platycodon)	6-9 gm.	*Radix Platycodi*
前 胡 Qian Hu (Peucedanum)	6-9 gm.	*Radix Peucedani*
茯 苓 Fu Ling (Poria)	6-9 gm.	*Poria*
生 薑 Sheng Jiang (Fresh ginger)	3-6 gm.	*Rhizoma Zingiberis Recens*
甘 草 Gan Cao (Licorice)	3-6 gm.	*Radix Glycyrrhizae*

Action:

1. To dispel external wind, heat and dampness (Diaphoretic)
2. Anti-inflammatory

Indication:

For a person with interior heat and toxin but with exterior symptom-complexes. The symptoms are: fever, with no perspiration. aversion to cold, headache, muscle-ache, stuffy-nose, cough with sputum, suppurative infection or carbuncles.

Tongue: with white and greasy coating
Pulse: floating and feeble; or floating and rapid; or deep and rapid

Application:

Common cold, influenza, carbuncles, suppurative infections, tonsillitis, parotitis.

Generic Name:

Lien Chiao Pai Tu Pien

Yín Qiáo Sàn 銀翹散

(Yin-Chiao-San)
(Powder of Lonicera Flower and Forsythia)

Constituents:

金銀花	Jin Yin Hua (Lonicera flower)	9-12 gm.	*Flos Lonicerae*
連 翹	Lian Qiao (Forsythia)	9-12 gm.	*Fructus Forsythiae*
牛蒡子	Niu Bang Zi (Arctium)	6-9 gm.	*Fructus Arctii*
薄 荷	Bo He (Mentha)	3-6 gm.	*Herba Menthae*
荊芥穗	Jing Jie Sui (Schizonepeta spike)	3-6 gm.	*Spica Schizonepetae*
淡豆豉	Dan Dou Chi (Prepared soybean)	9-15 gm.	*Semen Sojae Praepartatum*
桔 梗	Jie Geng (Platycodon)	6-9 gm.	*Radix Platycodi*
淡竹葉	Dan Zhu Ye (Bamboo leaf)	3-6 gm.	*Herba Lophatheri*
蘆 根	Lu Gen (Phragmites)	6-9 gm.	*Rhizoma Phragmitis*
甘 草	Gan Cao (Licorice)	3-6 gm.	*Radix Glycyrrhizae*

Action:

1. To dispel wind and heat (Diaphoretic)
2. To eliminate interior heat and toxin

Indication:

For the initial stage of febrile disease caused by wind and heat. The symptoms are: fever, slightly intolerant to wind and cold, headache, with difficulty in sweating or no sweating, thirst, cough, sore throat.

> Tongue: tip color red, with thin white or yellow coating
> Pulse: floating and rapid

Application:

Measles, influenza, acute tonsillitis, epidemic encephalitis B, parotiditis.

Modification:

1. With sore throat, add:

土牛膝 Tu Niu Xi (Achyranthes)	*Radix Achyranthis Asperae*
板藍根 Ban Lan Gen (Isatis root)	*Radix Isatidis*
馬 勃 Ma Bo (Lasiophaera)	*Lasiosphaerae seu Calvatia*

2. With thirst, add:

天花粉 Tian Hua Fen (Trichosanthes root)	*Radix Trichosanthis*

3. With heat and toxin, add:

大青葉 Da Qing Ye (Isatis leaf)	*Folium Isatidis*
板藍根 Ban Lan Gen (Isatis root)	*Radix Isatidis*

Generic Name:

Yinchiao Chieh Tu Pien (Yinchiao Tablet);
Lonicera and Forsythia Formula

Yòu Guī Wán　　右歸丸

(You-Kuei-Wan)
(Replenishing the Yang—(Right) Pills)

Constituents:

熟地黄	Shu Di Huang (Prep. rehmannia)	20-30 gm.	*Radix Rehmanniae Praeparatae*
制附子	Fu Zi (Aconite)	6-9 gm.	*Radix Aconitii Praeparatae*
肉　桂	Rou Gui (Cinnamon bark)	6-9 gm.	*Cortex Cinnamomi*
山茱萸	Shan Zhu Yu (Cornus)	10-15 gm.	*Fructus Corni*
枸杞子	Gou Qi Zi (Lycium fruit)	10-15 gm.	*Fructus Lycii*
山　藥	Shan Yao (Dioscorea)	15-20 gm.	*Rhizoma Dioscoreae*
杜　仲	Du Zhong (Eucommia)	10-15 gm.	*Cortex Eucommiae*
當　歸	Dang Gui (Chinese angelica)	10-15 gm.	*Radix Angelicae Sinensis*
菟絲子	Tu Si Zi (Cuscuta)	10-15 gm.	*Semen Cuscutae*
鹿角膠	Lu Jiao Jiao (Antler glue)	15-20 gm.	*Colla Cornus Cervi*

Action:

1. To replenish the *Yang* (vital function) of the kidney
2. To treat spermatorrhea

Indication:

For a person with deficiency of kidney *Yang* (vital function). The symptoms are: face pale, intolerance of cold, hands and feet cold, spontaneous perspiration, early ejaculation of sperms, impotence, knees and lower back sore and painful, dizziness, enuresis (incontinence of urine), spermatorrhea.

Tongue: pale
Pulse: deep, slow and weak

Application:

Spermatorrhea, chronic nephritis, diabetes, impotence.

Generic Name:

You Gui Wan

Yòu Guī Yǐn 右歸飲

(You-Kuei-Yin)
(Replenishing the Yang Decoction)

Constituents:

熱地黃	Shu Di Huang (Prep. rehmannia)	20-30 gm.	*Radix Rehmanniae Praeparatae*
附 子	Fu Zi (Aconite)	6-9 gm.	*Radix Aconitii Praeparatae*
肉 桂	Rou Gui (Cinnamon bark)	3-6 gm.	*Cortex Cinnamomi*
山茱萸	Shan Zhu Yu (Cornus)	10-15 gm.	*Fructus Corni*
枸杞子	Gou Qi Zi (Lycium fruit)	10-15 gm.	*Fructus Lycii*
山 藥	Shan Yao (Dioscorea)	10-15 gm.	*Rhizoma Dioscoreae*
杜 仲	Du Zhong (Ecuommia)	6-9 gm.	*Cortex Eucommiae*
炙甘草	Zhi Gan Cao (Baked licorice)	3-6 gm.	*Radix Glycyrrhizae Praeparatae*

Action:

To replenish the *Yang* (vital function) of the kidney

Indication:

For a person with kidney *Yang* (vital function) deficiency. The symptoms are: cold and pain in the knees and lower back, abdominal pain, fatigue, feet cold, urination clear and prolonged, impotence, early ejaculation of semens.

Tongue: whitish
Pulse: deep, thready and weak

Application:

Diabetes insipitus, chronic nephritis, chronic bronchitis, urinary retention.

Modification:

1. With diarrhea, add:
肉豆蔻 Rou Dou Kou (Nutmeg)   *Semen Myristicae*
2. With pain in lower abdomen, add:
吳茱萸 Wu Zhu Yu (Evodia fruit)   *Fructus Evodiae*
3. With leukorrhea, add:
補骨脂 Bu Gu Zhi (Psoralea)   *Fructus Psoraleae*
4. With anemia or stagnant blood flow, add:
當 歸 Dang Gui (Chinese angelica)   *Radix Angelicae Sinensis*
5. With acid regurgitation, add:
炮乾薑 Gan Jiang (Stir-baked dry ginger)   *Rhizoma Zingiberis*
6. With *Qi* (vital energy) deficiency, add:
人 參 Ren Shen (Ginseng)   *Radix Ginseng*
白 朮 Bai Zhu (White atractylodes)   *Rz. Atractylodis Macrocephalae*

Yù Dài Wán 愈帶丸

(Yu-Tai-Wan)
(Pills for Leukorrhea)

Constituents:

椿根皮	Chun Gen Pi (Ailanthus bark)	90 gm.	*Cortex Ailanthi*
黄柏	Huang Bai (Phellodendron)	12 gm.	*Cortex Phellodendri*
白芍藥	Bai Shao Yao (White peony)	30 gm.	*Radix Paeoniae Alba*
高良姜	Gao Liang Jiang (Galanga)	18 gm.	*Rhizoma Galangae*

Action:

1. To eliminate heat and dampness
2. To stop vaginal discharges

Indication:

For a person with leukorrhea due to heat and dampness. The symptoms are: leukorrhea, color yellow, thick and sticky, foul smell, urine color red and decreased in volume, mouth dry and bitter.

Tongue: red with yellow coating
Pulse: thready and rapid

Application:

Leukorrhea

Generic Name:

Yudai Wan

Yù Nǚ Jiān　　玉女煎

(Yu-Nu-Chien)
(The Fair Maiden Decoction)

Constituents:

生石膏 Shi Gao (Gypsum)	10-15 gm.	*Gypsum Fibrosum*
熟地黄 Shu Di Huang (Prep. rehmannia)	10-15 gm.	*Radix Rehmanniae Praeparatae*
麥門冬 Mai Men Dong (Ophiopogon)	3-6 gm.	*Radix Ophiopogonis*
知　母 Zhi Mu (Anemarrhena)	3-6 gm.	*Rhizoma Anemarrhenae*
懷牛膝 Huai Niu Xi (Achyranthes)	3-6 gm.	*Radix Achyranthis Bidentatae*

Action:

1. To eliminate the intense heat or fire from the stomach (Febrifugal)
2. To replenish the *Yin* (vital essence)

Indication:

For a person with deficiency of *Yin* (vital essence) and with heat in the stomach. The symptoms are: headache, toothache, loose teeth, gingivitis, thirst, dry throat, nose-bleeding.

Tongue: red and dry, with yellow and dry coating
Pulse: floating, full, slippery, gigantic

Application:

Toothache, gingivitis, periodontitis, glossitis, inflammation of the oral cavity, diabetes mellitus.

Contraindication:

For a person with diarrhea

Modification:

1. With hidrosis and thirst, add:
五味子 Wu Wei Zi (Schisandra fruit)　　　　*Fructus Schisandrae*
2. With difficulty in urination, add:
澤　瀉 Ze Xie (Alisma tuber)　　　　*Rhizoma Alismatis*
3. With excessive heat and fire, add:
梔　子 Zhi Zi (Gardenia fruit)　　　　*Fructus Gardeniae*
地骨皮 Di Gu Pi (Lycium bark)　　　　*Cortex Lycii Radicis*
4. With deficiency of *Yin* (Vital essence), add:
沙　參 Sha Shen (Glehnia root)　　　　*Radix Glehniae*
石　斛 Shi Hu (Dendrobium stem)　　　　*Herba Dendrobii*
5. With spitting blood, add:
代赭石 Dai Zhe Shi (Hematite)　　　　*Haematitum*
白茅根 Bai Mao Gen (Imperata rhizome)　　　　*Rhizoma Imperatae*

Generic Name:

Rehmannia and Gypsum Combination

Yù Píng Fēng Sàn   玉屏風散

(Yu-Ping-Feng-San)
(The Jade Screen Powder)

Constituents:

黄 芪	Huang Qi (Astragalus)	10-15 gm.	*Radix Astragali*
白 术	Bai Zhu (White atractylodes)	9-12 gm.	*Rhizoma Atractylodis Macrocephalae*
防 風	Fang Feng (Ledebouriella)	9-12 gm.	*Radix Ledebouriellae*

Action:

1. To replenish *Qi* (vital energy)
2. To consolidate the exterior defensive system
3. Anti-perspirant

Indication:

For a person with low body resistance and deficiency of vital energy. The symptoms are: intolerance of wind, spontaneous perspiration, face pale white, prone to catching cold.

     Tongue: light red
     Pulse: floating and feeble

Application:

Common cold, influenza, chronic rhinitis, allergic rhinitis.

Modification:

1. For severe spontaneous perspiration, add:

浮小麥	Fu Xiao Mai (Light wheat)	*Fructus Tritici Levis*
麻黄根	Ma Huang Gen (Ephedra root)	*Radix Ephedrae*
牡 蠣	Mu Li (Oyster shell)	*Concha Ostreae*

2. To expel pathogenic wind and cold factors from the muscles, add:

桂 枝	Gui Zhi (Cinnamon twig)	*Ramulus Cinnamomi*
白芍藥	Bai Shao Yao (White peony)	*Radix Paeoniae Alba*

3. For chronic or allergic rhinitis, add:

辛夷花	Xin Yi Hua (Magnolia flower)	*Flos Magnoliae*
蒼耳子	Cang Er Zi (Xanthium fruit)	*Fructus Xanthii*

Yù Zhēn Sàn 玉真散

(Yu-Chen-San)
(Powder for Tetanus)

Constituents:

白附子	Bai Fu Zi (Typhonium)	30 gm.	*Rhizoma Typhonii*
天南星	Tian Nan Xing (Arisaema)	30 gm.	*Rhizoma Arisaematis*
羌 活	Qiang Huo (Notopterygium)	30 gm.	*Radix Notopterygii*
防 風	Fang Feng (Ledebouriella)	30 gm.	*Radix Ledebouriellae*
白 芷	Bai Zhi (Angelica)	30 gm.	*Radix Angelicae Dahuricae*
天 麻	Tian Ma (Gastrodia)	30 gm.	*Rhizoma Gastrodiae*

Grind the above ingredients into powder. Take 6 gm. each time with wine.

Action:

1. To dispel exterior wind
2. Anti-spasmodic

Indication:

For a person with tetanus. The symptoms are: lock-jaw, mouth lips tightly closed, body stiffness, kyphosis, spasms of the muscles.

Pulse: wiry/taut and tight

Application:

Tetanus, kyphosis, lock-jaw.

Contraindication:

For a pregnant woman

Modification:

For the person with convulsions, add:

全 蠍	Quan Xie (Scorpion)	*Scorpio*
蜈 蚣	Wu Gong (Centipede)	*Scolopendra*

Yuè Bì Tāng　　越婢湯
(Yueh-Pi-Tang)
(Decoction for Edema)

Constituents:

麻 黄	Ma Huang (Ephedra)	6-9 gm.	*Herba Ephedrae*
石 膏	Shi Gao (Gypsum)	10-15 gm.	*Gypsum Fibrosum*
生 薑	Sheng Jiang (Fresh ginger)	3-6 gm.	*Rhizoma Zingiberis Recens*
甘 草	Gan Cao (Licorice)	3-6 gm.	*Radix Glycyrrhizae*
大 棗	Da Zao (Jujube)	3-5 gm.	*Fructus Ziziphus Jujubae*

Action:

1. To eliminate wind and water and heat in lung
2. Diuretic

Indication:

For a person with edema due to affection of wind and water. The symptoms are: with fever or no fever, perspiration or no perspiration, intolerance of wind, thirst, edema over the whole body, decreased urination.

Tongue: with white coating
Pulse: floating

Application:

Edema, nephritis, arthritis.

Modification:

1. With weak spleen, add:
白 术 Bai Zhu (White atractylodes)　　*Rz. Atractylodis Macrocephalae*
This formula is called Yue Bi Jia Zhu Tang (Atractylodes Combination)
（越婢加术湯）

2. With decreased urination, add:
白茅根 Bai Mao Gen (Imperata rhizome)　　*Rhizoma Imperatae*
3. With cough and asthma, add:
杏 仁 Xing Ren (Apricot seed)　　*Semen Armeniacae Amarum*
前 胡 Qian Hu (Peucedanum)　　*Radix Peucedani*
4. With sore throat, add:
牛蒡子 Niu Bang Zi (Arctium fruit)　　*Fructus Arctii*
金銀花 Jin Yin Hua (Lonicera flower)　　*Flos Lonicerae*
黄 芩 Huang Qin (Scutellaria)　　*Radix Scutellariae*

Generic Name:

Ma-huang and Gypsum Combination

Yuè Jū Wán   越鞠丸

(Yue-Chu-Wan)
(Pills to Relieve Stagnancy of All Kinds)

Constituents:

香 附 Xiang Fu (Cyperus)	10-15 gm.	Rhizoma Cyperi
蒼 术 Cang Zhu (Atractylodes)	10-15 gm.	Rhizoma Atractylodis
川 芎 Chuan Xiong (Ligusticum)	10-15 gm.	Rz. Ligustici Chuanxiong
神 曲 Shen Qu (Medicated leaven)	10-15 gm.	Massa Fermentata Medicinalis
栀 子 Zhi Zi (Gardenia fruit)	10-15 gm.	Fructus Gardeniae

Grind the above ingredients into powder, mix with water and made into pills of the size like a green bean. This formula can also be prepared in decoction.

Action:

1. To promote the circulation of *Qi* (vital energy)
2. To relieve the stagnancy of all kinds—*Qi*, blood, phlegm, fire, dampness and food.

Indication:

For a person with stagnancy of all kinds (*Qi*, blood, phlegm, fire, dampness and food). The symptoms are: epigastric fullness and oppression, abdominal distention, acid regurgitation, vomiting, indigestion, belching.

> Tongue: white with thin coating, or greasy or slippery
> Pulse: wiry/taut or running

Application:

Gastro-intestinal neurosis, gastric or duodenal ulcer chronic gastritis, infectious hepatitis, cholecystits, cholecystolithiasis, intercostal neuralgia.

Contraindication:

For a person with stagnancy or stasis due to weakness or asthenia.

Modification:

1. For dysmenorrhea or mental depression, add:

郁 金 Yu Jin (Curcuma root)   *Radix Curcumae*
佛手柑 Fo Shou Gan (Finger citron)   *Fructus Citri Sarcodactylis*

2. For a person with heat and stasis in the liver, with pain in the hypochondrium, yellow tongue coating, wiry and rapid pulse, add:

延胡索 Yan Hu Suo (corydalis tuber)   *Rhizoma Corydalis*

3. For abdominal pain due to coldness and inactive circulation of vital energy, add:

高良姜 Gao Liang Jiang (Galanga)   *Rhizoma Galangae*
香 附 Xiang Fu (Cyperus tuber)   *Rhizoma Cyperi*

Which is known as the Liang Fu Wan (良附丸)

Zēng Yè Tāng   增液湯

(Chen-Yi-Tang)
(Decoction to Increase Body Fluids)

Constituents:

玄 參	Xuan Shen (Scrophularia)	10-15 gm.	*Radix Scrophulariae*
麥門冬	Mai Men Dong (Ophiopogon)	10-15 gm.	*Radix Ophiopogonis*
生地黃	Sheng Di Huang (Raw rehmannia)	15-20 gm.	*Radix Rehmanniae*

Action:

To increase body fluids and eliminate dryness

Indication:

For a person with deficiency of *Yin* (vital essence), but with febrile disease of the Yang-ming channel, and lack of body fluids. The symptoms are: constipation, dry throat, thirst.

       Tongue: dark red with yellow coating, dry
       Pulse: sinking and weak

Application:

Colon tuberculosis, hemorrhoids, colon irritable, chronic pancreatitis, erysipelas.

Contraindication:

For a person with no constipation or no symptoms of *Yin* deficiency.

Modification:

   1. If constipation is severe, add:

大 黃	Da Huang (Rhubarb)	*Radix et Rhizoma Rhei*
芒 硝	Mang Xiao (Mirabilitum)	*Natrii Sulfas*

This formula is called Zeng Ye Cheng Qi Tang （增液承氣湯）

   2. For dipheria, add:

白芍藥	Bai Shao Yao (White peony)	*Radix Paeoniae Alba*
牡丹皮	Mu Dan Pi (Moutan bark)	*Cortex Moutan Radicis*
川貝母	Chuan Bei Mu (Tendrilled fritillary)	*Bulbus Fritillariae Cirrhosae*
薄 荷	Bo He (Mentha)	*Herba Menthae*
甘 草	Gan Cao (Licorice)	*Radix Glycyrrhizae*

This formula is called Yang Yin Qing Fei Tang （養陰清肺湯）

Zhèn Gān Xī Fēng Tāng　鎮肝熄風湯

(Chen-Kan-Hsi-Feng-Tang)
(Decoction to Subdue the Endogenous Wind in the Liver)

Constituents:

懷牛膝	Huai Niu Xi (Achyranthes)	10-15 gm.	*Radix Achyranthis Bidentatae*
代赭石	Dai Zhe Shi (Hematite)	10-15 gm.	*Haematitum*
龍　骨	Long Gu (Dragon's bone)	9-12 gm.	*Os Oraconis*
牡　蠣	Mu Li (Oyster shell)	9-12 gm.	*Concha Ostreae*
龜　板	Gui Ban (Tortoise plastron)	9-12 gm.	*Plastrum Testudinis*
玄　參	Xuan Shen (Scrophularia)	9-12 gm.	*Radix Scrophulariae*
天門冬	Tian Men Dong (Asparagus)	9-12 gm.	*Radix Asparagi*
白芍藥	Bai Shao Yao (White peony)	9-12 gm.	*Radix Paeoniae Alba*
茵陳蒿	Yin Chen Hao (Capillaris)	3-6 gm.	*Herba Artemisiae Capillaris*
川楝子	Chuan Lian Zi (Sichuan chinaberry)	3-6 gm.	*Fructus Meliae Toosendan*
麥　芽	Mai Ya (Malt)	3-6 gm.	*Fructus Hordei Germinatus*
甘　草	Gan Cao (Licorice)	3-6 gm.	*Radix Glycyrrhizae*

Action:

To subdue the endogenous wind in the liver channel.

Indication:

For a person with endogenous wind in the liver channel due to the hyperactivity of the liver *Yang* (vital function). The symptoms are: dizziness, vertigo, tinnitis, distention in the eyes, heat and pain in the brain, irritable heat in the heart, face red (like drunk), belching, deviation of the eyes and mouth, inability to control the body movement, unconscious, coma.

> Tongue: red
> Pulse: wiry/taut, long and forceful

Application:

Apoplexy, apoplectiform, hypertension, cerebral thrombosis, chromaffinoma, hyperthyroidism, pre-menstrual nervousness, glaucoma.

Modification:

1. With headache and vertigo, add:

夏枯草	Xia Ku Cao (Prunella spike)	*Spica Prunellae*
菊　花	Ju Hua (Chrysanthemum flower)	*Flos Chrysanthemi*

2. With profuse sputum, add:

天南星	Tian Nan Xing (Arisaema)	*Rhizoma Arisaematis*
川貝母	Chuan Bei Mu (Tendrilled fritillary)	*Bulbus Fritillariae Cirrhosae*

3. With kidney deficiency, add:

熟地黃	Shu Di Huang (Prep. rehmannia)	*Radix Rehmanniae Praeparatae*
山茱萸	Shan Zhu Yu (Cornus)	*Fructus Corni*

Zhèn Líng Dān   震靈丹

(Chen-Ling-Tan)
(Pills for Shocking the Spirits)

Constituents:

禹余糧	Yu Yu Liang (Limonite)	120 gm.	*Limonitum*
赤石脂	Chi Shi Zhi (Red halloysite)	120 gm.	*Halloysitum Rubrum*
紫石英	Zi Shi Ying (Fluorite)	120 gm.	*Fluoritum*
代赭石	Dai Zhe Shi (Hematite)	120 gm.	*Haematitum*
沒 藥	Mo Yao (Myrrh)	60 gm.	*Resina Myrrhae*
乳 香	Ru Xiang (Mastic)	60 gm.	*Resina Olibani*
五靈脂	Wu Ling Zhi (Pteropus dung)	60 gm.	*Faeces Trogopterorum*
硃 砂	Zhu Sha (Cinnabar)	30 gm.	*Cinnabaris*

Grind the above ingredients into powder. Mix with rice powder into pills. Take 3-6 gm. each time, 1-2 times daily.

Action:

1. To stop vaginal discharges and bleeding
2. To remove blood stasis and stimulate the production of new blood cells.

Indication:

For a person with leukorrhea and uterine bleeding due to deficiency of heart and kidney. The symptoms are: dizziness, low back pain, uterine bleeding, leukorrhea, night perspiration, chronic diarrhea.

     Tongue: pale
     Pulse: deep and feeble

Application:

Leukorrhea, uterine bleeding, chronic diarrhea.

Contraindication:

For a pregnant woman; for a person with leukorrhea due to heat and dampness.

Zhēn Rén Yǎng Zàng Tāng 真人養臟湯
(Chen-Jen-Yang-Chang-Tang)
(Visceras Nourishing Decoction with Ginseng)

Constituents:

人 參	Ren Shen (Ginseng)	6-9 gm.	Radix Ginseng
白 术	Bai Zhu (White atractylodes)	10-15 gm.	Rhizoma Atractylodis Macrocephalae
肉豆蔻	Rou Dou Kou (Nutmeg)	6-9 gm.	Semen Myristicae
肉 桂	Rou Gui (Cinnamon bark)	6-9 gm.	Cortex Cinnamomi
訶 子	He Zi (Terminalis fruit)	6-9 gm.	Fructus Chebulae
罌粟殼	Ying Su Ke (Opium poppy capsule)	10-15 gm.	Pericarpium Papaveris
當 歸	Dang Gui (Chinese angelica)	6-9 gm.	Radix Angelicae Sinensis
白芍藥	Bai Shao Yao (White peony)	9-12 gm.	Radix Paeoniae Alba
木 香	Mu Xiang (Saussurea)	9-12 gm.	Radix Saussureae
炙甘草	Zhi Gan Cao (Baked licorice)	3-6 gm.	Radix Glycyrrhizae Praeparatae

Action:

1. To warm and tonify the spleen and stomach
2. Astringent, anti-diarrhetic

Indication:

For a person with cold and weak spleen and stomach. The symptoms are: diarrhea or dysentery, tenesmus, abdominal pain (prefer warmth and pressure), decreased food intake, malaise.

Tongue: with white coating
Pulse: slow and thready

Application:

Chronic diarrhea, chronic colitis, chronic dysentery.

Contraindication:

For initial stage of diarrhea or dysentery.

Modification:

1. With prolapse of rectum, add:

黃 芪	Huang Qi (Astragalus)	Radix Astragali
升 麻	Sheng Ma (Cimicifuga rhizome)	Rhizoma Cimicifugae

2. With diarrhea and undigested food, cold limbs, add:

附 子	Fu Zi (Aconite)	Radix Aconitii Praeparatae
乾 薑	Gan Jiang (Dry ginger)	Rhizoma Zingiberis

Zhēn Wǔ Tāng　　真武湯

(Chen-Wu-Tang)
(Decoction of Zhen-Wu, the God Who Control Water)

Constituents:

炮附子	Pao Fu Zi (Baked aconite)	9-12 gm.	*Radix Aconiti Praeparatae*
白　术	Bai Zhu (White atractylodes)	10-15 gm.	*Rhizoma Atractylodis Macrocephalae*
茯　苓	Fu Ling (Poria)	10-15 gm.	*Poria*
白芍藥	Bai Shao Yao (White peony)	6-9 gm.	*Radix Paeoniae Alba*
生　薑	Sheng Jiang (Fresh ginger)	6-9 gm.	*Rhizoma Zingiberis Recens*

Action:

1. To replenish the *Yang* (vital function) of Spleen and kidney
2. To relieve water retention

Indication:

For a person with retention of water due to deficiency of *Yang* (vital function) of the spleen and kidney. The symptoms are: edema over the limbs and body, heavy and painful sensation in the four limbs, abdominal pain, intolerance of cold, diarrhea, difficulty in urination.

Tongue: with white and slippery coating
Pulse: deep and thready

Application:

Edema, rheumatoid arthritis, leukorrhea, chronic nephritis, rheumatic arthritis, cardiac failure, primary hyperaldosteronism, hypothyroidism, chronic enteritis, intestinal tuberculosis, ascites.

Modification:

1. For chronic eczema or other skin abscess, add:
    Ma Huang Lian Qiao Chi Xiao Dou Tang (麻黃連翹赤小豆湯)
    (Ma-huang, Forsythia and Phaseolus Combination)

麻　黃	Ma Huang (Ephedra)	*Herba Ephedra*
連　翹	Lian Qiao (Forsythia)	*Fructus Forsythiae*
赤小豆	Chi Xiao Dou (Phaseolus)	*Semen Phaseoli*

2. For arthritis, add:

桂　枝	Gui Zhi (Cinnamon twig)	*Ramulus Cinnamomi*

3. With increased peritoneal fluid and shortness of breath, add:

澤　瀉	Ze Xie (Alisma)	*Rhizoma Alismatis*
薏苡仁	Yi Yi Ren (Coix)	*Semen Coicis*
車前子	Che Qian Zi (Plantago seed)	*Semen Plantaginis*
商　陸	Shang Lu (Poke root)	*Radix Phytolaccae*

Generic Name:

Vitality Combination

Zhī Bǎi Dì Huáng Wán　　知柏地黄丸

(Chih-Po-Ti-Huang-Wan)
(Anemarrhena, Phellodendron and Pills of Six Herbs with Rehmannia)

Constituents:

知　母	Zhi Mu (Anemarrhena)	6-9 gm.	*Rhizoma Anemarrhenae*
黄　柏	Huang Bai (Phellodendron)	6-9 gm.	*Cortex Phellodendri*
熱地黄	Shu Di Huang (Prep. rehmannia)	20-25 gm.	*Radix Rehmanniae Praeparatae*
山茱萸	Shan Zhu Yu (Cornus)	10-15 gm.	*Fructus Corni*
山　藥	Shan Yao (Dioscorea)	10-15 gm.	*Rhizoma Dioscoreae*
澤　瀉	Ze Xie (Alisma)	9-12 gm.	*Rhizoma Alismatis*
牡丹皮	Mu Dan Pi (Moutan bark)	6-9 gm.	*Cortex Moutan Radicis*
茯　苓	Fu Ling (Poria)	9-12 gm.	*Poria*

Action:

To replenish the *Yin* (vital essence) of the kidney and to reduce the weak fire.

Indication:

For a person with upflaring of fire due to deficiency of *Yin* (vital essence) in the kidney. The symptoms are: tinnitus, spermatorrhea, tidal fever, steaming sensation in the bones, night perspiration, spontaneous seminal emission, teeth loose, gums swollen, painful and light red in color.

Tongue: red
Pulse: thready and rapid

Application:

Tinnitus, spermatorrhea, gingivitis, diabetes, chronic nephritis, chronic urinary tract infection.

Zhì Bǎo Dān　　至寶丹
(Chih-Pao-Dan)
(The Most Precious Pellets)

Constituents:

麝 香	She Xiang (Musk)	.1-.3 gm.	*Moschus*
冰 片	Bing Pian (Borneol)	.3-.5 gm.	*Borneolum*
安息香	An Xi Xiang (Benzoin)	1-3 gm.	*Benzoinum*
犀 角	Xi Jiao (Rhinoceros horn)	.5-1 gm.	*Cornus Rhinocerri*
牛 黃	Niu Huang (Bos calculus)	1-3 gm.	*Calculus Bovis*
玳 瑁	Dai Mao (Hawksbill shell)	3-6 gm.	*Carapax Eretmochelydis*
雄 黃	Xiong Huang (Realgar)	.2-.5 gm.	*Arsenic Disulfide*
硃 砂	Zhu Sha (Cinnabar)	.2-.5 gm.	*Cinnabaris*
琥 珀	Hu Po (Succinum)	3-6 gm.	*Succinum*
金 箔	Jin Bo (Gold sheets)		
銀 箔	Yin Bo (Silver sheets)		

Action:

1. To eliminate heat and toxin
2. Resuscitating
3. Anti-convulsive

Indication:

For a person with stroke, heat-stroke, coma or other febrile diseases. The symptoms are: high body temperature, delirium, shortness of breath, convulsion, coma.

> Tongue: red with yellow and greasy coating
> Pulse: slippery and rapid

Application:

Cerebral vascular accident, hepatic coma, Japanese encephalitis, epilepsy, coma.

Contraindication:

For coma due to exuberance of liver *Yang* (vital function).

Zhì Gān Cǎo Tāng (Fù Mài Tāng)
炙甘草湯 (復脈湯)
(Chih-Kan-Tsao-Tang) (Fu-Mai-Tang)
(Baked Licorice Decoction)

Constituents:

炙甘草	Zhi Gan Cao (Baked licorice)	9-12 gm.	*Radix Glycyrrhizae Praeparatae*
人　參	Ren Shen (Ginseng)	3-6 gm.	*Radix Ginseng*
生地黄	Sheng Di Huang (Fresh rehmannia)	15-20 gm.	*Radix Rehmanniae*
麥門冬	Mai Men Dong (Ophiopogon)	6-9 gm.	*Radix Ophiopogonis*
火麻仁	Huo Ma Ren (Cannabis seed)	9-12 gm.	*Fructus Cannabis*
阿　膠	E Jiao (Ass-hide glue)	6-9 gm.	*Colla Corii Asini*
桂　枝	Gui Zhi (Cinnamon)	6-9 gm.	*Ramulus Cinnamomi*
生　薑	Sheng Jiang (Fresh ginger)	6-9 gm.	*Rhizoma Zingiberis Recens*
大　棗	Da Zao (Jujube)	3-5 pc.	*Fructus Ziziphus Jujubae*

Action:

1. To replenish the *Qi* (vital energy) and blood
2. To nourish the *Yin* (vital essence) and increase the pulse rate

Indication:

For a person with deficiency of *Qi* (vital energy) and blood. The symptoms are: weakness, shortness of breath, palpitation, fatigue, insomnia, stool dry and hard formed.

Tongue: light red with thin coating
Pulse: slow and uneven, intermittent, or feeble and rapid

Application:

Coronary heart disease, rheumatic heart disease, viral myocarditis, arrhythmia, tuberculosis, hyperthyroidism, neurasthenia.

Modification:

1. For arrhythmia, add:
酸棗仁 Suan Zao Ren (Wild jujube seed)   *Semen Ziziphi Spinosae*
2. For severe palpitation, add:
磁　石 Ci Shi (Magnetite)   *Magnetitum*
硃　砂 Zhu Sha (Cinnabar)   *Cinnabaris*
3. For severe deficiency of lung *Yin* (vital essence), add:
百　合 Bai He (Lily bulb)   *Bulbus Lilii*
北沙參 Bei Sha Shen (Glehnia)   *Radix Glehniae*
and eliminate:
桂　枝 Gui Zhi (Cinnamon) and fresh ginger.

Generic Name:

Baked Licorice Combination

Zhǐ Jìng Sàn　　止痙散
(Chih-Ching-San)
(Anticonvulsant Powder)

Constituents:

全　蠍 Quan Xie (Scorpion)	10-20 gm.	*Scorpio*
蜈　蚣 Wu Gong (Centipede)	10-20 gm.	*Scolopendra*

Grind the above ingredients into powder. Take 1.5 to 2.5 gm. each time, 2-4 times daily.

Action:

1. Anticonvulsant
2. Analgesic

Indication:

For a person with convulsions of the limbs with pain.

Application:

Infantile convulsions, tetanus, trigeminal neuralgia, meningitis, migraine headache, arthralgia.

Modification:

1. For acute febrile diseases, use in combination with:
   Bai Hu Tang (Gypsum Combination) (白虎湯)
   Huang Lian Jie Du Tang (Coptis and Scute Combination) (黄連解毒湯)
2. For tetanus, use in combination with:
   Yu Zhen San (Powder for Tetanus) (玉真散)
3. For infantile convulsions and diarrhea, use in combination with:
   Fu Zi Li Zhong Tang (Aconite, Ginseng and Ginger Combination) (附子理中湯)

Zhǐ Sòu Sàn 止嗽散
(Chih-Sou-San)
(Cough Relieving Powder)

Constituents:

紫 苑 Zi Wan (Aster root)	6-9 gm.	*Radix Asteris*
百 部 Bai Bu (Stemona root)	6-9 gm.	*Radix Stemonae*
白 前 Bai Qian (Cynanchum root)	6-9 gm.	*Radix Cynanchumi*
陳 皮 Chen Pi (Citrus peel)	3-6 gm.	*Pericarpium Citri Reticulate*
荊 芥 Jing Jie (Schizonepeta)	6-9 gm.	*Herba Schizonepetae*
桔 梗 Jie Geng (Platycodon)	6-9 gm.	*Radix Platycodi*
甘 草 Gan Cao (Licorice)	3-6 gm.	*Radix Glycyrrhizae*

Action:

1. To relieve cough and sputum (Anti-tussive and expectorant)
2. To dispel the exterior wind attack on the lung

Indication:

For a person with flu from the external attack of wind on the lung. The symptoms are: cough with sputum, sore throat, fever, intolerance of wind.

Tongue: whitish with thin coating
Pulse: floating

Application:

Cough, whopping cough, flu, chronic tracheitis.

Modification:

1. For common cold with cough, add:

防 風 Fang Feng (Ledebouriella)	*Radix Ledebouriellae*
紫蘇葉 Zi Su Ye (Perilla leaf)	*Folium Perillae*
生 薑 Sheng Jiang (Fresh ginger)	*Rhizoma Zingiberis Recens*

2. For dry cough with thin sputum due to excessive heat in lung, add:

瓜 蔞 Gua Lou (Trichosanthes)	*Semen Trichosanthis*
貝 母 Bei Mu (Fritillary bulb)	*Bulbus Fritillariae*

3. For cough with excessive sputum (damp phlegm), add:

半 夏 Ban Xia (Pinellia tuber)	*Rhizoma Pinelliae*
茯 苓 Fu Ling (Poria)	*Poria*

Generic Name:

Platycodon and Schizonepeta Formula

Zhĭ Zhú Wán 枳术丸
(Chih-Chu-Wan)
(Pills of Immature Bitter Orange & White Atractylodes)

Constituents:

枳 實 Zhi Shi (Immature bitter orange)	30 gm.	*Fructus Aurantii Immaturus*
白 术 Bai Zhu (White atractylodes)	60 gm.	*Rhizoma Atractylodis Macrocephalae*

Grind the above two ingredients into powder and made into pills. Take 6-9 gm. each time with water.

Action:

1. To strengthen the function of the spleen
2. To disperse lumps

Indication:

For a person with abdominal fullness or distention due to asthenia of the spleen and stomach. The symptoms are: indigestion, acid regurgitation, abdominal fullness or distention.

Tongue: with yellow or greasy coating
Pulse: slippery

Application:

Indigestion, gastroenteritis

Modification:

1. With indigestion, add:
神 曲 Shen Qu (Medicated leaven)　　*Massa Fermentata Medicinalis*
麥 芽 Mai Ya (Malt)　　*Fructus Hordei Germinatus*
This formula is called Qu Mai Zhi Zhu Wan (曲麥枳术丸)

2. With oppression and fullness, add:
陳 皮 Chen Pi (Citrus peel)　　*Pericarpium Citri Reticulatae*
半 夏 Ban Xia (Pinellia)　　*Rhizoma Pinelliae*
This formula is called Ju Ban Zhi Zhu Wan (橘半枳术丸)

3. To improve digestion and appetite, add:
木 香 Mu Xiang (Saussurea)　　*Radix Saussureae*
砂 仁 Sha Ren (Cardamon)　　*Fructus Amomi*
This formula is called Xiang Sha Zhi Zhu Wan (香砂枳术丸)

Zhōu Chē Wán　　舟車丸

(Chou-Che-Wan)
(The Boat and Carriage Pills)

Constituents:

甘 遂	Gan Sui (Kansui)	30 gm.	*Radix Euphorbiae Kansui*
芫 花	Yuan Hua (Genkwa)	30 gm.	*Flos Genkwa*
大 蓟	Da Ji (Euphorbia)	30 gm.	*Herba Cirsii Japonici*
大 黄	Da Huang (Rhubarb)	60 gm.	*Radix et Rhizoma Rhei*
牵牛子	Qian Niu Zi (Pharbitis seed)	120 gm.	*Semen Pharbitidis*
木 香	Mu Xiang (Saussurea)	15 gm.	*Radix Saussureae*
陳 皮	Chen Pi (Citrus peel)	15 gm.	*Pericarpium Citri Reticulatae*
青 皮	Qing Pi (Green tangerine peel)	15 gm.	*Pericarpium Reticulatae Viridae*
輕 粉	Qing Fen (Calomel)	3 gm.	*Calomelos*
檳 榔	Bing Lang (Areca seed)	15 gm.	*Semen Arecae*

Grind the above ingredient into powder and mix with honey into pills of 1.5-3 gm. each. Take 2 small pills or 1 large pill each time, twice daily.

Action:

To dispel water and regulate the circulation of the vital energy (Water-dispelling purgative)

Indication:

For a person with edema and distention. The symptoms are: thirst, dyspnea, abdomen hard and distended, constipation, dysuria.

> Tongue: slippery
> Pulse: deep, rapid and forceful

Application:

Edema, ascites, liver cirrhosis.

Contraindication:

For a pregnant woman

Zhū Líng Tāng　　豬苓湯

(Chu-Ling-Tang)
(Decoction of Polyporus or Umbellate Pore Fungus)

Constituents:

豬　苓	Zhu Ling (Polyporus)	6-9 gm.	*Polyporus Umbellatus*
茯　苓	Fu Ling (Poria)	6-9 gm.	*Poria*
澤　瀉	Ze Xie (Alisma)	6-9 gm.	*Rhizoma Alismatis*
阿　膠	E Jiao (Ass-hide glue)	6-9 gm.	*Colla Corii Asini*
滑　石	Hua Shi (Talc)	6-9 gm.	*Talcum*

Melt E Jiao (阿膠) (ass-hide glue) separately and mix in with the decoction.

Action:

1. Diuretic
2. To eliminate heat and nourish the *Yin* fluid

Indication:

For a person with dysuria caused by stagnation of heat and water. The symptoms are: fever, thirst with preferance to drink, irritability, insomnia, cough, nausea, difficulty in urination; may also have hematuria and burning sensation in urination.

Application:

Urinary tract infection, nephritis, dysuria.

Contraindication:

For a person with no heat symptoms caused by deficiency of *Yin*, or with no blood in the urine.

Modification:

1. For acute urinary tract infection, add:

瞿　麥	Qu Mai (Dianthus)	*Herba Dianthi*
萹　蓄	Bian Xu (Polygonum)	*Herba Polygoni*

2. For hematuria, add:

白茅根	Bai Mao Gen (Imperata)	*Rhizoma Imperatae*
大　薊	Da Ji (Japanese thistle)	*Radix Euphorbiae*
小　薊	Xiao Ji (Small thistle)	*Herba Cephalanoploris*

Generic Name:

Polyporus Combination

Zhū Shā Ān Shén Wán　　珠砂安神丸

(Chu-Sha-An-Shen-Wan)
(Cinnabar Sedative Pills)

Constituents:

珠　砂	Zhu Sha (Cinnabar)	3-6 gm.	*Cinnabaris*
黃　連	Huang Lian (Coptis)	6-9 gm.	*Rhizoma Coptidis*
當　歸	Dang Gui (Chinese angelica)	6-9 gm.	*Radix Angelicae Sinensis*
生地黃	Sheng Di Huang (Fresh rehmannia)	6-9 gm.	*Radix Rehmanniae*
甘　草	Gan Cao (Licorice)	3-6 gm.	*Radix Glycyrrhizae*

Action:

1. Sedative (Tranquilizing)
2. To clear the fire of the heart (Febrifugal)
3. To nourish blood

Indication:

For a person with up-flaring of heart fire due to deficiency of blood and vital essence. The symptoms are: fidgetiness, insomnia, forgetfulness, palpitation, shortness of breath.

　　Tongue: red
　　Pulse: thready and rapid

Application:

Neurosis, neurasthenia, mental depression, psychosis.

Modification:

1. With heat and phlegm in the chest, add:

瓜蔞子 Gua Lou Zi (Trichosanthes fruit)　*Semen Trichosanthis*
竹　茹 Zhu Ru (Bamboo shavings)　*Caulus Bambusae in Taenis*

2. With fidgetiness and insomnia, add:

梔　子 Zhi Zi (Gardenia fruit)　*Fructus Gardeniae*
蓮子心 Lian Zi Xin (Lotus plumule)　*Plumula Nelumbinis*

Caution:

Cinnabar is toxic, do not take over the dosage nor take the pills for long period of time.

Generic Name:

Cinnabar Formula

Zhú Yè Shí Gāo Tāng 竹葉石膏湯
(Chu-Yeh-Shih-Kao-Tang)
(Decoction of Bamboo Leaf and Gypsum)

Constituents:

竹 葉 Zhu Ye (Bamboo leaf)	6-9 gm.	*Folium Bambusae*
石 膏 Shi Gao (Gypsum)	20-30 gm.	*Gypsum Fibrosum*
人 參 Ren Shen (Ginseng)	6-9 gm.	*Radix Ginseng*
麥門冬 Mai Men Dong (Ophiopogon)	6-9 gm.	*Radix Ophiopogonis*
半 夏 Ban Xia (Pinellia)	6-9 gm.	*Rhizoma Pinelliae*
粳 米 Jing Mi (Oryza)	15-30 gm.	*Semen Oryzae*
炙甘草 Zhi Gan Cao (Baked Licorice)	3-6 gm.	*Radix Glycyrrhizae Praeparatae*

Action:

1. To eliminate heat in the stomach
2. To relieve thirst and increase the secretion of body fluids.

Indication:

1. For a person with depletion of *Qi* (vital energy) and body fluids, yet still with interior heat. The symptoms are: mouth and lips dry, nausea, loss of appetite, indigestion, oppression in the chest. Tongue red with thin coating. Pulse thready and rapid.

2. For a person with deficiency of body fluids in the stomach. The symptoms are: upflaring fire of the stomach, ulceration of the oral cavity, thirst, nausea. Tongue dark red and dry. Pulse thready and rapid.

3. For diabetes with polyphagia.

4. For summer heat stroke.

Application:

Summer heat stroke, diabetes mellitus, gingivitis.

Generic Name:

Bamboo Leaves and Gypsum Combination

Zǐ Xuě Dān   紫雪丹

(Tzu-Hsueh-Tan)
(Purple Snowy Powder)

Constituents:

麝 香	She Xiang (Musk)	.3-.5 gm.	*Moschus*
羚羊角	Ling Yang Jiao (Antelope horn)	.5-1 gm.	*Cornu Antelopis*
犀 角	Xi Jiao (Rhinoceros horn)	.5-1 gm.	*Cornus Rhinoceri*
青木香	Qing Mu Xiang (Birthwort)	3-6 gm.	*Radix Aristolochiae*
沉 香	Chen Xiang (Aquilaria)	1-3 gm.	*Lignum Aquilariae Resinatum*
丁 香	Ding Xiang (Cloves)	1-2 gm.	*Flos Caryophylli*
石 膏	Shi Gao (Gypsum)	6-9 gm.	*Gypsum Fibrosum*
寒水石	Han Shui Shi (Calcite)	6-9 gm.	*Calcitum*
黄 金	Huang Jin (Gold)	10-15 gm.	*Gold*
磁 石	Ci Shi (Loadstone)	6-9 gm.	*Magnetitum*
滑 石	Hua Shi (Talc)	10-15 gm.	*Talcum*
扑 硝	Pu Xiao (Mirabilitum)	10-15 gm.	*Natrii sulfas*
硝 石	Xiao Shi (Saltpeter)	10-15 gm.	*Niter, KNO$_3$*
玄 參	Xuan Shen (Scrophularia)	10-15 gm.	*Radix Scrophulariae*
升 麻	Sheng Ma (Cimicifuga)	6-9 gm.	*Rhizoma Cimicifugae*
甘 草	Gan Cao (Licorice)	3-6 gm.	*Radix Glycyrrhizae*
硃 砂	Zhu Sha (Cinnabar)	1-2 gm.	*Cinnabaris*

Action:

1. To eliminate heat and toxin
2. Anti-convulsive and resuscitating

Indication:

For a person with febrile disease and coma. The symptoms are: high fever, irritability, delirium, coma, convulsion, mouth dry, lips dry and burning, urine amber in color, constipation.

Application:

Japanese encephalitis, epidemic cerebral-spinal meningitis, scarlet fever, measles.

Generic Name:

Rhinoceros and Antelope Horn Formula

Zuǒ Guī Wán   左歸丸
(Chuo-Kuei-Wan)
(Replenishing the Yin Fluid Pills)

Constituents:

熟地黃	Shu Di Huang (Prep. rehmannia)	50-60 gm.	*Radix Rehmanniae Praeparatae*
山 藥	Shan Yao (Dioscorea)	20-30 gm.	*Rhizoma Dioscoreae*
枸杞子	Gou Qi Zi (Lycium fruit)	20-30 gm.	*Fructus Lycii*
山茱萸	Shan Zhu Yu (Cornus)	20-30 gm.	*Fructus Corni*
菟絲子	Tu Si Zi (Cuscuta)	20-30 gm.	*Semen Cuscutae*
川牛膝	Chuan Niu Xi (Cyathula)	15-25 gm.	*Radix Cyathulae*
鹿角膠	Lu Jiao Jiao (Antler glue)	20-30 gm.	*Colla Cornus Cervi*
龜板膠	Gui Ban Jiao (Turtle shell glue)	20-30 gm.	*Colla of Plastrum Testudinis*

Action:

To replenish the *Yin* (vital essence) of liver and kidney.

Indication:

For a person with kidney *Yin* (vital essence) deficiency. The symptoms are: dizziness, forgetfulness, tinnitus, deafness, cheeks red, sensation of heat in the hands and feet, night sweat, insomnia, mouth and throat dry, loss of hair and teeth, spermatorrhea, infertility, uterine bleeding, amenorrhea.

> Tongue: red
> Pulse: thready and rapid

Application:

Lumbago, diabetes, Addison's disease, tuberculosis, spermatorrhea, infertility, amenorrhea.

Zuŏ Guī Yĭn　左歸飲

(Chuo-Kuei-Yin)
(Replenishing the *Yin* Fluid Decoction)

Constituents:

枸杞子	Gou Qi Zi (Lycium Fruit)	10-15 gm.	*Fructus Lycii*
熟地黃	Shu Di Huang (Prep. rehmannia)	20-30 gm.	*Radix Rehmanniae Praeparatae*
山茱萸	Shan Zhu Yu (Cornus)	6-9 gm.	*Fructus Corni*
山　藥	Shan Yao (Dioscorea)	10-15 gm.	*Rhizoma Dioscoreae*
茯　苓	Fu Ling (Poria)	9-12 gm.	*Poria*
炙甘草	Zhi Gan Cao (Baked licorice)	3-6 gm.	*Radix Glycyrrhizae Praeparatae*

Action:

To replenish the *Yin* (vital essence) and tonify the kidney.

Indication:

For a person with kidney *Yin* deficiency. The symptoms are: lumbago, nocturnal emission, night sweat, mouth and throat dry, thirst, preference to drink, dizziness.

> Tongue: red with no coating, mirrorlike
> Pulse: thready and rapid

Application:

Lumbago, diabetes, Addison's disease, tuberculosis.

Modification:

1. With heat in the lung and irritability, add:
麥門冬 Mai Men Dong (Ophiopogon)　　*Radix Ophiopogonis*
2. With heat in heart, dryness, add:
玄　參 Xuan Shen (Scrophularia)　　*Radix Scrophulariae*
3. With heat in the spleen, and continuous hunger, add:
白芍藥 Bai Shao Yao (White peony)　　*Radix Paeoniae Alba*
4. With heat in the kidney, profuse perspiration, add:
地骨皮 Di Gu Pi (Wolfberry bark)　　*Cortex Lycii Radicis*
5. With random flow of blood circulation and bleeding, add:
生地黃 Sheng Di Huang (Fresh rehmannia)　　*Radix Rehmanniae*
6. With stagnant blood flow, add:
牡丹皮 Mu Dan Pi (Moutan bark)　　*Cortex Moutan Radicis*
7. With blood deficiency, add:
當　歸 Dang Gui (Chinese angelica)　　*Radix Angelicae Sinensis*

Zuǒ Jīn Wán   左金丸
(Chuo-Chin-Wan)
(Coptis and Evodia Pills)

Constituents:

黄 連	Huang Lian (Coptis)	180 gm.	*Radix Coptidis*
吳茱萸	Wu Zhu Yu (Evodia)	30 gm.	*Fructus Evodiae*

Grind these ingredients into powder and make into pills. Take 2-3 gm. each time with water.

Action:

1. To purge the liver Fire
2. Antiemetic

Indication:

For a person with excess fire in the liver channel and heat in the stomach. The symptoms are: hypochondriac distention and pain, vomiting, belching, acid regurgitation, mouth dry or bitter.

> Tongue: red with yellow coating
> Pulse: wiry and rapid

Application:

Acute and chronic gastritis, acid regurgitation.

Modification:

1. For diarrhea or dysentery with abdominal pain and spasm, add:
白芍藥 Bai Shao Yao (White peony)   *Radix Paeoniae Alba*
2. For dysentery with bloody stool and tenesmus, add:
木 香 Mu Xiang (Saussurea)   *Radix Saussureae*
 and subtract:
吳茱萸 Wu Zhu Yu (Evodia)   *Fructus Evodiae*
This formula is called Xiang Lian Wan (香連丸)

APPLICATION OF

CHINESE HERBAL FORMULAS

BY

TCM AND WESTERN DIAGNOSIS

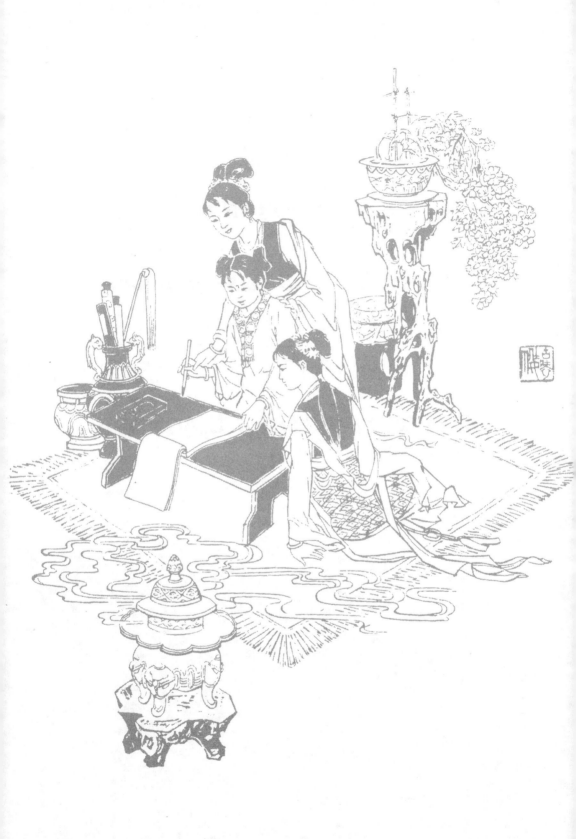

APPLICATION of CHINESE HERBAL FORMULAS
by TCM and WESTERN DIAGNOSIS

ABDOMINAL PAIN (腹痛)
1. Caused by Cold: (寒痛)
    Liang Fu Wan (良附丸)
    Tong Mai Si Ni Tang (通脈四逆湯)
2. Caused by Heat: (熱痛)
    Da Cheng Qi Tang (大承氣湯)
3. Caused by asthenia or deficiency: (虛痛)
    Xiao Jian Zhong Tang (小建中湯)
    Da Jian Zhong Tang (大建中湯)
    Fu Zi Li Zhong Tang (附子理中湯)
4. Caused by sthenia or excessiveness: (實痛)
    a. Due to stagnation of Qi and Blood stasis: (氣滯血瘀)
    Chai Hu Shu Gan Tang (柴胡舒肝湯)
    Shao Fu Zhu Yu Tang (少腹逐瘀湯)
    b. Due to stagnation of food: (飲食積滯)
    Bao He Wan (保和丸)

ABSCESS (膿腫)
1. Purulent abscess: (化膿期)
    Dang Gui Bu Xue Tang (當歸補血湯)
2. Chronic abscess: (慢性膿腫)
    Ba Zhen Tang (八珍湯)
    Shi Quan Da Bu Tang (十全大補湯)

ABSENT-MINDEDNESS (恍惚)
    San Piao Xiao San (桑螵蛸散)

ACCESSORY NASAL SINUSITIS (副鼻寶炎)
    Cang Er San (蒼耳散)
    Xin Yi San (辛夷散)

ACID REGURGITATION (反胃)
1. Caused by Cold: (寒症)
    Xiang Sha Liu Jun Zi Tang (香砂六君子湯)
2. Caused by Heat: (熱症)
    Zuo Jin Wan (左金丸)

ACNE VULGARIS (尋常性痤瘡、粉刺、青春豆)
    Wu Wei Xiao Du Yin (五味消毒飲)

ADDISON'S DISEASE (HYPOADRENOCORTICISM)
(阿狄森病、慢性腎上腺皮質功能減退症)
Da Bu Yin Wan (大補陰丸)
Liu Wei Di Huang Wan (六味地黃丸)
Zuo Gui Wan (左歸丸)
Zuo Gui Yin (左歸飲)

ADENITIS (腺炎)
Da Huang Mu Dan Pi Tang (大黃牡丹皮湯)
Gui Zhi Fu Ling Wan (桂枝茯苓丸)

AIDS (ACQUIRED IMMUNNE DEFICIENCY SYNDROME)
(愛滋病、獲得性免疫缺陷綜合症)
1. Initial Stage: (前軀期)
   Sheng Mai San (生脈散) & Zhi Bai Di Huang Wan (知柏地黃丸)
2. Stage of attack: (發病期)
   a. Hyperactivity of Fire due to Yin deficiency: (陰虛火旺)
      Da Ding Feng Zhu (大定風珠)
   b. Invasion of Heat into Ying (Nutrient) and Blood systems: (熱陷營血)
      Qing Wen Bai Du Yin (清瘟敗毒飲)

ALLERGY (過敏)
Xin Yi San (辛夷散)

ALOPECIA AREATA (BALDNESS) (禿髮、斑禿)
He Shou Wu Wan (何首烏丸)
Gui Pi Wan (歸脾丸)

AMEBIASIS (阿米巴病)
Long Dan Xie Gan Tang (龍膽瀉肝湯)
Huang Lian Jie Du Tang (黃連解毒湯)

AMOEBIC DYSENTERY (阿米巴痢疾)
Bai Tou Weng Tang (白頭翁湯)
Ge Gen Huang Qin Huang Lian Tang (葛根黃芩黃連湯)

AMENORRHEA (經閉)
1. Caused by deficiency of both Qi and Blood: (氣血虛弱)
   Ba Zhen Tang (八珍湯)
   Shi Quan Da Bu Tang (十全大補湯)
2. Caused by stagnation of Qi and Blood stasis: (氣滯血瘀)
   Xue Fu Zhu Yu Tang (血府逐瘀湯)
3. Caused by Blood stasis and accumulation of Cold: (寒凝血瘀)
   Wen Jing Tang (溫經湯)

ANEMIA (APLASTIC) （再生障礙性貧血）
1. Depletion of both Qi and Blood: （氣血虛弱）
   Ba Zhen Tang （八珍湯）
   Gui Pi Tang （歸脾湯）
2. Depletion of Spleen and Kidney Yang: （脾腎陽虛）
   Si Jun Zi Tang （四君子湯） & You Gui Wan （右歸丸）
3. Deficiency of Liver and Kidney Yin-fluid: （肝腎陰虛）
   Da Bu Yuan Jian （大補元煎）

ANEMIA (IRON DEFICIENCY) （缺鐵性貧血）
1. Insufficiency of Spleen Qi: （脾氣虛弱）
   Xiang Sha Liu Jun Zi Tang （香砂六君子湯）
2. Depletion of both Qi and Blood: （氣血虛弱）
   Ba Zhen Tang （八珍湯）
   Ren Shen Yang Ying Tang （人參養營湯）
3. Stagnation of Qi and Blood stasis: （氣滯血瘀）
   Xue Fu Zhu Yu Tang （血府逐瘀湯）

ANEMIA (NUTRITIONAL DEFICIENCY) （營養不良性貧血）
1. Blood deficiency: （血虛）
   Si Wu Tang （四物湯）
2. Deficiency of both Heart and Spleen: （心脾兩虛）
   Gui Pi Tang （歸脾湯）
3. Deficiency of both Liver and Kidney: （肝腎不足）
   Zuo Gui Wan （左歸丸）

ANGINA PECTORIS （心絞痛）
   Dan Shen Yin （丹參飲）
   Sheng Mai San （生脈散）
   Gua Lou Xie Bai Bai Jiu Tang （瓜蔞薤白白酒湯）
   Gua Lou Xie Bai Ban Xia Tang （瓜蔞薤白半夏湯）

ANOREXIA （厭食）
1. Dyspepsia （乳食壅滯）
   Bao He Wan （保和丸）
2. Weakness of both Spleen and Stomach: （脾胃虛弱）
   Xiang Sha Liu Jun Zi Tang （香砂六君子湯））
3. Deficiency of the Stomach Yin-fluid: （胃陰不足）
   Yi Wei Tang （益胃湯）

APHASIA （失語症）
   Di Huang Yin Zi （地黃飲子）

APOPLECTIFORM （類中風性的）
   Zhen Gan Xi Feng Tang （鎮肝熄風湯）

APOPLEXY（中風、卒中）
1. In the Channels and Collaterals:（中經絡）
    Qian Zheng San（牽正散）
    Zhen Gan Xi Feng Tang（鎮肝熄風湯）
2. In the internal visceras:（中臟腑）
  a. Syndrome of Tension:（閉証）
    Zhi Bao Dan（至寶丹）
    Su He Xiang Wan（蘇合香丸）
  b. Syndrome of Prostration:（脱証）
    Di Huang Yin Zi（地黄飲子）
3. Sequelae:（續發症）
  a. Hemiplegia:（半身不遂）
    (1) Deficiency of Qi and stagnation of Blood:（氣虛血滯）
      Bu Yang Huan Wu Tang（補陽還五湯）
    (2) Excuberance of Liver Yang:（肝陽上亢）
      Zhen Gan Xi Feng Tang（鎮肝熄風湯）
      Tian Ma Gou Teng Yin（天麻鉤藤飲）
  b. Difficulty of Speech:（語言困難）
    (1) Depletion of Kidney Essence:（腎虛精虧）
      Di Huang Yin Zi（地黄飲子）
    (2) Excuberance of Liver Yang:（肝陽上亢）
      Tian Ma Gou Teng Yin（天麻鉤藤飲）
      Zhen Gan Xi Feng Tang（鎮肝熄風湯）
  c. Deviation of the eye and mouth:（口眼歪斜）
    Qian Zheng San（牽正散）

APPENDICITIS:（闌尾炎）
    Da Cheng Qi Tang（大承氣湯）
    Da Huang Mu Dan Pi Tang（大黄牡丹皮湯）
    Si Ni San（四逆散）
    Xiao Cheng Qi Tang（小承氣湯）

APHONIA（失音症）
    Bei Mu Gua Lou San（貝母瓜蔞散）

ARRHYTHMIA（心率不齊）
    Jia Jian Fu Mai Tang（加減復脈湯）
    Sheng Mai San（生脈散）

ARTHRALGIA (BI SYNDROME)（關節痛、痺証）
1. Caused by Wind, Cold and Dampness:（風寒濕痺）
  a. Painfull:（痛痺）
    Wu Tou Tang（烏頭湯）
    Fu Zi Tang（附子湯）

b. Migratory: (行痹)
   Gui Zhi Shao Yao Zhi Mu Tang (桂枝芍藥知母湯)
c. Fixed: (着痹)
   Juan Bi Tang (蠲痹湯)
2. Caused by Heat: (熱痹)
   Bai Hu Jia Gui Zhi Tang (白虎加桂枝湯)
   Er Miao San (二妙散)
3. Chronic: (慢性)
   Du Huo Ji Sheng Tang (獨活寄生湯)

ARTHRITIS (SUPPURATIVE) (化膿性關節炎)
1. Initial stage: (初期)
   Wu Wei Xiao Du Yin (五味消毒飲)
2. Middle stage: (中期)
   Tou Nong San (透膿散)
3. Later stage: (晚期)
   Ba Zhen Tang (八珍湯)

ASCARIASIS (蛔蟲病)
   Bu Dai Wan (布袋丸)
   Wu Mei Wan (烏梅丸)

ASCITES (腹水)
   Shi Zao Tang (十棗湯)
   Wei Ling Tang (胃苓湯)
   Zhen Wu Tang (真武湯)
   Zhou Che Wan (舟車丸)

ASTHMA (哮喘)
1. Caused by Excessiveness: (實喘)
   a. Wind and Cold acting on the Lung: (風寒襲肺)
      Ma Huang Tang (麻黃湯)
      Gui Zhi Jia Hou Po Xing Ren Tang (桂枝加厚朴杏仁湯)
   b. Wind and Heat acting on the Lung: (風熱犯肺)
      Ma Xing Shi Gan Tang (麻杏石甘湯)
      Bai Hu Jia Ren Shen Tang (白虎加人參湯)
   c. Accumulation of phlegm in the Lung: (痰濁阻肺)
      San Zi Yang Qing Tang (三子養親湯) & Er Chen Tang (二陳湯)
2. Caused by Deficiency: (虛喘)
   a. Asthenia of the Lung: (肺虛)
      Sheng Mai San (生脈散)
      Bu Zhong Yi Qi Tang (補中益氣湯)
   b. Asthenia of the Kidney: (腎虛)
      Jin Kui Shen Qi Wan (金匱腎氣丸)
      Shen Jie San (參蚧散), Du Qi Wan (都氣丸)

ATHEROSCLEROSIS (see CORONARY ATHEROSCLEROSIS) (動脈粥樣硬化)

ATHETOSIS (手足徐動症)
    Da Ding Feng Zhu (大定風珠)

BACILLARY DYSENTERY (細菌性痢疾)
    Bai Tou Weng Tang (白頭翁湯)
    Ge Gen Huang Qin Huang Lian Tang (葛根黃芩黃連湯)

BALDNESS (see ALOPECIA AREATA)

BED-WETTING (遺尿)
    Suo Quan Wan (縮泉丸)

BELCHING (噯氣)
    Bao He Wan (保和丸)

BELL'S PALSY (FACIAL PARALYSIS) (面癱)
    Qian Zheng San (牽正散) & Bu Yang Huan Wu Tang (補陽還五湯)

BERI-BERI (腳氣)
    Ji Ming San (雞鳴散)

BI SYNDROME (see ARTHRALGIA) (痹症)

BILIARY ASCARIASIS (膽囊性蛔蟲病)
    Da Jian Zhong Tang (大建中湯)
    Si Ni San (四逆散)

BILIARY CALCULUS (膽結石)
    Da Chai Hu Tang (大柴胡湯)
    Shi Wei San (石葦散)

BLEEDING (出血) (血証)
1. Cough with Blood: (咳血)
   a. Wind and Heat acting on the Lung: (風熱傷肺)
      Sang Xing Tang (桑杏湯)
   b. Liver Fire acting on the Lung: (肝火犯肺)
      Xie Bai San (瀉白散)
      Xi Jiao Di Huang Tang (犀角地黃湯)
   c. Deficiency of Yin with Excess Fire: (陰虛火旺)
      Bai He Gu Jin Tang (百合固金湯)
2. Epistaxis: (衄血)
   a. Heat in the Lung: (肺熱)
      Sang Ju Yin (桑菊飲)

b. Heat in the Stomach: (胃熱)
   Yu Nu Jian (玉女煎)
c. Liver Fire: (肝火)
   Long Dan Xie Gan Tang (龍膽瀉肝湯)
d. Depletion of both Qi and Blood: (氣血虧虛)
   Shi Quan Da Bu Tang (十全大補湯)
   Gui Pi Tang (歸脾湯)

3. Spitting Blood: (吐血)
   a. Accumulation of Heat in the Stomach: (胃中積熱)
      Xie Xin Tang ((瀉心湯) & Shi Hui San (十灰散)
   b. Stomach attacked by Liver Fire: (肝火犯胃)
      Long Dan Xie Gan Tang (龍膽瀉肝湯)
      Xi Jiao Di Huang Tang (犀角地黃湯)

4. Blood in the stools: (便血)
   a. Deficiency of Spleen and Stomach with presence of Cold: (脾胃虛寒)
      Huang Tu Tang (黃土湯)
   b. Accumulation of Heat and Dampness: (實熱蘊蒸)
      Huai Hua San (槐花散)

5. Blood in the urine: (尿血)
   a. Deficiency of Yin with Excess Fire: (陰虛火旺)
      Zhi Bai Di Huang Wan (知柏地黃丸)
   b. Hyperactivity of the Heart Fire: (心火亢盛)
      Xiao Ji Yin Zi (小薊飲子)
   c. Deficiency of both Spleen and Kidney: (脾腎兩虧)
      Bu Zhong Yi Qi Tang (補中益氣湯)

6. Hemorrhoid bleeding: (痔瘡出血)
   Huai Hua San (槐花散)
   Huai Jiao Wan (槐角丸)

7. Uterine bleeding: (子宮出血)
   Huang Tu Tang (黃土湯)
   Jiao Ai Tang (膠艾湯)

8. Post-surgical bleeding: (手術後出血)
   Shen Fu Tang (參附湯)

9. Post-Partum bleeding: (產後出血)
   Dang Gui bu Xue Tang (當歸補血湯)

BLOOD- SHOT EYES (紅眼症)
   Dan Zhi Xiao Yao San (丹梔逍遙散)
   Long Dan Xie Gan Tang (龍膽瀉肝湯)
   Chai Ge Jie Ji Tang (柴葛解肌湯)
   Jing Fang Bai Du San (荊防敗毒散)

BLOODY STOOL (便血)
   Huang Tu Tang (黃土湯)
   Huai Hua San (槐花散)

BLOOD STASIS(YU SYNDROME)（血瘀）（瘀証）
1. Pathogenic heat in Blood:（邪熱入血）
      Xi Jiao Di Huang Tang（犀角地黄湯）
      An Gong Niu Huang Wan（安宫牛黄丸）
      Tao He Cheng Qi Tang（桃核承氣湯）
2. Presence of Cold in the Blood Vessels:（寒客血脈）
      Dang Gui Si Ni Tang（當歸四逆湯）
      Huang Qi Gui Zhi Wu Wu Tang（（黄芪桂枝五物湯）
3. Qi stagnation and Blood stasis:（氣滯血瘀）
   a. In the face and head:（瘀在頭面）
      Tong Qiao Huo Xue Tang（通竅活血湯）
   b. In the chest and hypochondriac region:（瘀停胸肋）
      Xue Fu Zhu Yu Tang（血府逐瘀湯）
   c. In the abdomen:（瘀接于腹）
      Ge Xie Zhu Yu Tang（膈下逐瘀湯）
   d. In the abdomen (lateral):（瘀在少腹）
      Shao Fu Zhu Yu Tang（少腹逐瘀湯）
   e. In the Channels and Collaterals:（瘀阻經絡）
      Tao Hong Si Wu Tang（桃紅四物湯）
4. Blood stasis with decreased Vital Energy:（血瘀正衰）
   a. With Qi Deficiency:（氣虚血瘀）
      Bu Yang Huan Wu Tang（補陽還五湯）
   b. With Deficiency of Yin and Yang, and with hard lumps:
     （陰陽虚，有積塊）
      Gui Zhi Fu Ling Wan（桂枝茯苓丸）

BLURRINESS OF VISION（視力模糊）
      Ci Zhu Wan（磁硃丸）
      Qi Ju Di Huang Wan（杞菊地黄丸）

BOILS（癤）
      Pu Ji Xiao Du Yin（普濟消毒飲）
      Tou Nong San（透膿散）
      Wu Wei Xiao Du Yin（五味消毒飲）

BORBORYGMUS（腹鳴）
      Ban Xia Xie Xin Tang（半夏瀉心湯）
      Huo Xiang Zheng Qi San（藿香正氣散）
      Tong Xie Yao Fang（痛瀉要方）

BREAST DISTENTION（乳房漲痛）
      Chai Hu Shu Gan San（柴胡舒肝散）
      Ge Xie Zhu Yu Tang（膈下逐瘀湯）

BRONCHIECTASIS （支氣管擴張）
    Si Sheng Wan （四生丸）
    Xing Su San （杏蘇散）

BRONCHIAL ASTHMA （支氣管哮喘）
1. With Cold Phlegm: （寒哮）
    Xiao Qing Long Tang （小青龍湯）
    Su Zi Jiang Qi Tang （蘇子降氣湯）
    She Gan Ma Huang Tang （射干麻黄湯）
2. With Heat in the Lung: （熱哮）
    Ding Chuan Tang （定喘湯）
    Ma Xing Shi Gan Tang （麻杏石甘湯） & San Zi Yang Qing Tang （三子養親湯）
3. With deficiency of Kidney: （腎虚）
    Du Qi Tang （都氣湯）
4. With deficiency of Lung and Kidney: （肺腎虚）
    Ren Shen Hu Tao Tang （人參胡桃湯）

BRONCHOGENIC CARCINOMA （支氣管癌）
1. With Qi stagnation and Blood stasis: （氣滯血瘀）
    Xue Fu Zhu Yu Tang （血府逐瘀湯）
2. With Toxin, Phlegm and Dampness: （痰濕毒蘊）
    Dao Tan Tang （導痰湯）
    Ting Li Da Zao Xie Fei Tang （葶藶大棗瀉肺湯）
3. With pathogenic Heat caused by deficiency of Yin: （陰虚毒熱）
    Sha Shen Mai Men Dong Tang （沙參麥門冬湯）
4. Deficiency of both Qi and Yin: （氣陰兩虚）
    Sheng Mai San （生脈散）

BRONCHITIS （支氣管炎）
1. Acute bronchitis: （急性支氣管炎）
  a. Wind and Cold acting on the Lung: （風寒束肺）
    San Niu Tang （三拗湯）
  b. Wind and Heat acting on the Lung: （風熱襲肺）
    Sang Ju Yin （桑菊飲）
  c. Heat and Dryness acting on the Lung: （燥熱傷肺）
    Sang Xin Tang （桑杏湯）
    Qing Zao Jiu Fei Tang （清燥救肺湯）
2. Chronic bronchitis: （慢性支氣管炎）
  a. Phlegm and Dampness acting on the Lung: （痰濕犯肺）
    Ban Xia Hou Po Tang （半夏厚朴湯）
  b. Exterior affection of Cold and interior accumulation of Heat: （外寒內熱）
    Ma Xing Shi Gan Tang （麻杏石甘湯）
  c. Exterior affection of Cold with interior accumulation of fluid:
    （外寒內飲）
    Xiao Qing Long Tang （小青龍湯）

2 d.   Stagnation of Heat and Phlegm: (痰熱蘊結)
        Xie Bai San (瀉白散)
        & Qing Qi Hua Tan Tang (清氣化痰湯)
   e.   Deficiency of both Lung and Spleen: (肺脾兩虛)
        Liu Jun Zi Tang (六君子湯)
        Bu Fei Tang (補肺湯)
   f.   Deficiency of both Lung and Kidney: (肺腎兩虛)
        Jin Kui Shen Qi Wan (金匱腎氣丸)

BRUCELLOSIS (UNDULANT FEVER) (布氏桿菌病、波動性發熱)
        Heat and Dampness in the Wei Portion (superficial defence system)
        and the Qi Portion (inner defense system) (實熱在衛分，氣分)
   a.   With more Dampness: (濕盛)
        San Ren Tang (三仁湯)
   b.   With more Heat: (熱盛)
        Gan Lu Xiao Du Yin (甘露消毒飲)

BUERGER'S DISEASE (THROMBOANGIITIS OBLITERANS) (血栓閉塞性脈管炎)
        Dang Gui Si Ni Tang (當歸四逆湯)
        Dang Gui Si Ni Jia Wu Zhu Yu Sheng Jiang Tang
        (當歸四逆加吳茱萸生薑湯)

CALCULUS (結石病)
1. Biliary calculus: (膽結石)
        Da Chai Hu Tang (大柴胡湯)
2. Calculus in the urinary tract: (尿道結石)
        San Jin Tang (三金湯)
        Shi Wei San (石葦散)
        Ba Zheng San (八正散)
3. All kinds of calculus: (各種結石)
        Shi Wei San (石葦散)

CARDIAC EDEMA (心性水腫)
        Fang Ji Fu Ling Tang (防己茯苓湯)
        Fang Ji Huang Qi Tang (防己黃芪湯)
        Ling Gui Zhu Gan Tang (苓桂术甘湯)
        Wei Ling Tang (胃苓湯)

CARBUNCLE (癰、疽)
        Pu Ji Xiao Du Yin (普濟消毒飲)
        Wu Wei Xiao Du Yin (五味消毒飲)
        Tou Nong San (透膿散)
        Ren Shen Xiao Du San (人參消毒散)
        Liu Shen Wan (六神丸)

CARDIAC FAILURE （心力衰竭）
1. To recuperate the depleted Yang: （回陽救逆）
   Si Ni Tang （四逆湯）
   Tong Mai Si Ni Tang （通脈四逆湯）
   Shen Fu Tang （參附湯）
2. To warm the Kidney and disperse Cold: （溫腎散寒）
   Zhen Wu Tang （真武湯）
3. With Lung deficiency: （肺虛）
   Sheng Mai San （生脈散）

CARTILAGE COSTALGIA （肋間神經痛）
   Xue Fu Zhu Yu Tang （血府逐瘀湯）

CATARACT （白內障）
   Ci Zhu Wan （磁硃丸）
   Si Wu Tang （四物湯）& Er Chen Tang （二陳湯）

CEREBRAL CONCUSSION （腦震盪）
   Tong Qiao Huo Xue Tang （通竅活血湯）
   Xue Fu Zhu Yu Tang （血府逐瘀湯）

CEREBRAL THROMBOSIS （腦血栓）
   Zhen Gan Xi Feng Tang （鎮肝熄風湯）

CEREBRAL VASCULAR ACCIDENT (CVA) （腦血管意外）
   Bu Yang Huan Wu Tang （補陽還五湯）
   Xiao Huo Luo Dan （小活絡丹）

CHEST PAIN （胸痛）
1. Blood stasis in the Heart: （心血瘀阻）
   Xue Fu Zhu Yu Tang （血府逐瘀湯）
   Dan Shen Yin （丹參飲）
2. Obstruction of Vital Energy and Function in the Chest: （胸陽痹阻）
   Gua Lou Xie Bai Ban Xia Tang （瓜蔞薤白半夏湯）
3. Accumulation of Heat and Phlegm in the Lung: （痰熱壅肺）
   Xiao Xian Xiong Tang （小陷胸湯）& Wei Jing Tang （葦莖湯）

CHICKENPOX （水痘）
   Yin Qiao San （銀翹散）

CHILLS AND FEVER （寒熱交戰）
   Xiao Chai Hu Tang （小柴胡湯）
   Da Yuan Yin （達原飲）
   Hao Qin Qing Dan Tang （蒿芩清膽湯）

CHLOASMA (YELLOW PIGMENTATION) (黃褐斑)
1. Stagnation of Liver Qi: (肝氣郁結)
    Xiao Yao San (逍遙散)
2. Deficiency of Liver and Kidney Yin-fluid: (肝腎陰虛)
    Zuo Gui Wan (左歸丸) & Si Wu Tang (四物湯)

CHOLELITHIASIS (膽石病)
    Dan Dao Pai Shi Tang (膽道排石湯)
    Shi Wei San (石葦散)

CHOLECYSTITIS (膽囊炎)
1. Acute cholecystitis: (急性膽囊炎)
    Da Chai Hu Tang (大柴胡湯)
    Da Cheng Qi Tang (大承氣湯)
    Yin Chen Hao Tang (茵陳蒿湯)
      & Long Dan Xie Gan Tang (龍膽瀉肝湯)
2. Chronic cholecystitis: (慢性膽囊炎)
    Da Chai Hu Tang (大柴胡湯)
    Shi Xiao San (失笑散)

CHOLERA (霍亂)
    Huo Xiang Zheng Qi San (藿香正氣散)
    Fu Zi Li Zhong Wan (附子理中丸)
    Li Zhong Wan (理中丸)

CHROMAFFINOMA (嗜鉻細胞瘤)
    Ling Yang Gou Teng Tang (羚羊鉤藤湯)
    Zhen Gan Xi Feng Tang (鎮肝熄風湯)

CLIMACTERIC SYNDROMES (MENOPAUSE) (更年期綜合症)
1. Stagnation of Liver Qi: (肝氣郁結)
    Dan Zhi xiao Yao San (丹梔逍遙散)
    Xiao Yao San (逍遙散)
2. Deficiency of Kidney Yin-fluid: (腎陰虛)
    Zuo Gui Yin (左歸飲)
3. Deficiency of Kidney Yang: (腎陽虛)
    You Gui Yin (右歸飲)

COLD SORES (凍瘡)
    Bi Yu San (碧玉散)

COLITIS (結腸炎)
1. Acute colitis: (急性結腸炎)
    Ge Gen Huang Qin Huang Lian Tang (葛根黄芩黄連湯)
    Bai Tou Weng Tang (白頭翁湯)

2. Chronic colitis: (慢性結腸炎)
　　Fu Zi Li Zhong Wan (附子理中丸)
　　Si Shen Wan (四神丸)
　　Zhen Ren Yang Zang Tang (真人養臟湯)
3. Allergenic colitis: (過敏性結腸炎)
　　Tong Xie Yao Fang (痛瀉要方)

COLON CARCINOMA (結腸癌)
1. Accumulation of Heat and Dampness: (濕熱蘊結)
　　Huai Jiao Wan (槐角丸)
2. Qi stagnation and blood stasis: (氣滯血瘀)
　　Ge Xia Zhu Yu Tang (膈下逐瘀湯)
3. Deficiency of Spleen and Kidney Yang (vital function): (脾腎陽虛)
　　Shen Ling Bai Zhu San (參苓白术散) & Si Shen Wan (四神丸)
4. Deficiency of Liver and Kidney Yin (vital essence): (肝腎陰虛)
　　Zhi Bai Di Huang Wan (知柏地黃丸)
5. Deficiency of both Qi and blood: (氣血兩虧)
　　Ba Zhen Tang (八珍湯)

COLON IRRITABLE (結腸過敏)
　　Wen Pi Tang (溫脾湯)
　　Zeng Ye Tang (增液湯)

COLON TUBERCULOSIS (結腸結核)
　　Zeng Ye Tang (增液湯)

COMA (昏迷)
1. Syndrome of Tension: (閉証)
　a.　Heat type: (熱閉)
　　　(1)　Heat in the Pericardium: (熱入心包)
　　　　　Qing Ying Tang (清營湯)
　　　　　Zhi Bao Dan (至寶丹)
　　　　　Zi Xue Dan (紫雪丹)
　　　　　An Gong Niu Huang Wan (安宮牛黃丸)
　　　(2)　Heat in the Stomach and Intestines: (熱結胃腸)
　　　　　Da Cheng Qi Tang (大承氣湯)
　　　(3)　Endogenous Liver Wind caused by heat: (熱動肝風)
　　　　　Ling Yang Gou Teng Tang (羚羊鉤藤湯) & Zi Xue Dan (紫雪丹)
　b.　Phlegm type: (痰閉)
　　　(1)　Interior obstruction by Phlegm and Dampness: (痰濕內阻)
　　　　　Su He Xiang Wan (蘇合香丸)
　　　(2)　Upward flaring of Fire and Phlegm: (痰火上蒙)
　　　　　Wen Dan Tang (溫胆湯) & Zhi Bao Dan (至寶丹)
　c.　Turbid type: (濁閉)
　　　　　Wen Pi Tang (溫脾湯) & Su He Xiang Wan (蘇合香丸)

2. Syndrome of Prostration: (脱証)
  a. Depletion of Yin (vital essence): (亡陰)
        Sheng Mai San (生脈散)
        Di Huang Yin Zi (地黄飲子)
  b. Depletion of Yang (vital function): (亡陽)
        Shen Fu Tang (參附湯)

COMMON COLD (see FLU) (感冒)

CONGESTIVE HEART FAILURE (充血性心力衰竭)
1. Deficiency of Qi and Yin (vital essence): (氣陰兩虛)
      Sheng Mai San (生脈散)
2. Blood stasis with obstruction of Water: (血瘀水阻)
      Ge Xia Zhu Yu Tang (膈下逐瘀湯) & Wu Ling San (五苓散)
3. Edema caused by defeiciency of Yang (vital function): (陽虛水泛)
      Zhen Wu Tang (真武湯)
4. Prostration of Yang Qi: (陽氣虛脱)
      Shen Jie San (參蚧散)

CONJUNCTIVITIS (ACUTE) (急性結膜炎)
1. Wind and Heat in the Lung channel: (肺經風熱)
      Xie Ban San (瀉白散)
      Sang Ju Yin (桑菊飲)
2. Pathogenic heat from the Lung and Spleen: (脾肺熱毒)
      Xie Fei San (瀉肺散)
3. Caused by Liver Fire: (肝火)
      Long Dan Xie Gan Tang (龍膽瀉肝湯)

CONSUMPTIVE DISEASE (虛勞)
1. Deficiency of Qi (vital energy): (氣虛)
      Shen Ling Bai Zhu San (參苓白术散)
      Bu Zhong Yi Qi Tang (補中益氣湯)
2. Deficiency of Blood: (血虛)
  a. In the Heart: (心血虛)
      Zhi Gan Cao Tang (炙甘草湯)
  b. In the Liver: (肝血虛)
      Si Wu Tang (四物湯)
      Gui Pi Tang (歸脾湯)
      Dang Gui Bu Xue Tang (當歸補血湯)
3. Deficiency of Yang (vital function): (陽虛)
  a. Of the Kidney: (腎陽虛)
      You Gui Wan (右歸丸)
      Jin Suo Gu Jin Wan (金鎖固金丸)
      Fu Gui Li Zhong Wan (附桂理中丸)
      Si Shen Wan (四神丸) ,Zhen Wu Tang (真武湯)

b. Of the Spleen: (脾陽虛)
     Fu Zi Li Zhong Tang (附子理中湯)
4. Deficiency of Yin (vital essence): (陰虛)
  a. Of the Lung: (肺陰虛)
     Bai He Gu Jin Tang (百合固金湯)
  b. Of the Heart: (心陰虛)
     Tian Wang Bu Xin Dan (天王補心丹)
  c. Of the Liver: (肝陰虛)
     Bu Gan Tang (補肝湯)
  d. Of the Kidney: (腎陰虛)
     Zuo Gui Wan (左歸丸)

CONSUMPTIVE PULMONARY DISEASE (消耗性肺病)
1. Caused by Heat and Asthenia: (虛熱)
     Mai Men Dong Tang (麥門冬湯)
     Qing Zao Jiu Fei Tang (清燥救肺湯)
2. Caused by Cold and Asthenia: (虛寒)
     Zhi Gan Cao Tang (炙甘草湯)

CONSTIPATION (便秘)
1. Excessive type: (實秘)
     Ma Zi Ren Wan (麻子仁丸)
2. Deficient type: (虛秘)
     Ji Chuan Jian (濟川煎)

CONVULSION (驚厥)
1. Infantile: (嬰兒期的)
     An Gong Niu Huang Wan (安宮牛黃丸)
     Zhi Jing San (止痙散)
2. Clonic: (陣攣性的)
     Da Ding Feng Zhu (大定風珠)
     San Jia Fu Mai Tang (三甲復脈湯)

CONVULSIVE DISEASE (驚厥病、痙症)
1. Caused by pathogenic factors in the Channels and Collaterals:
     (邪壅經絡)：Ge Gen Tang (葛根湯)
     Qiang Huo Sheng Shi Tang (羌活勝濕湯)
2. Caused by intensive Heat: (熱甚發痙)
     Zeng Ye Cheng Qi Tang (增液承氣湯)
     An Gong Niu Huang Wan (安宮牛黃丸)
     Ling Yang Gou Teng Tang (羚羊鉤藤湯)
     Zhi Bao Dan (至寶丹)
     Da Ding Feng Zhu (大定風珠)
3. Caused by deficiency of Qi and Blood: (氣血虧虛)
     Ba Zhen Tang (八珍湯)

4. Obstruction of Blood stasis: (瘀血內阻)
   Tong Qiao Huo Xue Tang (通竅活血湯)

COR PULMONALE (CHRONIC) (慢性肺氣腫)
1. Accumulation of Cold Phlegm: (寒痰壅盛)
   Ling Gui Zhu Gan Tang (苓桂朮甘湯) & Su Zi Jiang Qi Tang (蘇子降氣湯)
   Xiao Qing Long Tang (小青龍湯)
   Bu Fei Tang (補肺湯)
2. Accumulation of Heat and Phlegm in the Lung: (痰熱壅肺)
   Ma Xing Shi Gan Tang (麻杏石甘湯)
3. Accumulation of Phlegm due to deficiency of Lung and Kidney Qi:
   (肺腎氣虛，痰濁壅盛)
   Jin Kui Shen Qi Wan (金匱腎氣丸) & San Zi Yang Qing Tang (三子養親湯)

CORNEAL ULCER (SERPIGINOUS) (匐行性角膜潰瘍)
1. Excessive Heat in the Liver and Gallbladder: (肝膽熱盛)
   Long Dan Xie Gan Tang (龍膽瀉肝湯)
2. Excessive Heat in the Triple-burner: (三焦火盛)
   Da Cheng Qi Tang (大承氣湯) & Bai Hu Tang (白虎湯)

CORONARY ATHEROSCLEROSIS (動脈粥狀硬化)
1. Shi (Excessive) type: (實証)
   a. Obstruction of Yang with Chest pain: (胸陽痺阻)
      Gua Lou Xie Bai Gui Zhi Tang (瓜蔞薤白桂枝湯)
   b. Obstruction of Blood stasis in the Blood Vessels: (心脈瘀阻)
      Dan Shen Yin (丹參飲) & Tao Hong Si Wu Tang (桃紅四物湯)
   c. Obstruction of turbid Phlegm: (痰濁內阻)
      Su He Xiang Wan (蘇合香丸)
      Wen Dan Tang (溫胆湯)
2. Xu (Deficient) type: (虛証)
   a. Deficiency of both Qi and Yin: (氣陰兩虛)
      Sheng Mai San (生脈散)
   b. Asthenia of Kidney Yang: (腎陽虛弱)
      Jin Kui Shen Qi Wan (金匱腎氣丸)
   c. Prostration of Yang: (陽虛欲脫)
      Shen Fu Tang (參附湯)

CORONARY HEART DISEASE (冠心病)
1. Obstruction of the Chest Yang with pain: (胸陽痺阻)
   Gua Lou Xie Bai Ban Xia Tang (瓜蔞薤白半夏湯)
2. Blood stasis in the cardio-vascular system: (心脈瘀阻)
   Dan Shen Yin (丹參飲)
      & Tao Hong Si Wu Tang (桃紅四物湯)
3. Deficiency of both Qi and Yin-fluid: (氣陰兩虛)
   Sheng Mai San (生脈散)

4. Deficiency of both Blood and Yin-fluid: (陰血兩虛)
   Jia Jian Fu Mai Tang (加減復脈湯)
   Zhi Gan Cao Tang (炙甘草湯)
5. Resuscitating: (復甦)
   Su He Xiang Wan (蘇合香丸)

COUGH (咳嗽)
1. Cough caused by exterior affection: (外感咳嗽)
   a. Affection of Wind and Cold: (風寒咳嗽)
      Xin Su San (杏蘇散)
   b. Affection of Wind and Heat: (風熱咳嗽)
      Sang Ju Yin (桑菊飲)
   c. Affection of Heat and Dryness: (燥熱咳嗽)
      Sang Xing Tang (桑杏湯)
      Zhi Sou San (止嗽散)
2. Cough caused by internal injury: (內傷咳嗽)
   a. Phlegm and Dampness acting on the Lung: (痰濕犯肺)
      Er Chen Tang (二陳湯)
      Liu Jun Zi Tang (六君子湯)
      (Qian Jin) Wei Jing Tang (千金葦莖湯)
   b. Lung Xu (Asthenia): (肺虛咳嗽)
      Sha Shen Mai Men Dong Tang (沙參麥門冬湯)
      Shen Jie San (參蚧散)

CRAPULENCE (酗酒)
   Gua Di San (瓜蒂散)

CYSTITIS (膀胱炎)
   Ba Zheng San (八正散)
   Shi Wei San (石葦散)

DAMPNESS OBSTRUCTION (濕阻)
1. Dampness in the Splèen and Stomach: (濕困脾胃)
   Huo Xiang Zheng Qi San (藿香正氣散)
   Ping Wei San (平胃散)
2. Dampness and Heat in the Middle-burner: (濕熱中阻)
   Gan Lu Xiao Du Dan (甘露消毒丹)
3. Dampness caused by Asthenia of Spleen: (脾虛濕阻)
   Xiang Sha Liu Jun Zi Tang (香砂六君子湯)

DELIRIUM (譫妄)
   An Gong Niu Huang Wan (安宮牛黃丸)
   Qing Ying Tang (清營湯)
   Zi Xue Dan (紫雪丹)
   Xi Jiao Di Huang Tang (犀角地黄湯)

DEAFNESS (耳聾)

Ci Zhu Wan (磁硃丸)

Er Long Zuo Ci Wan (耳聾左慈丸)

Tong Qiao Huo Xue Tang (通竅活血湯)

DEPRESSIVE SYNDROME (YU ZHENG) (郁証)

1. Shi (Excess) type: (實症)
   a. Stagnation of Liver Qi: (肝氣郁結)

      Chai Hu Shu Gan Tang (柴胡舒肝湯)

      Yue Qu Wan (越麴丸)
   b. Transformation of Qi Stagnation into Fire: (氣郁化火)

      Dan Zhi Xiao Yao San (丹梔逍遙散) & Zuo Jin Wan (左金丸)
   c. Stagnation of Qi and Phlegm: (氣滯痰郁)

      Ban Xia Hou Po Tang (半夏厚朴湯)

      Wen Dan Tang (溫胆湯)
2. Xu (Deficiency) type: (虛症)
   a. With melancholia: (疣郁傷神)

      Gan Mai Da Zao Tang (甘麥大棗湯)
   b. Deficiency of both Heart and Spleen: (心脾兩虛)

      Gui Pi Tang (歸脾湯)

DERMATITIS (CONTACT) (接觸性皮膚炎)

1. With Heat and Toxin: (熱毒型)

   Pu Ji Xiao Du Yin (普濟消毒飲)
2. With Heat and Dampness: (濕熱型)

   Long Dan Xie Gan Tang (龍膽瀉肝湯)

DIABETES INSIPITUS (尿崩病)

1. Deficiency of Kidney Yin-fluid: (腎陰虛)

   Liu Wei Di Huang Wan (六味地黃丸)
2. Deficiency of Kidney Yang: (腎陽虛)

   You Gui Yin (右歸飲)

   Jin Kui Shen Qi Wan (金匱腎氣丸)

DIABETES MELLITUS (糖尿病)

1. Heat and Drought in the Lung and Stomach: (肺胃燥熱)

   Bai Hu Jia Ren Shen Tang (白虎加人參湯)

   Yu Nu Jian (玉女煎)

   & Yi Wei Tang (益胃湯)
2. Depletion of Kidney Yin: (腎陰虧損)

   Liu Wei Di Huang Wan (六味地黃丸)
3. Depletion of both Yin and Yang: (陰陽兩虛)

   Jin Kui Shen Qi Wan (金匱腎氣丸)
4. In the Upper-burner: (上消)

   Bai Hu Jia Ren Shen Tang (白虎加人參湯)

5. In the Middle-burner: （中消）
   Yu Nu Jian （玉女煎）
6. In the Lower-burner: （下消）
   a. Depletion of Kidney Yin: （腎陰虧虛）
   Liu Wei Di Huang Wan （六味地黃丸）
   b. Depletion of both Yin and Yang: （陰陽兩虛）
   Jin Kui Shen Qi Wan （金匱腎氣丸）

DIARRHEA （腹瀉）
1. Caused by exterior pathogenic factors: （感受外邪）
   a. By Wind and Cold; or Cold and Dampness: （風寒/寒濕）
   Huo Xiang Zheng Qi San （藿香正氣散）
   Wei Ling Tang （胃苓湯）
   b. By Heat and Dampness; or Summer Heat and Dampness: （濕熱/暑濕）
   Ge Gen Huang Qin Huang Lian Tang （葛根黃芩黃連湯）
2. Caused by Indigestion: （食滯腸胃）
   Bao He Wan （保和丸）
3. Caused by Liver Qi acting on the Spleen: （肝氣乘脾）
   Tong Xie Yao Fang （痛瀉要方）
4. Caused by Asthenia of both Spleen and Stomach: （脾胃虛弱）
   Shen Ling Bai Zhu San （參苓白术散）
   Fu Zi Li Zhong Wan （附子理中丸）
   Bu Zhong Yi Qi Tang （補中益氣湯）
5. Caused by Asthenia of Kidney Yang: （腎陽虛衰）
   Si Shen Wan （四神丸）
   Tao Hua Tang （桃花湯）

DIFFERENTIATION according to "SHANG HAN LUN" (Treatise on Febrile Disease) （傷寒論辯證）
---in accordance with the six Channels: （六經辯證）
1. Syndrome of the Tai Yang Channel: （太陽病辯證）
   a. In the Tai Yang Channels: （太陽經証）
      (1) Deficiency in the Exterior: （表虛）
          Gui Zhi Tang （桂枝湯）
      (2) Excessiveness in the Exterior: （表實）
          Ma Huang Tang （麻黃湯）
   b. In the Tai Yang Visceras: （太陽腑証）
      (1) Retention of Water: （蓄水証）
          Wu Ling San （五苓散）
      (2) Retention of Blood: （蓄血証）
          Tao Ren Cheng Qi Tang （桃仁承氣湯）
2. Syndrome of the Yang Ming Channel: （陽明病辯證）
   a. In the Yang Ming Channel: （陽明經証）
      Bai Hu Tang （白虎湯）
      Bai Hu Jia Ren Shen Tang （白虎加人參湯）

  b. In the Yang Ming Viscera: (陽明腑証)
     Da Cheng Qi Tang (大承氣湯)
 3. Syndrome of the Shao Yang Channel: (少陽病辯證)
     Xiao Chai Hu Tang (小柴胡湯)
 4. Syndrome of the Tai Yin Channel: (太陰病辯證)
     Li Zhong Tang (理中湯)
 5. Syndrome of the Shao Yin Channel: (少陰病辯證)
  a. With Cold: (寒化証)
     Si Ni Tang (四逆湯)
  b. With Heat: (熱化証)
     Huang Lian E Jiao Tang (黄連阿膠湯)
 6. Syndrome of Jue Yin Channel: (厥陰証辯證)
  a. With parasite infestation: (蛔厥証)
     Wu Mei Wan (烏梅丸)
  b. With cold, headache and dry vomiting: (寒逆、干嘔、頭疼症)
     Wu Zhu Yu Tang (吳茱萸湯)

DIFFERENTIATION according to "WEN BIN LUN" (Treatise on Epidemic Febrile Disease) (溫病論辯證)

---in accordance with the 4 conditions: (衛氣營血)

1. In the WEI (superficial defensive) system: (衛分証)
    Yin Qiao San (銀翹散)
    Sang Ju Yin (桑菊飲)
2. In the QI (inner defensive) system: (氣分証)
  a. Heat in the Lung: (熱壅於肺)
    Ma Xing Shi Gan Tang (麻杏石甘湯)
  b. Heat in the Chest: (熱郁胸膈)
    Zhi Zi Chi Tang (梔子豉湯)
    Liang Ge San (涼膈散)
  c. Heat in the Yang Ming Channel: (熱熾陽明)
    Bai Hu Tang (白虎湯)
  d. Heat in the Intestines: (熱結腸道)
    Da Cheng Qi Tang (大承氣湯)
  e. Heat and Dampness in the three burners: (濕熱蘊結三焦)
    Gan Lu Xiao Du Dan (甘露消毒丹)
3. In the YING (constructive or nutrient) system: (營分証)
  a. Heat causing the depletion of Yin fluid: (熱傷營陰)
    Qing Ying Tang (清營湯)
  b. Heat in the Pericardium: (熱入心包)
    Zhi Bao Dan (至寶丹)
4. In the XUE (Blood system): (血分証)
  a. Heat causing the random flow of blood: (血熱妄行)
    Xi Jiao Di Huang Tang (犀角地黄湯)
  b. Flaring of fire in the Qi and Xue System: (氣血兩燔)
    Qing Wen Bai Du Yin (清瘟敗毒飲)

c. Depletion of Yin leading to endogenous Wind: (傷陰動風)
San Jia Fu Mai Tang (三甲復脈湯)

DIFFERENTIATION according to ZANG-FU (Internal Visceras) (臟腑辩證)
1. Heart: (心病辩證)
   a. Xu (Deficiency) syndrome: (虛証)
      (1) Deficiency of Heart Qi/Yang: (心氣虛/心陽虛)
         Yang Xin Tang (養心湯)
      (2) Deficiency of Heart Blood/Yin: (心血虛/心陰虛)
         (a) Deficiency of Blood: (心血虛)
            Si Wu Tang (四物湯)
         (b) Deficiency of Yin: (心陰虛)
            Tian Wang Bu Xin Dan (天王補心丹)
   b. Shi (Excessive) syndrome: (實証)
      (1) Flaring up of the Heart Fire: (心火上炎)
         Dao Chi San (導赤散)
         San Huang Xie Xin Tang (三黄瀉心湯)
      (2) Obstruction of blood stasis: (心血瘀阻)
         Gua Lou Xie Bai Ban Xia Tang (瓜蔞薤白半夏湯)
         & Xue Fu Zhu Yu Tang (血府逐瘀湯)
      (3) Melancholia caused by fire and phlegm: (痰火疣心)
         Meng Shi Gun Dan Wan (礞石滾痰丸)
2. Small Instestine: (小腸病辩證)
  Obstruction of the flow of Qi causing pain: (小腸氣痛)
     Ju He Wan (橘核丸)
3. Liver: (肝病辩證)
   a. Xu (Deficiency) syndrome: (虛証)
   Insufficiency of Liver Blood: (肝血不足)
   Si Wu Tang (四物湯)
   b. Shi (Excessive) syndrome: (實証)
      (1) Flaring of Liver Fire: (肝火上炎)
         Dang Gui Long Hui Wan (當歸龍薈丸)
      (2) Stagnation of Liver Qi: (肝氣郁結)
         Chai Hu Shu Gan Yin (柴胡舒肝飲)
         Ban Xia Hou Po Tang (半夏厚朴湯)
         Ge Xia Zhu Yu Tang (膈下逐瘀湯)
      (3) Liver Qi attacking the stomach: (肝氣犯胃)
         Si Ni San (四逆散) & Zuo Jin Wan (左金丸)
      (4) Endogenous Wind in Liver: (肝風內動)
         (a) Wind caused by sthenic Liver Yang: (肝陽化風)
            Tian Ma Gou Teng Yin (天麻鉤藤飲)
         (b) Wind caused by intensive Heat: (熱極生風)
            Ling Jiao Gou Teng Tang (羚角鉤藤湯)
         (c) Wind caused by blood deficiency: (血虛生風)
            Bu Gan Tang (補肝湯)

(5) Heat and Dampness in Liver and Gall-bladder: (肝膽濕熱)
Da Chai Hu Tang (大柴胡湯)
Long Dan Xie Gan Tang (龍膽瀉肝湯)

(6) Stagnation of Cold in the Liver channel: (寒滯肝脈)
Nuan Gan Jian (暖肝煎)

4. Gallbladder: (膽囊病辯證)
Stagnation of Phlegm in the Gall-bladder: (膽郁痰扰)
Wen Dan Tang (溫胆湯)

5. Spleen: (脾病辯證)
   a. Xu (Deficiency) syndrome: (虛証)
      (1) Deficiency of Spleen Qi: (脾氣虛)
          Shen Ling Bai Zhu San (參苓白术散)
      (2) Downward flow of the Spleen Qi: (脾氣下陷)
          Bu Zhong Yi Qi Tang (補中益氣湯)
      (3) Blood is not controlled by the Spleen: (脾不統血)
          Gui Pi Tang (歸脾湯)
          Huang Tu Tang (黄土湯)
      (4) Deficiency of the Spleen and Stomach with cold: (脾胃虛寒)
          Li Zhong Tang (理中湯)
   b. Shi (Excessive) syndrome: (實証)
      (1) Dampness in the Spleen: (濕邪困脾)
          Wei Ling Tang (胃苓湯)
      (2) Heat and Dampness in Spleen and Stomach: (脾胃濕熱)
          Yin Chen Hao Tang (茵陳蒿湯)

6. Stomach: (胃病辯證)
   a. Deficiency of the Stomach Yin (fluid): (胃陰不足)
      Yi Wei Tang (益胃湯)
   b. Excessive fire in the Stomach: (胃火熾盛)
      Qing Wei San (清胃散)
   c. Stagnation of food in the Stomach: (食滯胃腕)
      Bao He Wan (保和丸)

7. Lung: (肺病辯證)
   a. Xu (Deficiency) syndrome: (虛証)
      (1) Deficiency of Lung Qi: (肺氣虛)
          Bu Fei Tang (補肺湯)
      (2) Deficiency of Lung Yin (fluid): (肺陰虛)
          Bai He Gu Jin Tang (百合固金湯)
   b. Shi (Excessive) syndrome: (實証)
      (1) Wind and Cold acting on the Lung: (風寒束肺)
          Xin Su San (杏蘇散)
      (2) Wind and Heat acting on the Lung: (風熱犯肺)
          Sang Ju Yin (桑菊飲)
      (3) Heat and Phlegm obstructing the Lung: (痰熱壅肺)
          Ma Xing Shi Gan Tang (麻杏石甘湯)
          Wei Jing Tang (葦莖湯)

(4)   Turbid Phlegm obstructing the Lung: （痰濁阻肺）
       Er Chen Tang （二陳湯）& Su Zi Jiang Qi Tang （蘇子降氣湯）

8. Large Intestine: （大腸病辯證）
  a. Shi (Excessive syndrome): （實証）
    Heat and Dampness in the Large Intestine: （大腸濕熱）
    Shao Yao Tang （芍藥湯）
    Bai Tou Weng Tang （白頭翁湯）
    Ge Gen Qin Lian Tang （葛根芩連湯）& Si Ling Tang （四苓湯）
  b. Xu (Deficiency) syndrome: （虛証）
    (1)   Depletion of body fluid in the Large Intestine: （大腸津虧）
       Zeng Ye Tang （增液湯）& Run Chang Wan （潤腸丸）
    (2)   Prolapse of the Intestine: （腸虛滑脫）
       Zhen Ren Yang Zang Tang （真人養臟湯）

9. Kidney: （腎病辯證）
  a. Deficiency of Kidney Yang: （腎陽虛）
    You Gui Wan （右歸丸）
    Jin Kui Shen Qi Wan （金匱腎氣丸）
  b. Deficiency of Kidney Yin: （腎陰虛）
    Zuo Gui Wan （左歸丸）
    Liu Wei Di Huang Wan （六味地黃丸）
  c. Kidney is not able to control the flow of Qi wih symptoms of dyspnea
    （腎不納氣）: Shen Jie San （參蚧散）
    Ren Shen Hu Tao Tang （人參胡桃湯）
  d. Depletion of Kidney Essence: （腎精不足）
    He Che Da Zao Wan （河車大造丸）
  e. Inconsolidation of Kidney Qi: （腎氣不固）
    Jin Suo Gu Jing Wan （金鎖固經丸）
    Suo Quan Wan （縮泉丸）

10. Urinary Bladder: （膀胱病辯證）
    Heat and Dampness in the Urinary Bladder: （膀胱濕熱）
    Ba Zheng San （八正散）

DIFFICULTY OF SPEECH: （語言困難）
    Bu Yang Huan Wu Tang （補陽還五湯）
    Qian Zheng San （牽正散）

DIPHTHERIA: （白喉病）
    Liu Shen Wan （六神丸）
    Yang Yin Qing Fei Tang （養陰清肺湯）

DISTENTION （鼓脹）
1. Xu (Deficiency) syndrome: （虛脹）
  a. Deficiency of Spleen and Kidney Yang （脾腎陽虛）
    Fu Zi Li Zhong Tang （附子理中湯）& Wu Ling San （五苓散）
    Jin Kui Shen Qi Wan （金匱腎氣丸）

   b. Deficiency of Liver and Kidney Yin: (肝腎陰虛)
       Liu Wei Di Huang Wan (六味地黃丸)
       Yi Guan Jian (一貫煎) & Ge Xia Zhu Yu Tang (膈下逐瘀湯)

2. Shi (Excessive) syndrome: (實脹)
   a. Stagnation of Qi and Dampness: (氣滯濕阻)
       Chai Hu Shu Gan San (柴胡舒肝散) & Wei Ling Tang (胃苓湯)
   b. Stagnation of Heat and Dampness: (濕熱蘊結)
       Yin Chen Hao Tang (茵陳蒿湯)
       Zhou Che Wan (舟車丸)
   c. Blood Stasis in Liver and Spleen: (肝脾血瘀)
       Shi Zao Tang (十棗湯)
       Zhou Che Wan (舟車丸)

DIZZINESS (see Vertigo) (眩暈)

DUODENAL ULCER (see Ulcer) (十二指腸潰瘍)

DYSENTERY (痢疾)

1. Caused by Heat and Dampness: (濕熱痢)
     Shao Yao Tang (芍藥湯)
     Jing Fang Bai Du San (荊防敗毒散)
     Ge Gen Qin Lian Tang (葛根芩連湯)
2. Caused by Toxin: (疫毒痢)
     Bai Tou Weng Tang (白頭翁湯)
3. Caused by Cold and Dampness: (寒濕痢)
     Wei Ling Tang (胃苓湯)
4. Caused by Cold and Deficiency: (虛寒痢)
     Li Zhong Tang (理中湯)
     Tao Hua Tang (桃花湯)
     Zhen Ren Yang Zang Tang (真人養臟湯)
5. Intermittent Dysentery: (休息痢)
     Wen Pi Tang (溫脾湯)
     Xiang Sha Liu Jun Zi Tang (香砂六君子湯)

DYSMENORRHEA (經痛)

1. Stagnation of Qi and Blood: (氣滯血瘀)
     Ge Xia Zhu Yu Tang (膈下逐瘀湯)
2. Stagnation of Cold and Dampness: (寒濕凝滯)
     Shao Fu Zhu Yu Tang (少腹逐瘀湯)
3. Depletion of Liver and Kidney: (肝腎虧損)
     Tiao Gan Tang (調肝湯)

DYSURIA (癃閉)

1. Stagnation of Heat and Dampness: (濕熱壅積)
     Ba Zheng San (八正散), Dao Chi San (導赤散)

2. Downward flow of Qi in the Middle-burner: （中氣下陷）
   　　Bu Zhong Yi Qi Tang （補中益氣湯）
3. Deficiency of Kidney Qi: （腎氣不充）
   　　Shen Qi Wan （腎氣丸）

ECLAMPSIA　GRAVIDARUM （妊娠痛症）
1. Up-flaring of the endogenous Wind: （肝風內動）
   　　Ling Yang Gou Teng Tang （羚羊鉤藤湯）
2. Up-flaring of the Fire and Phlegm: （痰火上擾）
   　　Niu Huang Qing Xin Wan （牛黃清心丸）

ECZEMA （濕疹）
   　　Long Dan Xie Gan Tang （龍膽瀉肝湯）
   　　Wei Ling Tang （胃苓湯）
   　　Gui Zhi Tang （桂枝湯）
   　　Jia Wei Er Miao San （加味二妙散）
   　　Zhen Wu Tang （真武湯）
   　　& Ma Huang Lian Qiao Chi Xiao Dou Tang （麻黃連翹赤小豆湯）

EDEMA （水腫）
1. Yang type of edema: （陽水）
   a. Overflooding of Wind and Water: （風水泛濫）
   　　Yue Bi Jia Zhu Tang （越婢加术湯）
   　　Fang Ji Huang Qi Tang （防己黃芪湯）
   　　Wu Ling San （五苓散）
   　　Wu Pi Yin （五皮飲）
   b. Soaked in Water and Dampness: （水濕浸跡）
   　　Wu Ling San （五苓散）
   　　& Wu Pi Yin （五皮飲）
   c. Excessive Heat and Dampness: （濕熱壅盛）
   　　Ji Jiao Li Huang Wan （己椒藶黃丸）
   　　Ting Li Da Zao Xie Fei Tang （葶藶大棗瀉肺湯）
2. Ying type of edema: （陰水）
   a. Insufficiency of Spleen Yang: （脾陽不振）
   　　Shen Ling Bai Zhu San （參苓白术散）
   b. Decrease of Kidney Yang: （腎陽衰微）
   　　Zhen Wu Tang （真武湯）

EMPHYSEMA （肺氣腫）
   　　Ren Shen Hu Tao Tang （人參胡桃湯）
   　　San Zi Yang Qing Tang （三子養親湯）
   　　She Gan Ma Huang Tang （射干麻黃湯）
   　　Shen Jie San （參蚧散）
   　　Du Qi Wan （都氣丸）

ENCEPHALITIS （腦炎）
　　　An Gong Niu Huang Wan （安宮牛黃丸）
　　　Qing Wen Bai Du Yin （清瘟敗毒飲）
　　　Qing Ying Tang （清營湯）
　　　Zhi Bao Dan （至寶丹）
　　　Zi Xue Dan （紫雪丹）

ENDOMETRIOSIS （子宮內膜移位病）
　　　Gui Zhi Fu Ling Wan （桂枝茯苓丸）
　　　Shi Xiao San （失笑散）

ENTERITIS （腸炎）
　　　Tong Xie Yao Fang （痛瀉要方）
　　　Wei Ling Tang （胃苓湯）
　　　Wu Ling San （五苓散）
　　　Zhen Wu Tang （真武湯）

ENURESIS （遺尿）
1. With Cold and Deficiency of Kidney: （下元虛寒）
　　　Sang Piao Xiao San （桑螵蛸散）
　　　Jin Suo Gu Jing Wan （金鎖固經丸）
2. Deficiency of Qi of Lung and Spleen: （脾肺氣虛）
　　　Suo Quan Wan （縮泉丸）　&　Bu Zhong Yi Qi Tang （補中益氣湯）
3. With Heat and Dampness in the Liver channel: （肝經濕熱）
　　　Long Dan Xie Gan Tang （龍膽瀉肝湯）

EPIGASTRIC PAIN （胃脘痛、腹上部疼痛）
1. Pathogenic cold attacking the Stomach: （寒邪犯胃）
　　　Liang Fu Wan （良附丸）
　　　Xiang Su San （香蘇散）
2. Stagnation of Food: （飲食停滯）
　　　Bao He Wan （保和丸）
　　　Xiao Cheng Qi Tang （小承氣湯）
3. Liver Qi attacking the Stomach: （肝氣犯胃）
　　　Chai Hu Shu Gan San （柴胡舒肝散）
4. Stagnation of Heat in Liver and Stomach: （肝胃郁熱）
　　　Hua Gan Jian （化肝煎）
　　　Xiao Yao San （逍遙散）
5. Pain caused by Deficiency of Stomach Yin: （陰虛胃痛）
　　　Yang Wei Tang （養胃湯）&　Shao Yao Gan Cao Tang （芍藥甘草湯）
　　　Zuo Jin Wan （左金丸）
6. Blood Stasis: （瘀血停滯）
　　　Shi Xiao San （失笑散）&　Dan Shen Yin （丹參飲）
　　　Xie Xin Tang （瀉心湯）
　　　Huang Tu Tang （黃土湯）

7. Deficiency of Spleen and Stomach with Cold: (脾胃虛寒)
   Huang Qi Jian Zhong Tang (黃芪建中湯)
   Da Jian Zhong Tang (大建中湯)
   Xiang Sha Liu Jun Zi Tang (香砂六君子湯)

EPIGASTRIC UPSET (嘈雜)
1. Heat in Stomach: (胃熱)
   Wen Dan Tang (溫胆湯)
2. Deficiency of Stomach: (胃虛)
   Si Jun Zi Tang (四君子湯)
3. Deficiency of Blood: (血虛)
   Gui Pi Tang (歸脾湯)

EPILEPSY (癲癇)
1. Liver Fire with Heat and Phlegm: (肝火痰熱)
   Long Dan Xie Gan Tang (龍膽瀉肝湯)
2. Deficiency of Liver and Kidney Yin: (肝腎陰虛)
   Zuo Gui Wan (左歸丸)
   He Che Da Zao Wan (河車大造丸)
3. Defiency of Spleen and Stomach: (脾胃虛弱)
   Liu Jun Zi Tang (六君子湯)
4. With Blood stasis: (血瘀)
   Tong Qiao Huo Xue Tang (通竅活血湯)

EPISTAXIS (鼻衄)
   Huang Lian Jie Du Tang (黃連解毒湯)
   Shi Hui San (十灰散)
   Si Sheng Wan (四生丸)

ERYSIPELAS (丹毒)
1. Excessive Wind, Heat and Fire (風熱火熾)
   Pu Ji Xiao Du Yin (普濟消毒飲)
2. Stagnation of Fire in the Liver channel: (肝經郁火)
   Long Dan Xie Gan Tang (龍膽瀉肝湯)
3. Heat and Toxin in the Ying (Nutrient) system: (熱毒入營)
   Qing Wen Bai Du Yin (清瘟敗毒飲)
4. Heat and Toxin in the Heart and Stomach: (心胃熱毒)
   Xie Xin Tang (瀉心湯)
5. With deficiency of Yin-fluid: (陰虛)
   Zeng Ye Tang (增液湯)
   Yi Wei Tang (益胃湯)

ESOPHAGEAL CARCINOMA (食管癌)
1. Obstruction of Qi and Phlegm: (痰氣交阻)
   Xuan Fu Dai Zhe Tang (旋覆代赭湯)

2. Heat and Toxin depleting the Yin: (熱毒傷陰)
    Sha Shen Mai Men Dong Tang (沙參麥門冬湯)
3. Depletion of Qi and Blood: (氣血兩虛)
    Ba Zhen Tang (八珍湯)

ESOPHAGIOSPASM (食管痙攣)
    Ban Xia Hou Po Tang (半夏厚朴湯)

FATIGUE (疲勞)
1. Deficiency of Qi and Blood: (氣血兩虛)
    Ba Zhen Tang (八珍湯)
    Shi Quan Da Bu Tang (十全大補湯)
2. Deficiency of Blood: (血虛)
    Dang Gui Bu Xue Tang (當歸補血湯)
3. Deficiency of Heart Yin: (心陰虛)
    Zhi Gan Cao Tang (炙甘草湯)
    Tian Wang Bu Xin Dan (天王補心丹)
4. Deficiency of Kidney Yang: (腎陽虛)
    You Gui Yin (右歸飲)

FEVER (發燒、發熱)
1. Internal fever caused by Deficiency of Yin: (陰虛內熱)
    Qing Gu San (清骨散)
    Da Bu Yin Wan (大補陰丸)
    Zhi Bai Di Huang Wan (知柏地黄丸)
2. Depletion of both Qi and Blood: (氣虛血虧)
    Bu Zhong Yi Qi Tang (補中益氣湯)
    Qing Shu Yi Qi Tang (清暑益氣湯)
3. Deficiency of Blood: (血虛)
    Gui Pi Tang (歸脾湯)
    Dang Gui Bu Xue Tang (當歸補血湯)
4. Fever caused by Deficiency of Yang: (陽虛發熱)
    Jin Kui Shen Qi Wan (金匱腎氣丸)
5. Stagnation of Heat in the Liver Channel: (肝經郁熱)
    Dan Zhi Xiao Yao San (丹梔逍遙散)
    Yue Qu Wan (越麴丸)
6. Interior Blood Stasis: (瘀血內結)
    Xue Fu Zhu Yu Tang (血府逐瘀湯)

FIDGETINESS (煩躁)
    Huang Lian E Jiao Tang (黄連阿膠湯)
    San Huang Si Wu Tang (三黄四物湯)
    Suan Zao Ren Tang (酸棗仁湯)
    Xie Xin Tang (瀉心湯)

FILARIASIS (絲蟲病)
1. Heat and Dampness in the Liver Channel: (肝經濕熱)
    Long Dn Xie Gan Tang (龍膽瀉肝湯)
2. Heat and Dampness in the Urinary Bladder: (膀胱濕熱)
    Ba Zheng San (八正散)
3. Depletion of Kidney Yin: (腎陰虧損)
    Zhi Bai Di Huang Wan (知柏地黃丸)
4. Interior accumulation of Cold and Dampness: (寒濕內聚)
    Wu Ling San (五苓散)

FLACCIDITY of BONES and MUSCLES (骨骼肌肉鬆弛)
    Hu Qian Wan (虎潛丸)
    Qing E Wan (青娥丸)

FLU (感冒)
1. Wind and Cold: (風寒感冒)
    Cong Chi Tang (葱豉湯)
    Jing Fang Bai Du San (荊防敗毒散)
2. Wind and Heat: (風熱感冒)
    Yin Qiao San (銀翹散)
    Sang Xing Tang (桑杏湯)
    Xin Jia Xiang Ru Yin (新加香薷飲)
3. Exterior Cold with interior Heat: (表寒裡熱)
    Ma Xing Shi Gan Tang (麻杏石甘湯)
4. With weak constitution: (體虛感冒)
  a. With Deficiency of Qi: (氣虛感冒)
    Shen Su Yin (參蘇飲)
    Yu Ping Feng San (玉屏風散)
  b. Deficiency of Yin (陰虛感冒)
    Jia Jian Wei Rui Tang (加減葳蕤湯)

FLUID RENTENTION (Yin Zheng) (飲証)
1. Shi (excessive) syndrome: (實証)
  a. Retention of fluid in the Stomach and Intestines: (飲留胃腸)
    Ji Jiao Li Huang Wan (己椒藶黃丸)
  b. Retention of fluid in the Chest and Hypochondria: (飲留胸肋)
    Shi Zao Tang (十棗湯)
    Ting Li Da Zao Xie Fei Tang (葶藶大棗瀉肺湯)
  c. Retention of fluid in the Lung and Chest: (飲犯胸肺)
    Xiao Qing Long Tang (小青龍湯)
    Ling Gan Wu Wei Jiang Xin Tang (苓甘五味薑辛湯)
    Ting Li Da Zao Xie Fei Tang (葶藶大棗瀉肺湯)
  d. Retention of fluid in the 4 limbs: (飲溢四肢)
    Xiao Qing Long Tang (小青龍湯)
    Da Qing Long Tang (大青龍湯)

2. Xu (Deficiency) syndrome: (虛証)
   a. Deficiency of Spleen and Stomach Yang: (脾胃陽虛)
       Ling Gui Zhu Gan Tang (苓桂术甘湯)
   b. Deficiency of Kidney Yang: (腎陽虛弱)
       Jin Kui Shen Qi Wan (金匱腎氣丸)
       Zhen Wu Tang (真武湯)
       Wu Ling San (五苓散)

FLUKE INFESTATION (吸蟲蛭感染)
1. Stagnation of Liver and Deficiency of Spleen: (肝郁脾虛)
       Xiao Yao San (逍遙散)
2. Stagnation of Qi and Blood Stasis: (氣滯血瘀)
       Ge Xia Zhu Yu Tang (膈下逐瘀湯)
         & Liu Jun Zi Tang (六君子湯)
3. Stagnation of Heat and Dampness: (濕熱蘊結)
       Da Chai Hu Tang (大柴胡湯) & Yin Chen Hao Tang (茵陳蒿湯)

FOOD POISONING (食物中毒)
       Gua Di San (瓜蒂散)

FORGETFULLNESS (健忘症)
       Gui Pi Tang (歸脾湯)
       Ren Shen Yang Ying Tang (人參養營湯)
       Sang Piao Xiao San (桑螵蛸散)
       Tian Wang Bu Xin Dan (天王補心丹)
       Zuo Gui Wan (左歸丸)

FREQUENT URINATION (尿頻)
1. Accumulation of Heat and Dampness: (濕熱互結)
       Ba Zheng San (八正散)
       Bi Xie Fen Qing Yin (草薢分清飲)
2. Deficiency of Heart and Kidney: (心腎虛)
       Sang Piao Xiao San (桑螵蛸散)
3. Deficiency of Spleen and Kidney: (脾腎虛)
       Suo Quan Wan (縮泉丸)

FROSTBITE (凍瘡)
1. Accumulation of Cold and Blood stasis: (寒凝血瘀)
       Gui Zhi Tang (桂枝湯)
       Dang Gui Si Ni Tang (當歸四逆湯)
       Dang Gui Si Ni Jia Wu Zhu Yu Sheng Jiang Tang
       (當歸四逆加吳茱萸生薑湯)
2. Type of Heat transferance from Cold: (寒凝化熱)
       Huang Lian Jie Du Tang (黃連解毒湯)

FURUNCLE (癤)
  Huang Lian Jie Du Tang (黃連解毒湯)
  Liu Shen Wan (六神丸)
  Niu Huang Jie Du Pian (牛黃解毒片)
  Wu Wei Xiao Du Yin (五味消毒飲)
  Fang Feng Tong Sheng San (防風通聖散)

GALLSTONE (膽結石)
  San Jin Tang (三金湯)
  Shi Wei San (石葦散)

GASTRECTASIS (胃擴張)
  Fu Gui Li Zhong Wan (附桂理中丸)
  Fu Zi Li Zhong Wan (附子理中丸)
  Li Zhong Wan (理中丸)

GASTRIC CARCINOMA (胃癌)
1. Upset Liver and Stomach: (肝胃不和)
  Chai Hu Shu Gan San (柴胡舒肝散)
   & Xuan Fu Dai Zhe Tang (旋覆代赭湯)
  Yi Wei Tang (益胃湯)
2. Obstruction of Phlegm and Blood Stasis: (痰瘀互結)
  Ge Xia Zhu Yu Tang (膈下逐瘀湯)
3. Deficiency of Spleen and Stomach with cold syndrome: (脾胃虛寒)
  Li Zhong Tang (理中湯) & Liu Jun Zi Tang (六君子湯)

GASTRIC NEUROSIS (胃神經官能症)
  Ping Wei San (平胃散)
  Si Ni San (四逆散)
  Wei Ling Tang (胃苓湯)

GASTRIC ULCER (see Ulcer) (胃潰瘍)

GASTROPTOSIS (胃下垂)
  Bu Zhong Yi Qi Tang (補中益氣湯)
  Li Zhong Wan (理中丸)

GASTRITIS (Chronic) (慢性胃炎)
1. Stagnation of Liver and Stomach Qi: (肝胃氣滯)
  Si Ni San (四逆散)
  Zuo Jin Wan (左金丸)
  Shi Xiao San (失笑散)
  Ban Xia Xie Xin Tang (半夏瀉心湯)
2. Hyperactivity of Liver Qi attacking the Stomach: (肝氣犯胃)
  Chai Hu Shu Gan San (柴胡舒肝散)

3. Heat in Stomach with Deficiency of Yin: (胃熱陰虛)
    Yu Nu Jian (玉女煎)
    Yang Wei Tang (養胃湯)
4. Deficiency of both Spleen and Stomach: (脾胃虛弱)
    Xiang Sha Liu Jun Zi Tang (香砂六君子湯)
    Huang Qi Jian Zhong Tang (黃芪建中湯)

GASTROENTERITIS (腸胃炎)

1. Accumulation of Cold and Heat: (寒熱互結)
    Ban Xia Xie Xin Tang (半夏瀉心湯)
2. Accumulation of Heat and Water: (水熱互結)
    Sheng Jiang Xie Xin Tang (生薑瀉心湯)
3. Accumulation of Heat and Dampness: (濕熱互結)
    San Ren Tang (三仁湯)
4. Deficiency of Spleen and Stomach with Cold: (脾胃虛寒)
    Li Zhong Wan (理中丸)
    Fu Zi Li Zhong Wan (附子理中丸)
5. With Heat in the upper body and Cold in the lower body:
    (上熱下寒)
    Huang Lian Tang (黃連湯)
6. With Deficiency of Spleen and Stomach Qi: (脾胃氣虛)
    Gan Cao Xie Xin Tang (甘草瀉心湯)

GASTRO-INTESTINAL BLEEDING (胃腸出血)
    Huang Tu Tang (黃土湯)

GASTRO-INTESTINAL FLU (胃腸感染)
    Bao He Wan (保和丸)

GASTRO-INTESTINAL NEUROSIS (胃腸神經官能症)
    Ban Xia Hou Po Tang (半夏厚朴湯)
    Xuan Fu Dai Zhe Tang (旋覆代赭湯)
    Yi Guan Jian (一貫煎)
    Yue Qu Wan (越麴丸)

GASTROINTESTINAL SPASM (胃腸痙攣)
    Dang Gui Jian Zhong Tang (當歸健中湯)
    Xio Jian Zhong Tang (小建中湯)

GINGIVITIS (牙齦炎)
    Bai Hu Tang (白虎湯)
    Yu Nu Jian (玉女煎)
    Zhi Bai Di Huang Wan (知柏地黃丸)
    Zhu Ye Shi Gao Tang (竹葉石膏湯)

GLAUCOMA （青光眼）
　　Ci Zhu Wan （磁硃丸）
　　Qi Ju Di Huang Wan （杞菊地黃丸）
　　Zhen Gan Xi Feng Tang （鎮肝熄風湯）

GLOBUS HYSTERICUS （梅核氣）
　　Ban Xia Hou Po Tang （半夏厚朴湯）

GLOMERULAR NEPHRITIS (CHRONIC) （血管球性腎炎）
1. Retention of Water and Dampness caused by Deficiency of Spleen Yang:
　　（脾陽虛弱，水濕逗留）
　　Huang Qi Bu Zhong Tang （黃芪補中湯）
2. Retention of Water and Dampness caused by Deficiency of Spleen and
　Kidney Yang （脾腎陽虛，水濕泛濫）
　　Wei Ling Tang （胃苓湯）
　　Si Mo Tang （四磨湯）& Wu Ling San （五苓散）
　　Ji Jiao Li Huang Wan （己椒藶黃丸）
　　She Gan Ma Huang Tang （射干麻黃湯）
3. Depletion of Liver and Kidney Yin with exuberance of Liver Yang:
　　（肝腎陰虧，肝陽上亢）
　　Di Huang Yin Zi （地黃飲子）
　　Qi Ju Di Huang Wan （杞菊地黃丸）
4. Depletion of Qi and Blood of both Spleen and Kidney:
　　（脾腎兩虧，氣血不足）
　　Da Bu Yuan Jian （大補元煎）
5. Failure of Spleen and Kidney with interior turbid Yin:
　　（脾腎衰敗，濁陰內盛）
　　Wen Pi Tang （溫脾湯）

GLOSSITIS （舌炎）
　　Yu Nu Jian （玉女煎）

GOITER （甲狀腺種）
　　Dao Tan Tang （導痰湯）
　　Xiao Luo Wan （消瘰丸）

GONORRHEA （淋病）
　　Bi Xie Fen Qing Yin （萆薢分清飲）
　　Er Miao San （二妙散）

HEADACHE （頭痛）
1. Affection of exterior factors: （外感頭痛）
　a.　Caused by Wind and Cold （風寒頭痛）
　　　Chuan Xiong Cha Tiao San （川芎茶調散）
　　　Wu Zhu Yu Tang （吳茱萸湯）

b. Caused by Wind and Heat:（風熱頭痛）
Ju Hua Cha Tiao San（菊花茶調散）
Huang Lian Shang Qing Wan（黄連上清丸）
c. Caused by Wind and Dampness:（風濕頭痛）
Qiang Huo Sheng Shi Tang（羌活勝濕湯）
2. Affection of interior factors:（內傷頭痛）
a. Caused by Liver Yang:（肝陽頭痛）
Tian Ma Gou Teng Yin（天麻鉤藤飲）
b. Caused by Kidney Deficiency:（腎虛頭痛）
Da Bu Yuan Jian（大補元煎）
You Gui Wan（右歸丸）
c. Deficiency of Qi and Blood:（氣血虧虛）
Ba Zhen Tang（八珍湯）
d. Caused by turbid Phlegm:（痰濁頭痛）
Ban Xia Bai Zhu Tian Ma Tang（半夏白术天麻湯）
e. Caused by Blood stasis:（瘀血頭痛）
Tong Qiao Huo Xue Tang（通竅活血湯）

HEAT-STROKE（中暑）

Qing Shu Yi Qi Tang（清暑益氣湯）
Zhu Ye Shi Gao Tang（竹葉石膏湯）
Xiang Ru San（香薷散）
Xin Jia Xiang Ru San（新加香薷散）

HEMATEMESIS（嘔血）

Shi Hui San（十灰散）

HEMATURIA（血尿症））

Xiao Ji Yin Zi（小薊飲子）
Xi Jiao Di Huang Tang（犀角地黄湯）

HEMIPLEGIA（半身不遂）

Bu Yang Huan Wu Tang（補陽還五湯）
Qian Zheng San（牽正散）

HEMOPTYSIS（咯血）

Ba Xian Chang Shou Wan（八仙長壽丸）
Bai He Gu Jin Tang（百合固金湯）
Qing Zao Jiu Fei Tang（清燥救肺湯）
Shi Hui San（十灰散），Xie Bai San（瀉白散）

HEMORRHAGIC FEVER（出血性發熱）

1. Febrile stage:（發熱期）
a. Pathogenic factors attacking the Wei (superficial defensive) system
（溫邪擊衛）: Yin Qiao San（銀翹散）

    b.   Heat in the Yang Ming Channel: (陽明熱熾)
          Bai Hu Tang (白虎湯)
    c.   Flaring of Fire in the Qi (secondary defensive) and Ying (nutrient) system
          (氣營兩燔): Qing Wen Bai Du Yin (清瘟敗毒飲)

2. Stroke stage, with low blood pressure: (休克期，低血壓)
    a.   Prostration of Heat: (熱厥)
          Bai Hu Tang (白虎湯) & Sheng Mai San (生脈散)
    b.   Prostration of Cold: (寒厥)
          Shen Fu Tang (參附湯)

3. Dysuria stage: (少尿期)
    a.   Deficiency of Kidney Yin, causing false Fire inside:
          (腎陰虧損，虛火內生)
          Zhi Bai Di Huang Wan (知柏地黃丸)
    b.   Pathogenic factors in the Pericardium, with endogenous Liver Wind:
          (邪陷心包，肝風內動)
          Xi Jiao Di Huang Tang (犀角地黃湯)
          & Ling Yang Gou Teng Tang (羚羊鉤藤湯)
    c.   Retention of Fluid in the Lung: (飲邪壅肺)
          Ting Li Da Zao Xie Fei Tang (葶藶大棗瀉肺湯)

4. Polyuria stage: (多尿期)
    a.   Inconsolidation of Kidney Qi: (腎氣不固)
          Ba Xian Chang Shou Wan (八仙長壽丸) & Suo Quan Wan (縮泉丸)
    b.   Intensive Heat in the Lung and Stomach: (肺胃熱盛)
          Sha Shen Mai Men Dong Tang (沙參麥門冬湯)

5. Recovery stage: (恢復期)
    a.   Depletion of Kidney Yin: (腎陰虧損)
          Liu Wei Di Huang Wan (六味地黃丸)
    b.   Loss of Spleen Yang: (脾陽不振)
          Shen Ling Bai Zhu San (參苓白术散)
    c.   Insufficient Stomach Yin Fluid: (腎陰未復)
          Yi Wei Tang (益胃湯)

HEMORRHOID (痔瘡)
          Huai Hua San (槐花散)
          Huai Jiao Wan (槐角丸)

HEPATIC COMA (肝昏迷)
          Xi Jiao Di Huang Tang (犀角地黃湯)
          Zhi Bao Dan (至寶丹)

HEPATITIS (肝炎)
1. With Heat and Dampness: (濕熱薰蒸)
          Yin Chen Hao Tang (茵陳蒿湯)
          Ma Huang Lian Qiao Chi Xiao Dou Tang (麻黃連翹赤小豆湯)
          Gan Lu Xiao Du Dan (甘露消毒丹)

2. Stagnation of Liver Qi: (肝氣郁滯)
   Chai Hu Shu Gan Tang (柴胡舒肝湯)
3. Dampness in the Spleen: (濕邪困脾)
   Wei ling Tang (胃苓湯)
4. Depletion of Liver Yin: (肝陰虧損)
   Yi Guan Jian (一貫煎)
5. With intensive Heat and Toxin: (熱毒熾盛)
   An Gong Niu Huang Wan (安宮牛黃丸)
   Zhi Bao Dan (至寶丹)

HEPATO-CIRRHOSIS (肝硬化)
1. Stagnation of Liver Qi and asthenia of Spleen: (肝郁脾虛)
   Xiao Yao San (逍遙散)
2. Obstruction of Blood in Liver: (肝血瘀阻)
   Xue Fu Zhu Yu Tang (血府逐瘀湯)
3. Retention of Water in the body: (水濕內阻)
   Wei Ling Tang (胃苓湯)

HEPATOCUTICULAR DEGENERATION (WILSON'S DISEASE) (肝豆狀核變性病)
   Da Ding Feng Zhu (大定風珠)

HERNIA (疝)
   Ju He Wan (橘核丸)
   Tian Tai Wu Yao San (天台烏藥散)

HERPES ZOSTER (帶狀疱疹)
1. With Heat and Dampness: (濕熱型)
   Long Dan Xie Gan Tang (龍膽瀉肝湯)
2. With stagnaion of Qi and Blood: (瘀滯型)
   Chai Hu Shu Gan Tang (柴胡舒肝湯)

HICCOUGH (打嗝)
1. Shi (excessive) syndrome: (實証)
   a. With Coldness in the Stomach: (胃中寒冷)
      Ding Xiang San (丁香散)
   b. With Stomach Fire upflaring: (胃火上逆)
      Xiao Cheng Qi Tang (小承氣湯)
      Zhu Ye Shi Gao Tang (竹葉石膏湯)
   c. With reverse flow of Qi and obstruction of Phlegm: (氣逆痰阻)
      Xuan Fu Dai Zhe Tang (旋覆代赭湯)
      Er Chen Tang (二陳湯)
2. Xu (deficiency) syndrome: (虛証)
   a. Deficiency of Spleen and Stomach Yang: (脾胃陽虛)
      Li Zhong Tang (理中湯)
      Bu Zhong Yi Qi Tang (補中益氣湯)

b. Deficiency of Stomach Yin: (胃陰不足)
   Yi Wei Tang (益胃湯)

HORDEOLUM (麥粒腫)
   Yin Qiao San (銀翹散)
   Yin Qiao Bai Du San (銀翹敗毒散)

HYPERALDOSTERONISM (CONN'S SYNDROME)(原發性醛甾酮過多症)
   Jin Kui Shen Qi Wan (金匱腎氣丸)
   Zhen Wu Tang (真武湯)

HYPERLIPOPROTEINEMIA (高脂蛋白血症)
   Long Dan Xie Gan Tang (龍膽瀉肝湯)

HYPERTENSION (高血壓)
1. Excessive Liver Fire: (肝火亢盛)
   Long Dan Xie Gan Tang (龍膽瀉肝湯)
2. Hyperactivity of Liver Yang: (肝陽上亢)
   Tian Ma Gou Teng Yin (天麻鈎藤飲)
2. Deficiency of Yin with excurberance of Yang: (陰虛陽亢)
   Qi Ju Di Huang Wan (杞菊地黃丸)
3. Depletion of both Yin and Yang (陰陽兩虛)
   Er Xian Tang (二仙湯)
4. Excessive accumulation of Phlegm and Dampness: (痰濕壅盛)
   Ban Xia Bai zhu Tian Ma Tang (半夏白术天麻湯)

HYPERTHYROIDISM (甲狀腺機能亢進)
1. Obstruction and stagnation of Qi and Phlegm: (氣滯痰凝)
   Hai Zao Yu Wu Tang (海藻玉壺湯)
2. Excessive Liver Fire: (肝火亢盛)
   Long Dan Xie Gan Tang (龍膽瀉肝湯)
3. Deficiency of Heart and Liver Yin: (心肝陰虛)
   Tian Wang Bu Xin Dan (天王補心丹) & Yi Guan Jian (一貫煎)

HYPOCALCEMIA (低鈣血症)
   San Jia Fu Mi Tang (三甲復脈湯)

HYPOCHONDRIAC PAIN (肋骨痛)
1. Stagnation of Liver Qi: (肝氣郁結)
   Chai Hu Shu Gan San (柴胡舒肝散)
   Zuo Jin Wan (左金丸)
2. Blood Stasis: (瘀血停着)
   Xuan Fu Hua Tang (旋覆花湯)
   Fu Yuan Huo Xue Tang (復元活血湯)
   Ge Xia Zhu Yu Tang (膈下逐瘀湯)

3. Heat and Dampness in Liver and Gall Bladder: (肝膽濕熱)
   Long Dan Xie Gan Tang (龍膽瀉肝湯)
4. Deficiency of Liver Yin: (肝陰不足)
   Yi Guan Jian (一貫煎)

HYPOTHYROIDISM (甲狀腺機能減退)
Jin Kui Shen Qi Wan (金匱腎氣丸)
Zhen Wu Tang (真武湯)

HYSTERIA (癔病)
Gan Mai Da Zao Tang (甘麥大棗湯)

HYSTEROMYOMA (子宮肌瘤)
Gui Zhi Fu Ling Wan (桂枝茯苓丸)

HYSTEROPTOSIS (子宮下垂)
Bu Zhong Yi Qi Tang (補中益氣湯)

IMPETIGO (膿皰病)
Huang Lian Jie Du Tang (黃連解毒湯)
Wu Wei Xiao Du Yin (五味消毒飲)

IMPOTENCE (陽萎)
1. Diminishing Fire of the Ming-men: (命火衰微)
   Wu Zi Yan Zong Wan (五子衍宗丸)
2. Depletion of Heart and Spleen: (心脾受損)
   Gui Pi Tang (歸脾湯)
3. Kidney damaged by Fear and Fright: (恐懼傷腎)
   Da Bu Yuan Jian (大補元煎)
4. Heat and Dampness in the lower-burner: (濕熱下注)
   Zhi Bai Di Huang Wan (知柏地黃丸)

INCONTINENCE of URINATION (尿失禁)
Bu Yang Huan Wu Tang (補陽還五湯)

INDIGESTION (消化不良)
1. Caused by Stagnation of Food: (飲食停滯)
   Bao He Wan (保和丸)
2. Stagnation of Qi: (氣滯)
   Yue Qu Wan (越麴丸)
3. Stagnation of Liver Qi: (肝氣郁結)
   Chai Hu Shu Gan San (柴胡舒肝散)
4. Deficiency of Spleen and Stomach: (脾胃虛弱)
   Liu Jun Zi Tang (六君子湯)
   Shen Ling Bai Zhu San (參苓白术散)

INFANTILE DIARRHEA (小兒腹瀉)
Shen Ling Bai Zhu San (參苓白术散)

INFANTILE MALNUTRITION (小兒營養不良)
Bai Zhu San (白术散)

INFANTILE PARALYSIS (小兒麻痹症)
Bu Yang Huan Wu Tang (補陽還五湯)

INFANTILE CONVULSION (小兒驚厥)
Zhi Jing San (止痙散)

INFERTILITY (不孕、不育症)
1. Stagnation of Blood: (血瘀)
   Gui Zhi Fu Ling Wan (桂枝茯苓丸)
2. Accumulation of Cold in the Channels: (寒凝經絡)
   Wen Jing Tang (溫經湯)
3. Deficiency of Kidney Yin: (腎陰虛)
   Zuo Gui Wan (左歸丸)
4. Deficiency of Kidney Yang: (腎陽虛)
   You Gui Wan (右歸丸)
5. Diminishing Fire of the Ming-men: (命火衰微)
   Wu Zi Yan Zong Wan (五子衍宗丸)

INFLAMMATION (炎症)
Jing Fang Bai Du San (荊防敗毒散)
Si Miao Yong An Tang (四妙勇安湯)
Yin Qiao Bai Du San (銀翹敗毒散)

INFLUENZA (see FLU) (感冒)

INGUINAL HERNIA (腹股溝疝)
Dao Qi Tang (導氣湯)
Tian Tai Wu Yao San (天台烏藥散)

INJURY (損傷)
Qi Li San (七釐散)
Xue Fu Zhu Yu Tang (血府逐瘀湯)

INSOMNIA (失眠、不寐)
1. Shi (excessive) syndrome: (實証)
   a. Stagnation of Liver into Fire: (肝瘀化火)
      Long Dan Xie Gan Tang (龍膽瀉肝湯)
   b. Accumulation of Heat and Phlegm: (痰熱內擾)
      Wen Dan Tang (溫胆湯)

2. Xu (deficiency) syndrome: (虛証)
   a. Deficiency of Yin and excess of Fire: (陰虛火旺)
      Huang Lian E Jiao Tang (黃連阿膠湯)
      Zhu Sha An Shen Wan (硃砂安神丸)
      Tian Wang Bu Xin Dan (天王補心丹)
   b. Depletion of both Heart and Spleen: (心脾兩虛)
      Gui Pi Tang (歸脾湯)
      Yang Xin Tang (養心湯)
   c. Deficiency of Heart and Gallbladder Qi: (心膽氣虛)
      Suan Zao Ren Tang (酸棗仁湯)

INTERCOSTAL NEURALGIA (肋間神經痛)
1. Accumulation of Heat and Water: (水熱互結)
      Da Xian Xiong Tang (大陷胸湯)
2. Blood Stasis: (血瘀)
      Fu Yuan Huo Xue Tang (復元活血湯)
3. Stagnation of Qi: (氣滯)
      Yue Qu Wan (越麴丸)
4. Disharmony between Liver and Spleen: (肝脾不和)
      Si Ni San (四逆散)

INTESTINAL ABSCESS: (腸膿腫)
      Da Huang Mu Dan Pi Tang (大黃牡丹皮湯)

INTESTINAL OBSTRUCTION (ACUTE) (腸堵塞、腸梗阻)
      Da Chai Hu Tang (大柴胡湯)
      Da Cheng Qi Tang (大承氣湯)
      Da Xian Xiong Tang (大陷胸湯)
      Gan Sui Tong Jie Tang (甘遂通結湯)

INTESTINAL TUBERCULOSIS (腸結核)
1. Deficiency of Spleen and Kidney: (脾腎虛弱) —潰瘍型
      Shen Ling Bai Zhu San (參苓白朮散) & Si Shen Wan (四神丸)
2. Blood Stasis: (瘀血內結) —增生型
      Shao Fu Zhu Yu Tang (少腹逐瘀湯)

IRON DEFICIENCY ANEMIA (see ANEMIA) (缺鐵性貧血)

IRREGULAR MENSTRUATION (see MENSTRUATION) (月經失調)

JAUNDICE (黃疸)
1. Yang type: (陽黃)
   a. Accumulation of Heat and Dampness: (濕熱蘊蒸)
      (1) Heat more than Dampness: (熱重于濕)
          Yin Chen Hao Tang (茵陳蒿湯)

a. (2) Dampness more than Heat: (濕重于熱)
　　　 Yin Chen Wu Ling San (茵陳五苓散)
　　(3) Both Heat and Dampness: (濕熱並重)
　　　 Gan Lu Xiao Du Dan (甘露消毒丹)
　　(4) With Exterior symptoms: (兼表症)
　　　 Ma Huang Lian Qiao Chi Xiao Dou Tang (麻黃連翹赤小豆湯)
b. With intense Heat and Toxin: (濕熱熾盛)
　　An Gong Niu Huang Wan (安宮牛黃丸)
c. Obstruction of the Bile Duct: (膽道阻滯)
　　Da Chai Hu Tang (大柴胡湯)
　　Wu Mei Wan (烏梅丸)
2. Ying type: (陰黃)
　a. Obstruction of Cold and Dampness: (寒濕阻遏)
　　 Yin Chen Zhu Fu Tang (茵陳术附湯)
　b. Deficiency of Blood and Spleen: (脾虛血虧)
　　 Huang Qi Jian Zhong Tang (黃芪建中湯)
　c. With Blood Stasis: (瘀血停積)
　　 Ge Xia Zhu Yu Tang (膈下逐瘀湯)

JAUNDICE (NEONATAL) (初生兒黃疸)
1. Neontal jaundice due to Heat and Dampness: (濕熱胎黃)
　　 Yin Chen Hao Tang (茵陳蒿湯)
2. Neonatal jaundice due to Cold and Dampness: (寒濕胎黃)
　　 Yin Chen Hao ＆ Li Zhong Tang (茵陳理中湯)
3. Neonatal jaundice due to Blood stasis: (瘀血胎黃)
　　 Xue Fu Zhu Yu Tang (血府逐瘀湯)

KERATITIS (角膜炎)
1. Asthenia of Liver with Heat in Lung: (肝虛肺熱)
　　 Si Wu Tang (四物湯) ＆ Xie Bai San (瀉白散)
2. Heat and Drought in the Lung channel: (肺經燥熱)
　　 Qing Zao Jiu Fei Tang (清燥救肺湯)

KNEE INJURY (膝損傷)
1. Ligamentous injury of the knee joint: (膝關節韌帶損傷)
　　 Fu Yuan Huo Xue Tang (復元活血湯)
2. Meniscus injury of knee: (半月板損傷)
　　 Fu Yuan Huo Xue Tang (復元活血湯)

KYPHOSIS (駝背、脊柱後凸)
　　 Yu Zhen San (玉真散)

LEPTOSPIROSIS: (細螺旋體病)
1. Pathogenic factors in the Wei and Qi systems: (邪在衛氣)
　　 Yin Qiao San (銀翹散)

2. Heat and Dampness in the three burners: (暑濕彌漫三焦)
 San Shi Tang (三石湯)
3. Summer Heat and Dampness turned into acute jaundice:
 (暑濕郁蒸，發為急黃)
 Qing Wen Bai Du Yin (清瘟敗毒飲) & Yin Chen Hao Tang (茵陳蒿湯)
4. Summer Heat injuring the Lung: (暑熱傷肺)
 Bai Hu Tang (白虎湯)
 & (Qian Jin) Wei Jing Tang (千金葦莖湯)
5. Heat into the Pericardium, with endogenous Liver Wind:
 (熱入心包，肝風內動)
 Qing Ying Tang (清營湯)
 & Ling Yang Gou Teng Tang (羚羊鉤藤湯)

LARYNGITIS (喉炎)
1. Acute laryngitis: (急性喉炎)
 Yin Qiao San (銀翹散)
 Yin Qiao Bai Du San (銀翹敗毒散)
2. Chronic laryngitis: (慢性喉炎)
 a. Deficiency of Lung and Kidney Yin-fluid: (肺腎陰虛)
 Bai He Gu Jin Tang (百合固金湯)
 Yang Yin Qing Fei Tang (養陰清肺湯)
 b. Deficiency of Lung and Spleen Qi: (肺脾氣虛)
 Bu Zhong Yi Qi Tang (補中益氣湯)

LEUKEMIA (ACUTE) (急性白血病)
1. Intense Heat and Toxin: (熱毒熾盛)
 Xi Jiao Di Huang Tang (犀角地黃湯)
 Zi Xue Dan (紫雪丹)
 Zhi Bao Dan (至寶丹)
2. Deficiency of Liver and Kidney Yin: (肝腎陰虛)
 Da Bu Yuan Jian (大補元煎)
3. Deficiency of Kidney Yang: (腎陽虛)
 You Gui Wan (右歸丸)

LEUKEMIA (CHRONIC) (慢性白血病)
1. Obstruction of Phlegm and Blood Stasis: (瘀血痰阻)
 Ge Xia Zhu Yu Tang (膈下逐瘀湯)
2. Deficiency of both Qi and Blood: (氣血兩虛)
 Ren Shen Yang Ying Tang (人參養營湯)
 Ba Zhen Tang (八珍湯)
3. Deficiency of Liver and Kidney Yin: (肝腎陰虛)
 Da Bu Yuan Jian (大補元煎)
4. Intense Heat and Toxin: (熱毒熾盛)
 Xi Jiao Di Huang Tang (犀角地黃湯)

LEUKOCYTOPENIA and GRANULOCYTOPENIA
（白細胞減少、粒狀白血球過少症）
1. Deficiency of both Qi and Yin: （氣陰兩虧）
   Sheng Mai San （生脈散）
2. Deficiency of Spleen and Kidney Yang: （脾腎陽虛）
   Fu Zi Li Zhong Tang （附子理中湯） ＆ You Gui Wan （右歸丸）
3. Weakness of both Spleen and Stomach: （脾胃虛弱）
   Si Jun Zi Tang （四君子湯）＆ Huang Qi Jian Zhong Tang （黃芪建中湯）

LEUKORRHEA （帶下病）
1. With Heat and Dampness: （濕熱帶下）
   Jia Wei Er Miao San （加味二妙散）
   Yu Dai Wan （愈帶丸）
   Er Miao San （二妙散）
2. Deficiency of Yin with excess Fire: （陰虛火旺）
   Gu Jing Wan （固經丸）
3. Deficiency of Heart and Kidney: （心腎虛）
   Zhen Ling Dan （震靈丹）
4. Stagnation of Liver Qi: （肝氣郁結）
   Xiao Yao San （逍遙散）
   Long Dan Xie Gan Tang （龍膽瀉肝湯）

LIVER CARCINOMA (PRIMARY) （肝癌）
1. Stagnation of Qi and Blood Stasis: （氣滯血瘀）
   Xiao Yao San （逍遙散）＆ Tao Hong Si Wu Tang （桃紅四物湯）
2. Stagnation of Heat, Toxin and Dampness: （濕熱瘀毒）
   Yin Chen Hao Tang （茵陳蒿湯）＆ Ge Xia Zhu Yu Tang （膈下逐瘀湯）
3. Heat and Toxin causing the depletion of Yin: （熱毒傷陰）
   Xi Jiao Di Huang Tang （犀角地黃湯）
4. Deficiency of Liver and Kidney Yin: （肝腎陰虛）
   Liu Wei Di Huang Wan （六味地黃丸）

LIVER CIRRHOSIS （肝硬化）
1. Stagnation of Liver Qi and deficiency of Spleen: （肝郁脾虛）
   Chai Hu Shu Gan Tang （柴胡舒肝湯）＆ Si Jun Zi Tang （四君子湯）
2. Stagnation of Qi and Blood: （氣滯血瘀）
   Hua Yu Tang （化瘀湯）
3. Interior Obstruction of Water and Dampness: （水濕內阻）
   Wei Ling Tang （胃苓湯）
4. Deficiency of Spleen and Kidney Yang: （脾腎陽虛）
   Fu Zi Li Zhong Tang （附子理中湯）＆ Wu Ling San （五苓散）
5. Deficiency of Liver and Kidney Yin: （肝腎陰虛）
   Yi Guan Jian （一貫煎）
   ＆ Zhu Ling Tang （豬苓湯）

LOBAR PNEUMONIA（大葉肺炎）
1. Pathogenic factors affecting the Lung:（邪犯肺衛）
    Yin Qiao San（銀翹散）
2. Accumulation of Heat and Phlegm in the Lung:（痰熱壅肺）
    Ma Xing Shi Gan Tang（麻杏石甘湯）& Wei Jing Tang（葦莖湯）
3. Depletion of Qi and Yin, with remaining Heat and Phlegm:
    （氣陰兩虧、痰熱未清）
    Zhu Ye Shi Gao Tang（竹葉石膏湯）
4. Prostration of Yang Qi:（陽氣虛脱）
    Shen Fu Tang（參附湯）
    Sheng Mai San（生脈散）

LOCHIA（惡露）
    Sheng Hua Tang（生化湯）

LOCK-JAW（牙關緊閉）
    Su He Xiang Wan（蘇合香丸）
    Yu Zhen San（玉真散）

LOSS of HAIR and TEETH（脱髮、掉牙）
    Zuo Gui Wan（左歸丸）

LOSS of SMELL（失嗅覺）
    Xin Yi San（辛夷散）

LUMBAGO（腰背痛、腰肌痛）
1. Caused by Cold and Dampness:（寒濕腰痛）
    Gan Jiang Ling Zhu Tang（乾薑苓术湯）
    Du Huo Ji Sheng Tang（獨活寄生湯）
2. Caused by Heat and Dampness:（濕熱腰痛）
    Jia Wei Er Miao San（加味二妙散）
3. Caused by Kidney Deficiency:（腎虚腰痛）
    Qing E Wan（青娥丸）
    a. With deficiency of Yang（陽虚）, add:
    You Gui Wan（右歸丸）
    b. With deficiency of Yin,（陰虚）, add:
    Zuo Gui Wan（左歸丸）

LUNG ABSCESS（肺膿腫）
1. Initial stage:（初期）
    Yin Qiao San（銀翹散）
2. Abscess stage:（成癰期）
    (Qian Jin) Wei Jing Tang（千金葦莖湯）
3. Purulent stage:（潰膿期）
    Jie Geng Tang（桔梗湯）& Wei Jing Tang（葦莖湯）

4. Recovery stage: (恢復期)
    Qing Zao Jiu Fei Tang (清燥救肺湯)

LUPUS (see SYSTEMIC LUPUS ERYTHEMATOSUS) (狼瘡)

LYMPHADENITIS (淋巴腺炎)
    Pu Ji Xiao Du Yin (普濟消毒飲)
    Xiao Luo Wan (消瘰丸)

LYMPHANGITIS (ACUTE) (急性淋巴管炎)
    Huang Lian Jie Du Tang (黃連解毒湯)
    Wu Wei Xiao Du Yin (五味消毒飲)

MACULA (斑點)
    Huang Lian Jie Du Tang (黃連解毒湯)
    Qing Wen Bai Du Yin (清瘟敗毒飲)
    Xi Jiao Di Huang Tang (犀角地黃湯)
    Qing Ying Tang (清營湯)

MALARIA (瘧)
1. Regular malaria: (正瘧)
    Xiao Chai Hu Tang (小柴胡湯)
2. Warm marlaria (more fever, less chill) (溫瘧)
    Bai Hu Jia Gui Zhi Tang (白虎加桂枝湯)
    Bai Hu Jia Ren Shen Tang (白虎加人參湯)
3. Cold malaria (only chill, no fever): (寒瘧)
    Chai Hu Gui Jiang Tang (柴胡桂薑湯)
4. Malignant malaria: (瘴瘧)
  a. Heat type: (熱瘴)
    Zi Xue Dan (紫雪丹)
  b. Cold type: (寒瘴)
    Huo Xiang Zheng Qi San (藿香正氣散)
    Su He Xiang Wan (蘇合香丸)
5. Alternate Chills and Fever: (寒熱往來)
    Da Yuan Yin (達原飲)

MALNUTRITION (INFANTILE) (小兒營養不良)
    Bai Zhu San (白朮散)
    Bu Dai Wan (布袋丸)

MANIA (躁狂)
1. Upflaring of Fire and Phlegm: (痰火上擾)
    An Gong Niu Huang Wan (安宮牛黃丸)
2. With Convulsions: (抽搐，肝風內動)
    Ling Yang Gou Teng Tang (羚羊鉤藤湯)

3. Depletion of Yin by excessive Fire:（火盛傷陰）
Xue Fu Zhu Yu Tang（血府逐瘀湯）

MASS（ABDOMINAL）（積聚、腹部塊質）
1. Soft mass (with no fixed spot or shape):（聚証）
   a. Stagnation of Liver Qi:（肝郁氣滯）
      Mu Xiang Shun Qi San（木香順氣散）
      Zuo Jin Wan（左金丸）
      Gan Mai Da Zao Tang（甘麥大棗湯）
   b. Stagnation of Food and Phlegm:（食滯痰阻）
      Xiang Sha Liu Jun Zi Tang（香砂六君子湯）
2. Lumps (with fixed spot and shape):（積証）
   a. Obstruction of Blood and stagnation of Qi:（氣郁血阻）
      Wu Ji San（五積散）
   b. Stagnation of Qi and Blood Stasis:（氣結血瘀）
      Ge Xia Zhu Yu Tang（膈下逐瘀湯）
   c. Caused by deficiency of genuine Qi:（正虛瘀結）
      Ba Zhen Tang（八珍湯） & Hua Ji Wan（化積丸）

MASTADENITIS（急性乳腺炎）
     Tou Nong San（透膿散）
      & Wu Wei Xiao Du Yin（五味消毒飲）

MEASLES:（痲疹）
     Sheng Ma Ge Gen Tang（升麻葛根湯）
     Xie Bai San（瀉白散）
     Yin Qiao San（銀翹散）

MENIERE'S DISEASE（美尼爾氏病、耳性眩暈病）
1. Hyperactivity of the Liver Yang:（肝陽上亢）
     Tian Ma Gou Teng Yin（天麻鉤藤飲）
2. With turbid Phlegm in the middle-burner:（痰濁中阻）
     Ban Xia Bai Zhu Tian Ma Tang（半夏白术天麻湯）
3. With asthenia of both Spleen and Kidney:（脾腎虛弱）
     Bu Zhong Yi Qi Tang（補中益氣湯）
      & Zhen Wu Tang（真武湯）
     Er Long Zuo Ci Wan（耳聾左慈丸）

MENINGITIS（腦膜炎）
     An Gong Niu Huang Wan（安宮牛黃丸）
     Liang Ge San（涼膈散）
     Qing Ying Tang（清營湯）
     Zi Xue Dan（紫雪丹）
     Qing Wen Bai Du Yin（清瘟敗毒飲）

MENOPAUSE (停經、經絕期)
1. Deficiency of Kidney Yin: (腎陰虛)
   Zuo Gui Yin (左歸飲)
2. Deficiency of Kidney Yang: (腎陽虛)
   You Gui Yin (右歸飲)
3. Deficiency of both Yin and Yang: (陰陽皆虛)
   Er Xian Tang (二仙湯)
4. Stagnation of Liver Qi: (肝氣郁結)
   Xiao Yao San (逍遙散)

MENSTRUATION (月經、行經)
1. Irregular menstruation: (月經先後無定期)
   a. Stagnation of Liver Qi: (肝郁)
      Xiao Yao San (逍遙散)
   b. Stagnation of Liver acting on the Spleen: (肝郁侵脾)
      Shen Ling Bai Zhu San (參苓白术散)
   c. Kidney asthenia: (腎虛)
      Gu Yin Jian (固陰煎)
2. Early menstruation: (月經先期)
   a. Heat in the Blood: (血熱)
      Dan Zhi Xiao Yao San (丹梔逍遙散)
   b. Deficiency of Qi: (氣虛)
      Gui Pi Tang (歸脾湯)
      Bu Zhong Yi Qi Tang (補中益氣湯)
3. Delayed menstruation: (月經後期)
   a. Coldness in the blood: (血寒)
      Wen jing Tang (溫經湯)
   b. Deficiency of Blood: (血虛)
      Ren Shen Yang Ying Tang (人參養营湯)
   c. Stagnation of Qi: (氣滯)
      Jia Wei Wu Yao Tang (加味烏药湯)
   d. Blood stasis: (血瘀)
      Tao Hong Si Wu Tang (桃紅四物湯)
4. Prolonged menstruation: (經期延長)
   a. Deficiency of Qi: (氣虛)
      Gui Pi Tang (歸脾湯)
   b. Heat in the Blood: (血熱)
      Gu Jing Wan (固經丸)

MORNING SICKNESS (晨吐、孕嘔)
   Xiang Sha Liu Jun Zi Tang (香砂六君子湯)

MUMPS (流行性腮腺炎)
   Qiang Lan Tang (羌籃湯)

MUSCLE-ACHE (肌肉疼痛)
1. Exterior Wind and Cold, with interior Heat: (風寒裡熱)
    Chai Ge Jie Ji Tang (柴葛解肌湯)
    Jiu Wei Qiang Huo Tang (九味羌活湯)
2. Wind and Dampness: (風濕)
    Qiang Huo Sheng Shi Tang (羌活勝濕湯)
3. Qi stagnation and Blood stasis: (氣滯血瘀)
    Shen Tong Zhu Yu Tang (身痛逐瘀湯)

MUSCULAR ATROPHY (肌肉萎縮)
    Da Ding Feng Zhu (大定風珠)
    Bu Zhong Yi Qi Tang (補中益氣湯)

MUSHROOM POISONING (蘑菇中毒，傘菌中毒)
    Gua Di San (瓜蒂散)

MYASTHENIA GRAVIS (重症肌無力)
    Bu Zhong Yi Qi Tang (補中益氣湯)

MYCARDIAL INFARCTION (心肌梗塞)
    Sheng Mai San (生脈散)

MYOCARDITIS (心肌炎)
1. Deficiency of Qi and Yin: (氣陰兩虛)
    Sheng Mai San (生脈散)
    Zhi Gan Cao Tang (炙甘草湯)
    Jia Jian Fu Mai Tang (加減復脈湯)
2. Deficiency of Yang with edema: (陽虛水泛)
    Zhen Wu Tang (真武湯)
3. Deficiency of Yang with Prostration: (陽虛欲脫)
    Shen Fu Long Mu Tang (參附龍牡湯)

NASAL-SINUSITIS (鼻竇炎)
1. Acute nasal-sinusitis: (急性鼻竇炎)
    a. Wind and Heat acting on the Lung channel: (肺經風熱)
       Cang Er San (蒼耳散)
        & Yin Qiao San (銀翹散)
    b. Intense Heat in the Gallbladder channel: (膽經熱盛)
       Long Dan Xie Gan Tang (龍膽瀉肝湯)
    c. Heat and Dampness in the Spleen channel: (脾經濕熱)
       Gan Lu Xiao Du Dan (甘露消毒丹)
2. Chronic nasal-sinusitis: (慢性鼻竇炎)
    Cang Er San (蒼耳散)
     & Xin Yi San (辛夷散)

NAUSEA and VOMITING (惡心，嘔吐)
    Huo Xiang Zheng Qi San (藿香正氣散)
    Ping Wei San (平胃散)
    Xiang Sha Liu Jun Zi Tang (香砂六君子湯)
    Wen Dan Tang (溫胆湯)

NEPHRITIS (ACUTE) (急性腎炎)
1. Edema with exterior affection of Wind: (風水泛濫)
    Yue Bi Jia Zhu Tang (越婢加术湯)
      & Ma Huang Lian Qiao Chi Xiao Dou Tang (麻黄連翹赤小豆湯)
2. Edema with heavy sensation: (水濕浸漬)
    Wu Ling San (五苓散) & Wu Pi Yin (五皮飲)
3. Edema with intense Heat and Toxin: (熱毒)
    Wu Wei Xiao Du Yin (五味消毒飲)
4. Hematuria caused by Heat and Dampness: (濕熱壅盛)
    Xiao Ji Yin Zi (小薊飲子)

NEPHRITIS (CHRONIC) (慢性腎炎)
1. With edema caused by over-flooding of Water: (水腫期，水濕泛濫)
    Zhen Wu Tang (真武湯)
2. With no edema, but with retention of Water and Dampness:
    (無水腫期，水濕逗留)
    Huang Qi Bu Zhong Tang (黃芪補中湯)
3. With hypertension, caused by deficiency of Liver and Kidney Yin,
    and exuberance of Liver Yang: (高血壓，下虛上盛)
    Di Huang Yin Zi (地黄飲子)
4. With uremia caused by increase of pathogenic factors and weakened
    body resistance: (尿毒症期，正虛邪實)
    Wen Pi Tang (溫脾湯)
5. Latent stage, with deficiency of Spleen and Kidney:
    (隱匿期，脾腎兩虛)
    Da Bu Yuan Jian (大補元煎)

NEPHROTIC SYNDROME (腎病綜合症)
1. Deficiency of Spleen and Kidney Yang: (脾腎陽虛)
    Zhen Wu Tang (真武湯)
2. Deificiency of Kidney Qi: (腎氣虧虛)
    You Gui Wan (右歸丸)

NEURASTHENIA (神經衰弱)
1. Deficiency of Heart and Spleen: (心脾虧虛)
    Gui Pi Tang (歸脾湯)
2. Deficiency of yin with excess of Fire: (陰虛火旺)
    Suan Zao Ren Tang (酸棗仁湯)
      & Zhu Sha An Shen Wan (硃砂安神丸)

3. Deficiency of Gall-bladder with Heat and Phlegm: (膽虛痰熱)
    Wen Dan Tang (溫胆湯)

NEUROSIS (神經官能症)
1. Stagnaion of Liver Qi: (肝氣郁結)
    Chai Hu Shu Gan San (柴胡舒肝散)
2. Hyperactivity of Fire due to Yin-fluid deficiency: (陰虛火旺)
    Huang Lian E Jiao Tang (黄連阿膠湯)
       & Tian Wang Bu Xin Dan (天王補心丹)
3. Up-flaring of Heart Fire: (心火上炎)
    Zhu Sha An Shen Wan (硃砂安神丸)

NIGHT PERSPIRATION (盜汗)
    Ba Xian Chang Shou Wan (八仙長壽丸)
    Da Bu Yin Wan (大補陰丸)

NIGHTMARE (夢魘)
    Gui Pi Tang (歸脾湯)

NOCTURIA (夜尿)
    Jin Kui Shen Qi Wan (金匱腎氣丸)
    Suo Quan Wan (縮泉丸)

NOCTURNAL EMISSION (夢遺，遺精)
    Jin Suo Gu Jing Wan (金鎖固經丸)
    Gui Lu Er Xin Jiao (龜鹿二仙膠)
    Da Bu Yin Wan (大補陰丸)

NOSE BLEEDING (鼻出血)
1. Wind and Heat acting on the Lung: (風熱犯肺)
    Yin Qiao San (銀翹散)
    Si Sheng Wan (四生丸)
    Sang Ju Yin (桑菊飲)
2. Intense Heat in the Stomach: (胃熱熾盛)
    Xi Jiao Di Huang Tang (犀角地黄湯)
    Yu Nu Jian (玉女煎)
3. Up-flaring of Liver Fire: (肝火上炎)
    Long Dan Xie Gan Tang (龍膽瀉肝湯)
4. Deficiency of Liver and Kidney Yin-fluid: (肝腎陰虛)
    Zhi Bai Di Huang Wan (知柏地黄丸)
5. Spleen loss the control of blood flowing in the vessels: (脾不統血)
    Gui Pi Tang (歸脾湯)
6. Deficiency of Spleen Yang: (脾陽虛)
    Huang Tu Tang (黄土湯)

OBESITY (肥胖症)
  Dao Tan Tang (導痰湯)
  Fang Feng Tong Sheng San (防風通聖散)

OBSTRUCTED BACKFLOW of LYMPH DUCTS (淋巴管回流梗阻)
  Pu Ji Xiao Du Yin (普濟消毒飲)

OPHTHALMALGIA (眼痛)
  Qi Ju Di Huang Wan (杞菊地黄丸)

OPISTHOTONOS (角後弓反張)
  Ling Yang Gou Teng Tang (羚羊鉤藤湯)

OPTIC NEURITIS (視神經炎)
  Liu Wei Di Huang Wan (六味地黄丸)
  Long Dan Xie Gan Tang (龍膽瀉肝湯)
  Ming Mu Di Huang Wan (明目地黄丸)

ORAL ULCERATION (口腔潰瘍)
  Niu Huang Jie Du Pian (牛黄解毒片)
  Xie Xin Tang (瀉心湯)

ORCHIDIPTOSIS (睪丸下垂)
  Ju He Wan (橘核丸)

OSTEOMYELITIS (PYOGENIC) (化膿性骨髓炎)
1. Early stage: (初期)
  Wu Wei Xiao Du Yin (五味消毒飲)
   & Huang Lian Jie Du Tang (黄連解毒湯)
2. Purulent stage: (化膿期)
  Tuo Li Xiao Du Yin (托裡消毒飲)

OTITIS MEDIA (中耳炎)
1. Acute catarrhal otitis media: (急性卡他性中耳炎)
 a. Pathogenic Wind attacking on the ear: (風邪犯耳)
  Yin Qiao San (銀翹散)
  Xin Yi San (辛夷散)
 b. Accumulation of Dampness in the ear: (濕聚清竅)
  Si Ling San (四苓散)
2. Chronic catarrhal otitis media: (慢性卡他性中耳炎)
  Tong Qiao Huo Xue Tang (通竅活血湯)
3. Acute suppurative otitis media: (急性化膿性中耳炎)
 a. External pathogenic Heat and Toxin on the ear: (風熱邪毒外襲)
  Yin Qiao San (銀翹散)
  Cang Er San (蒼耳散)

b. Heat and Dampness in Liver and Gallbladder: （肝膽濕熱）
　　Long Dan Xie Gan Tang （龍膽瀉肝湯）
4. Chronic suppurative otitis media: （慢性化膿性中耳炎）
　　Sheng Ling Bai Zhu San （參苓白术散）
　　Zhi Bai Di Huang Wan （知柏地黃丸）

OVARIAN CYST （卵巢囊腫）
　　Gui Zhi Fu Ling Wan （桂枝茯苓丸）

PALPITATION （心悸）
1. Irritability: （心神不寧）
　　Wen Dan Tang （溫胆湯）
2. Deficiency of Blood: （心血不足）
　　Gui Pi Tang （歸脾湯）
　　Sheng Mai San （生脈散）
　　Zhi Gan Cao Tang （炙甘草湯）
3. Deficiency of Yin with excess Fire: （陰虛火旺）
　　Tian Wang Bu Xin Dan （天王補心丹）
　　Zhu Sha An Shen Wan （硃砂安神丸）
　　Zhi Bai Di Huang Wan （知柏地黃丸）
4. Deficiency of Heart Yang: （心陽不足）
　　Gui Zhi Gan Cao Long Gu Mu Li Tang （桂枝甘草龍骨牡蠣湯）
5. Retention of fluid: （飲邪上犯）
　　Ling Gui Zhu Gan Tang （苓桂术甘湯）
　　Zhen Wu Tang （真武湯）

PANCREATITIS （胰腺炎）
1. Stagnation of Qi and retention of Food: （氣滯食積）
　　Qing Yi Tang （清胰湯）
2. Excessive Heat in Spleen and Stomach: （脾胃實熱）
　　Qing Yi Tang （清胰湯） ＆ Da Cheng Qi Tang （大承氣湯）
3. Heat and Dampness in Liver and Gall-bladder: （肝膽濕熱）
　　Qing Yi Tang （清胰湯）＆ Long Dan Xie Gan Tang （龍膽瀉肝湯）
　　Yin Chen Hao Tang （茵陳蒿湯）＆ Chai Hu Shu Gan Tang （柴胡舒肝湯）
4. Stagnation of Heat in Liver and Stomach: （肝胃郁熱）
　　Da Chai Hu Tang （大柴胡湯）＆ Xiao Cheng Qi Tang （小承氣湯）
5. Stagnation of Qi and Blood stasis: （氣滯血瘀）
　　Si Ni San （四逆散）＆ Shao Fu Zhu Yu Tang （少腹逐瘀湯）
6. Weakened body resistance with prevailing pathogenic factors: （正虛邪陷）
　　Fu Zi Li Zhong Tang （附子理中湯）＆ Ge Xia Zhu Yu Tang （膈下逐瘀湯）

PARALYSIS (WEI ZHENG) （痿証、麻痹）
1. Depletion of Fluid by Heat in the Lung: （肺熱傷津）
　　Qing Zao Jiu Fei Tang （清燥救肺湯）
　　Yi Wei Tang （益胃湯）

2. Accumulation of Heat and Dampness: (濕熱浸淫)
   Jia Wei Er Miao San (加味二妙散)
3. Deficiency of Spleen and Stomach with Cold: (脾胃虛寒)
   Shen Ling Bai Zhu San (參苓白术散)
4. Deficiency of Liver and Kidney: (肝腎虧虛)
   Hu Qian Wan (虎潛丸)

PARASITIC INFESTATION (寄生虫感染)
   Bu Dai Wan (布袋丸)
   Wu Mei Wan (烏梅丸)

PAROTITIS (腮腺炎)
1. Virulent pathogens from the exterior: (瘟毒在表)
   Yin Qiao San (銀翹散)
   Ying Qiao Bai Du San (銀翹敗毒散)
   Jing Fang Bai Du San (荊防敗毒散)
2. Accumulation of Heat and Toxin: (熱毒瘟結)
   Pu Ji Xiao Du Yin (普濟消毒飲)

PERICARDITIS (心包炎)
   Ji Jiao Li Huang Wan (己椒藶黄丸)

PELVIC INFLAMMATION (盆腔炎)
   Da Huang Mu Dan Pi Tang (大黄牡丹皮湯)
   Long Dan Xie Gan Tang (龍膽瀉肝湯)
   Tao He Cheng Qi Tang (桃核承氣湯)
   Gui Zhi Fu Ling Wan (桂枝茯苓丸)

PEPTIC ULCER (消化性潰瘍、十二指腸潰瘍)
1. With cold and asthenia: (虛寒)
   Huang Qi Jian Zhong Tang (黄芪建中湯)
2. With stagnation of Qi: (氣滯)
   Si Ni San (四逆散)
3. With Blood stasis: (血瘀)
   Shi Xiao San (失笑散) & Dan Shen Yin (丹參飲)

PERIODONTITIS (牙周炎)
   Niu Huang Jie Du Pian (牛黄解毒片)
   Yu Nu Jian (玉女煎)

PERITONITIS (腹膜炎)
1. Deficiency of Qi and Yin: (氣陰兩虛)
   Si Jun Zi Tang (四君子湯) & Qing Gu San (清骨散)
2. Obstruction of Blood flow with stasis: (瘀血阻滯)
   Xue Fu Zhu Yu Tang (血府逐瘀湯)

PERSPIRATION DISORDERS (HAN ZHENG) (汗証)

1. Spontaneous perspiration: (自汗)
   a. Imbalance between Ying (Nutrient) and Wei (superficial defensive) system:
      (營衛不和)
      Gui Zhi Tang (桂枝湯)
   b. Deficiency of Lung Qi: (肺氣不足)
      Yu Ping Feng San (玉屏風散)
   c. Interior Heat: (熱淫于內)
      Bai Hu Tang (白虎湯)
2. Night perspiration: (盜汗)
   a. Deficiency of Heart Blood: (心血不足)
      Gui Pi Tang (歸脾湯)
   b. Deficiency of Yin with excess Fire: (陰虛火旺)
      Dang Gui Liu Huang Tang (當歸六黃湯)
      Ba Xian Chang Shou Wan (八仙長壽丸)
3. Perspiration in shock: (脫汗)
      Shen Fu Tang (參附湯)
4. Perspiration with shivering: (戰寒)
      Zhen Ye Cheng Qi Tang (真液承氣湯)
      Liang Ge San (涼膈散)
5. Perspiration with stickiness and yellow color: (黃汗)
      Yin Chen Wu Ling San (茵陳五苓散)
      Ma Huang Lian Qiao Chi Xiao Dou Tang (麻黃連翹赤小豆湯)

PHARYNGITIS (咽炎)

      Niu Huang Jie Du Pian (牛黃解毒片)
      Pu Ji Xiao Du Yin (普濟消毒飲)
      Qiang Lan Tang (羌籃湯)

PHLEGM DISORDERS (TAN ZHENG) (痰証)

1. Shi (Excessive) syndrome: (實痰)
   a. Turbid phlegm in the Lung: (痰濁壅肺)
      Xing Su San (杏蘇散)
      Su Zi Jiang Qi Tang (蘇子降氣湯)
   b. Obstruction of Phlegm in the Middle-burner: (痰阻中焦)
      Er Chen Tang (二陳湯)
   c. Stagnation of Phlegm, causing dyspnea and oppression in the chest:
      (痰郁互結)
      Wen Dan Tang (溫胆湯)
   d. Obstruction of Phlegm and Wind, causing tremor or spasm in the face
      or extremities: (風痰閉阻)
      Qian Zheng San (牽正散)
2. Xu (deficiency) syndrome: (虛痰)
   a. Deficiency of Lung: (肺虛痰戀)
      Bu Fei E Jiao San (補肺阿膠散)

b. Deficiency of Spleen: (脾虛痰盛)
    Liu Jun Zi Tang (六君子湯)
c. Deficiency of Kidney: (腎虛痰犯)
    Jin Kui Shen Qi Wan (金匱腎氣丸)
    Jin Shui Liu Jun Jian (金水六君煎)
d. Deficiency of Lung and Kidney Yin: (肺腎陰虛)
    Sheng Mai San (生脈散)

PHLEGMON (ACUTE) (急性蜂窩織炎)

1. Initial and pyogenic stage: (初期及釀膿期)
    Wu Wei Xiao Du Yin (五味消毒飲)
2. Ulcerous stage: (潰膿後期)
    Tuo Li Xiao Du Yin (托裡消毒飲)

PHRENOSPASM (膈痙攣)

    Ding Xiang Shi Di Tang (丁香柿蒂湯)

PHTHIASIS (see PULMONARY TUBERCULOSIS) (癆瘵)

PIGMENTARY DEGENERATION of RETINA (色素性視網膜炎)

1. Diminished Fire of the Ming-men (Gate of Life): (命門火衰)
    You Gui Yin (右歸飲)
2. Asthenia of both Liver and Kidney: (肝腎兩虛)
    Ming Mu Di Huang Wan (明目地黃丸)

PLEURITIS (PLEURISY) (胸膜炎)

1. Accumulation of Heat and Phlegm: (痰熱蘊結)
    Chai Hu Xian Xiong Tang (柴胡陷胸湯)
    Da Qing Long Tang (大青龍湯)
2. Retention of Fluid in chest: (飲留肋下)
    Ting Li Da Zao Xie Fei Tang (葶藶大棗瀉肺湯)
    Shi Zao Tang (十棗湯)
3. Deficiency of Yin: (陰虛邪戀)
    Qing Gu San (清骨散)
    & Xiao Xian Xiong Tang (小陷胸湯)

PNEUMONIA (INFANTILE) (小兒肺炎)

1. Wind and Heat acting on the Lung: (風熱閉肺)
    Ma Xing Shi Gan Tang (麻杏石甘湯)
2. Heat and Phlegm obstructing the Lung: (痰熱閉肺)
    Ting Li Da Zao Xie Fei Tang (葶藶大棗瀉肺湯)

PNEUMONIA (LOBAR and LOBULAR) (大葉肺炎、下葉肺炎)

1. Pathogenic factors attacking the Lung: (邪犯肺衛)
    Yin Qiao San (銀翹散)

2. Accumulation of Heat and Phlegm in the Lung: (痰熱壅肺)
  Ma Xing Shi Gan Tang (麻杏石甘湯)
3. Pathogenic Heat in the Ying (Nutrient) system: (邪熱入營)
  Qing Ying Tang (清營湯)
4. Depletion of Yin fluid: (陰液枯竭)
  San Jia Fu Mai Tang (三甲復脈湯) & Qing Ying Tang (清營湯)
5. Prostration of Yang Qi with shock: (陽氣虛脫)
  Shen Fu Tang (參附湯)
6. Deficiency of Qi and Yin: (氣陰不足，邪退正虛)
  Yi Gong San (異功散) & Sang Xing Tang (桑杏湯)

PNEUMONIA (MYCOPLASMA) (支原菌肺炎)
1. With Wind, Cold and Dampness: (風寒夾濕)
  Xing Su San (杏蘇散)
2. Wind and Heat acting on the Lung: (風熱犯肺)
  Sang Ju Yin (桑菊飲)
3. Pathogenic factors in the Shao-yang Channel: (邪在少陽)
  Xiao Chai Hu Tang (小柴胡湯)
4. Pathogenic factor in the Lung and Stomach: (邪蘊肺胃)
  Bai Hu Tang (白虎湯) & Wei Jing Tang (葦莖湯)

PNEUMOSILICOSIS (肺矽炎、矽病)
1. Loss of purifying and descending function of the Lung: (肺失清肅)
  Sang Xing Tang (桑杏湯)
2. Stagnation of Phlegm: (痰瘀凝滯)
  Hai Zao Yu Hu Tang (海藻玉壺湯)
3. Depletion of Qi and Yin: (氣陰兩虧)
  Qing Zao Jiu Fei Tang (清燥救肺湯)

POLYRADICULITIS (INFECTIOUS) (傳染性多神經根炎)
1. Obstruction of the channels and collaterals by Heat and Dampness:
  (濕熱阻絡)
  San Miao San (三妙散)
2. Deficiency of the Liver and Kidney Yin-fluid: (肝腎陰虛)
  Hu Qian Wan (虎潛丸)
3. Deficiency of both Qi and Blood: (氣血兩虛)
  Ba Zhen Tang (八珍湯)

POSTPARTUM BLEEDING (產後出血)
  Dang Gui Bu Xue Tang (當歸補血湯)
  Jiao Ai Tang (膠艾湯)

POSTPARTUM CARE (產後調理)
  Sheng Hua Tang (生化湯)

POSTPARTUM FEVER (產後發熱)
 Dang Gui Jian Zhong Tang (當歸健中湯)
 Huang Qi Jian Zhong Tang (黃芪建中湯)
 Xiao Jian Zhong Tang (小建中湯)

PREMENSTRUAL TENSION SYNDROME (經前期緊張症)
1. Stagnation of the Liver Qi: (肝郁氣滯)
 Chai Hu Shu Gan San (柴胡舒肝散)
 Xiao Yao San (逍遙散)
2. Asthenia of both Heart and Spleen: (心脾兩虛)
 Gui Pi Tang (歸脾湯)

PROLAPSE of ANUS and UTERUS (脱肛、子宮下垂)
 Bu Zhong Yi Qi Tang (補中益氣湯)

PROSTATE HYPERPLASIA (前列腺增生)
 Ba Zheng San (八正散)

PROSTATITIS (前列腺炎)
 Ba Zheng San (八正散)
 Long Dan Xie Gan Tang (龍膽瀉肝湯)
 Bi Xie Fen Qing Yin (萆薢分清飲)

PROSTRATION (虛脱、衰竭)
 Da Ding Feng Zhu (大定風珠)
 Shen Fu Tang (參附湯)
 Si Ni Tang (四逆湯)
 Tong Mai Si Ni Tang (通脈四逆湯)

PRURITUS (CUTANEOUS) (皮膚瘙痒症)
1. With Wind and Drought: (風燥)
 Dang Gui Yin Zi (當歸飲子)
2. With Heat and Dampness: (濕熱)
 Long Dan Xie Gan Tang (龍膽瀉肝湯)

PSORIASIS (銀屑病)
 Dang Gui Yin Zi (當歸飲子)
 Xi Jiao Di Huang Tang (犀角地黃湯)
  & Bai Hu Tang (白虎湯)
 Chai Ge Jie Ji Tang (柴葛解肌湯)

PUERPERAL ECLAMPSIA (子癇、產驚)
 Ling Yang Gou Teng Tang (羚羊鉤藤湯)
 Tian Ma Gou Teng Tang (天麻鉤藤湯)

PULMONARY EMPHYSEMA (肺氣腫)
      Bei Mu Gua Lou San (貝母瓜蔞散)
      She Gan Ma Huang Tang (射干麻黃湯)
      Ling Gan Wu Wei Jiang Xin Tang (苓甘五味薑辛湯)
      Dao Tan Tang (導痰湯)
      San Zi Yang Qing Tang (三子養親湯)

PULMONARY ABSCESS (肺膿腫)
1. Initial stage: (初期)
      Yin Qiao San (銀翹散)
2. Abscess forming stage: (成癰期)
      Qian Jin Wei Jing Tang (千金葦莖湯)
3. Ulcerous stage: (潰膿期)
      Jie Geng Tang (桔梗湯)
4. Recovery stage: (恢復期)
      Sha Shen Mai Men Dong Tang (沙參麥門冬湯) & Sheng Mai San (生脈散)

PULMONARY ATELECTASIS (肺不張、肺膨脹不全)
      Mai Men Dong Tang (麥門冬湯)

PULMONARY TUBERCULOSIS (肺結核)
1. Depletion of Lung Yin: (肺陰虧損)
      Bai He Gu Jin Tang (百合固金湯)
2. Deficiency of Yin with excess Fire: (陰虛火旺)
      Qing Hao Bie Jia Tang (青蒿鱉甲湯)

PURPURA (ALLERGIC) (過敏性紫癜)
1. Affection of external Wind and Heat: (外感風熱)
      Yin Qiao Bai Du San (銀翹敗毒散)
2. Bleeding due to Heat in the Blood system: (血熱妄行)
      Xi Jiao Di Huang Tang (犀角地黃湯)
3. Failure of the Spleen to control the Blood flow: (脾不攝血)
      Gui Pi Tang (歸脾湯)

PURPURA (THROMBOCYTOPENIC) (see THROMBOCYTOPENIC PURPURA)
      (血小板減少性紫癜)

PURULENT ABSCESS (膿腫)
      Dang Gui Bu Xue Tang (當歸補血湯)
      Ba Zhen Tang (八珍湯)

PSYCHOSIS (精神病)
1. Depressive syndrome: (癲症)
  a. Stagnation of Qi and Phlegm: (痰氣郁結)
      Dao Tan Tang (導痰湯)

    b. Deficiency of Heart and Spleen: (心脾兩虛)
        Yang Xin Tang (養心湯)
2. Mania/Madness: (狂症)
    a. Upflaring of Fire and Phlegm: (痰火上擾)
        An Gong Niu Huang Wan (安宮牛黃丸)
        Dang Gui Long Hui Wan (當歸龍薈丸)
    b. Depletion of Yin by excessive Fire: (火盛傷陰)
        Xue Fu Zhu Yu Tang (血府逐瘀湯)

PYELITIS (腎盂炎)
    Long Dan Xie Gan Tang (龍肝瀉肝湯)

PYLORIC OBSTRUCTION (INCOMPLETE) (幽門梗阻)
    Xuan Fu Dai Zhe Tang (旋覆代赭湯)

PYELONEPHRITIS (腎盂腎炎)
1. Heat and Dampness in the Urinary Bladder: (膀胱濕熱)
    Ba Zheng San (八正散))
2. Stagnation of Dampness in the Liver and Gall-bladder: (肝膽郁熱)
    Long Dan Xie Gan Tang (龍膽瀉肝湯)
    a. With Wind and Heat: (風熱)
        Yin Qiao San (銀翹散)
    b. With high fever but no perspiration: (高熱無汗)
        Zhi Chi Tang (梔豉湯)
    c. With chills and fever: (寒熱往來)
        Xiao Chai Hu Tang (小柴胡湯)
3. Deficiency of Kidney Yin, with retention of Heat and Dampness:
    (腎陰不足，濕熱留戀)
    Zhi Bai Di Huang Wan (知柏地黃丸)
4. Deficiency of Spleen and Kidney: (脾腎兩虛，餘邪未清)
    Shen Ling Bai Zhu San (參苓白术散) & Er Xian Tang (二仙湯)

RENAL TUBERCULOSIS (腎結核)
1. Heat and Dampness in Urinary Bladder: (濕熱膀胱)
    Dao Chi San (導赤散)
2. Deficiency of Yin with excess Fire: (陰虛火旺)
    Da Bu Yin Wan (大補陰丸)
    Zhi Bai Di Huang Wan (知柏地黃丸)
3. Deficiency of Spleen and Kidney: (脾腎兩虛)
    Bu Zhong Yi Qi Tang (補中益氣湯)

RESTLESSNESS (坐立不安)
    Tian Wang Bu Xin Dan (天王補心丹)
    Wen Dan Tang (溫胆湯)

RETARDED GROWTH of CHILDREN（兒童發育不良）
He Che Da Zao Wan（河車大造丸）
Liu Wei Di Huang Wan（六味地黄丸）
Tiao Gan Tang（調肝湯）

RETCH（乾嘔）
Ban Xia Xie Xin Tang（半夏瀉心湯）
Fu Zi Xie Xin Tang（附子瀉心湯）
Ju Pi Zhu Ru Tang（橘皮竹茹湯）

RETENTION of LOCHIA（惡露）
Sheng Hua Tang（生化湯）

RETINITIS（網膜炎）
Ci Zhu Wan（磁硃丸）
Liu Wei Di Huang Wan（六味地黄丸）
Qi Ju Di Huang Wan（杞菊地黄丸）

RHEUMATIC FEVER（風濕熱病）
1. With Heat and Wind in the Ying (Nutrient) and Wei (Inner Defensive) systems:
   （風熱入營衛）
   Bai Hu Jia Gui Zhi Tang（白虎加桂枝湯）
2. With Heat in the Ying (Nutrient) and vascular Blood system:（熱入營血）
   Xi Jiao Di Huang Tang（犀角地黄湯）
3. With Wind, Cold and Dampness:（風寒濕証）
   Juan Bi Tang（蠲痺湯）
4. Deficiency of Yin with interior Heat:（陰虛內熱）
   Qing Gu San（清骨散）
5. Depletion of Heart Yang:（心陽衰弱）
   Sheng Mai San（生脈散）
   Shen Fu Tang（參附湯）

RHEUMATIC HEART DISEASE（心臟風濕病）
1. Obstruction of Blood stasis in the vessels:（心脈瘀阻）
   Tao Hong Yin（桃紅飲）
2. Deficiency of Qi and Blood:（氣血兩虧）
   Gui Pi Tang（歸脾湯）
3. Deficiency of Heart and Kidney Yang:（心腎陽虛）
   Zhen Wu Tang（真武湯）

RHEUMATISM（風濕病）
1. With pathogenic Heat:（熱邪偏盛）
   Bai Hu Jia Gui Zhi Tang（白虎加桂枝湯）
2. With Heat and Dampness:（濕熱蘊蒸）
   Xuan Bi Tang（宣痺湯）

3. With Cold and Dampness: (寒濕偏盛)
   Juan Bi Tang (蠲痹湯)
4. Deficiency of Qi and Yin: (氣陰兩虛)
   Sheng Mai San (生脈散)

RHINITIS (鼻炎)
1. Acute rhinitis: (急性鼻炎)
   a. Affection of exterior Wind and Cold: (風寒外襲)
      Xin Yi San (辛夷散)
   b. Affection of exterior Wind and Heat: (風熱外襲)
      Sang Ju Yin (桑菊飲) & Cang Er Zi San (蒼耳子散)
2. Chronic rhinitis: (慢性鼻炎)
      Yu Ping Feng San (玉屏風散)
      Cang Er Zi San (蒼耳子散) & Tao Hong Si Wu Tang (桃紅四物湯)
3. Allergic rhinitis: (過敏性鼻炎)
      Cang Er Zi San (蒼耳子散) & Bu Zhong Yi Qi Tang (補中益氣湯)
      Yu Ping Feng San (玉屏風散)
4. Atrophic rhinitis: (萎縮性鼻炎)
   a. Dryness of the Lung due to deficiency of Yin-fluid: (陰虛肺燥)
      Yang Yin Qing Fei Tang (養陰清肺湯)
   b. Asthenia of both Lung and Kidney: (肺腎虛弱)
      Bai He Gu Jin Tang (百合固金湯)

ROSACEA (酒齇鼻)
      Si Wu Tang (四物湯)
      Tong Qiao Huo Xue Tang (通竅活血湯)

RUNNING PIGGIES (流鼻涕)
      Xuan Fu Dai Zhe Tang (旋覆代赭湯)

SCAPULOHUMERAL PERIARTHRITIS (肩關節周圍炎)
      Juan Bi Tang I (蠲痹湯 I)
      Juan Bi Tang II (蠲痹湯 II)

SCARLET FEVER (猩紅熱)
      Zi Xue Dan (紫雪丹)

SCHISTOSOMIASIS (血吸虫病、分體吸虫病)
1. Retention of Heat and Dampness: (濕熱留戀)
      Liu Shen Wan (六神丸)
      San Ren Tang (三仁湯)
2. Stagnation of Liver Qi and deficiency of Spleen: (肝郁脾虛)
      Xiao Yao San (逍遙散)
3. Interior obstruction of Blood stasis: (瘀血內阻)
      Hua Yu Tang (化瘀湯)

4. Retention of Water and Dampness: (水濕停滯)
     Wu Ling San （五苓散）
5. Deficiency of Liver and Kidney Yin: (肝腎陰虛)
     Qi Qu Di Huang Wan （杞菊地黄丸）
6. Depletion of Kidney Yang: (腎陽虧損)
     You Gui Wan （右歸丸）
     Shi Quan Da Bu Tang （十全大補湯）

SCHIZOPHRENIA （精神分裂症）
1. Deficiency of Heart and Spleen: (心脾兩虛)
     Yang Xin Tang （養心湯） & Gan Mai Da Zao Tang （甘麥大棗湯）
2. Stagnation of Qi and Phlegm: (痰氣郁結)
     Dao Tan Tang （導痰湯）
3. Excessive Liver Fire and Phlegm: (肝火痰盛)
     Dang Gui Long Hui Wan （當歸龍薈丸）

SCIATICA （坐骨神經痛）
     Du Huo Ji Sheng Tang （獨活寄生湯）
     Qiang Huo Sheng Shi Tang （羌活勝濕湯）

SCLERITIS (ANTERIOR) （前鞏膜炎）
     Xie Bai San （瀉白散）
     Yang Yin Qing Fei Tang （養陰清肺湯）

SCLERODERMA （硬皮病）
1. With Blood stasis: (血瘀型)
     Tao Hong Si Wu Tang （桃紅四物湯）
2. With Blood stasis and deficiency of Kidney: (腎虛血瘀)
     You Gui Wan （右歸丸） & Tao Hong Si Wu Tang （桃紅四物湯）
3. With Blood stasis and deficiency of Spleen: (脾虛血瘀)
     Gui Pi Tang （歸脾湯）

SCLERODERMA NEONATORUM （初生兒硬皮病）
1. Insufficiency of Yang Qi: (陽氣虛衰)
     Shen Fu Tang （參附湯）
2. Blood stagnation due to Cold: (寒凝血滯)
     Dang Gui Si Ni Tang （當歸四逆湯）
3. Retention of Cold and Dampness in the Spleen: (寒濕困脾)
     Fu Zi Li Zhong Tang （附子理中湯）

SCLEROSIS of FUNICULUS LATERALIS （脊髓側索硬化）
     Da Ding Feng Zhu （大定風珠）

SCROTAL ECZEMA （陰囊濕疹）
     Long Dan Xie Gan Tang （龍膽瀉肝湯）

SCROTAL HYDROCELE (陰囊水囊腫)
  Wei Ling Tang (胃苓湯)
  Wu Ling San (五苓散)

SCROTAL HERNIA (陰囊疝氣)
  Tian Tai Wu Yao San (天台烏药散)

SEPTICEMIA (敗血病)
  Xi Jiao Di Huang Tang (犀角地黄湯)
  Huang Lian Jie Du Tang (黄連解毒湯)
  Qing Wen Bai Du Yin (清瘟敗毒飲)

SICK SINUS SYNDROME (FIBROSIS of SINOATRIAL NODE)
(PERSISTENT SINUS BRADYCARDIA)
  (病態竇房結綜合征) (持續性竇性心動過緩)
1. Deficiency of Heart and Kidney Yang: (心腎陽虛)
  Ma Huang Fu Zi Xi Xin Tang (麻黄附子細辛湯)
2. Deficiency of both Qi and Yin-fluid: (氣陰兩虛)
  Zhi Gan Cao Tang (炙甘草湯)

SINUSITIS (竇炎)
  Cang Er San (蒼耳散)
  Xin Yi San (辛夷散)

SORE THROAT (咽喉痛)
  Yin Qiao San (銀翹散)
  Liu Shen Wan (六神丸)
  Pu Ji Xiao Du Yin (普濟消毒飲)

SPONTANEOUS PERSPIRATION (see PERSPIRATION) (自汗)

STIFF NECK and SHOULDER (頸肩背僵硬、僵直)
  Gui Zhi Jia Ge Gen Tang (桂枝加葛根湯)
  Ge Gen Tang (葛根湯)
  Chai Ge Jie Ji Tang (柴葛解肌湯)

SPERMATORRHEA (遺精、精溢)
1. Deficiency of Yin with excess Fire: (陰虛火旺)
  Zhi Bai Di Huang Wan (知柏地黄丸)
  Zuo Gui Wan (左歸丸)
2. Deficiency of Kidney Yang: (腎陽虛，腎虛不藏)
  Jin Suo Gu Jing Wan (金鎖固經丸)
  You Gui Wan (右歸丸)
3. Interior accumulation of Heat and Dampness: (濕熱內蘊)
  Bi Xie Fen Qing Yin (萆薢分清飲)

4. Inbalance of the physiological function of Heart and Kidney: (心腎不交)
   Sang Piao Xiao San (桑螵蛸散)

SPRAIN/STRAIN of the LUMBAR MUSCLE (腰肌損傷)
   Du Huo Ji Sheng Tang (獨活寄生湯)
   Zhi Bai Di Huang Wan (知柏地黄丸)
   Liu Wei Di Huang Wan (六味地黄丸)

STOMATITIS (ULCERATIVE) (口腔潰瘍)
   Dao Chi San

STRABISMUS (斜視)
   Bu Zhong Yi Qi Tang (補中益氣湯)

STROKE (see APOPLEXY) (中風)

STUFFY NOSE (鼻塞)
   Cong Chi Tang (葱豉湯)
   Xin Yi San (辛夷散)

SUMMER HEAT STROKE (中暑)
   Qing Shu Yi Qi Tang I (清暑益氣湯I)
   Qing Shu Yi Qi Tang II (清暑益氣湯II)

SUPPURATIVE ARTHRITIS (化膿性關節炎)
1. Early stage: (初期)
   Wu Wei Xiao Du Yin (五味消毒飲)
2. Middlt stage: (中期)
   Tou Nong San (透膿散)
3. Late stage: (晚期)
   Ba Zhen Tang (八珍湯)

SUPPURATIVE INFECTION (化膿性感染)
   Ren Shen Bai Du San (人參敗毒散)
   Yin Qiao Bai Du San (銀翹敗毒散)

SYNCOPE (暈厥、厥証)
1. Related with Qi: (氣厥)
   a. Shi (excessive) syndrome: (實証)
      Wu Mo Yin Zi (五磨飲子)
   b. Xu (deficieny) syndrome: (虛証)
      Xiang Sha Liu Jun Zi Tang (香砂六君子湯)
2. Related with Blood: (血厥)
   a. Shi (excessive) syndrome: (實証)
      Tong Yu Jian (通瘀煎)

   b. Xu (deficiency) syndrome: (虛証)
       Du Shen Tang (獨參湯)
       Ren Shen Yang Ying Tang (人參養營湯)
3. Related with Phlegm: (痰厥)
       Dao Tan Tang (導痰湯)
4. Related with Food: (食厥)
       Bao He Wan (保和丸)
       Xiao Cheng Qi Tang (小承氣湯)
5. Related with Summer Heat: (暑厥)
       Niu Huang Qing Xin Wan (牛黃清心丸)
       Zi Xue Dan (紫雪丹)
       Bai Hu Jia Ren Shen Tang (白虎加人參湯)
       Qing Shu Yi Qi Tang (清暑益氣湯)

SYSTEMIC LUPUS ERYTHEMATOSUS (系統性紅斑狼瘡)

1. With intense Heat and Toxin: (熱毒熾盛)
       Qing Wen Bai Du Yin (清瘟敗毒飲)
2. Accumulation of internal Heat due to Yin deficiency: (陰虛內熱)
       Qing Hao Bie Jia Tang (青蒿鱉甲湯)
       & Da Bu Yin Wan (大補陰丸)
3. Deficiency of Spleen and Kidney Yang: (脾腎陽虛)
       Er Xian Tang (二仙湯)
       & Wu Ling San (五苓散)

SYSTEMIC PYOGENIC INFECTION (ACUTE) (系統性膿性感染)

1. Intense Heat in Qi and Ying systems: (氣營兩燔)
       Bai Hu Tang (白虎湯)   Huang Lian Jie Du Tang (黃連解毒湯)
2. Invasion of Heat into the Ying and Blood systems: (熱入營血)
       Xi Jiao Di Huang Tang (犀角地黃湯)
       & Huang Lian Jie Du Tang (黃連解毒湯)
3. Depletion of Heat due to excessive Heat: (熱盛亡陰)
       Xi Jiao Di Huang Tang (犀角地黃湯)
       & Huang Lian Jie Du Tang (黃連解毒湯)
       & Sheng Mai San (生脈散)
4. Depletion of Yang with symptoms of cold extremities due to excessive Heat:
    (熱厥亡陽)
       Shen Fu Tang (參附湯)

TESTITIS (睾丸炎)

       Ju He Wan (橘核丸)
       Pu Ji Xiao Du Yin (普濟消毒飲)

TETANUS (破傷風)

       Yu Zhen San (玉真散)
       Zhi Jing San (止痙散)

THERMOPLEGIA (熱射病、中暑)
    Qing Shu Yi Qi Tang (清暑益氣湯)
    Sheng Mai San (生脈散)

THIRST (渴)
    Mai Men Dong Tang (麥門冬湯)
    Qing Shu Yi Qi Tang (清暑益氣湯)
    Sha Shen Mai Men Dong Tang (沙參麥門冬湯)
    Zeng Ye Tang (增液湯)

THREATENED ABORTION (先兆流產)
    Jiao Ai Tang (膠艾湯)
    Si Wu Tang (四物湯)
    Tai Shan Pan Shi San (泰山盤石散)

THROMBOANGIITIS OBLITERANS (血栓性閉塞性脈管炎)
    Dang Gui Si Ni Jia Wu Zhu Yu Sheng Jiang Tang
    (當歸四逆加吳茱萸生薑湯)
    Dang Gui Si Ni Tang (當歸四逆湯)
    Si Miao Yong An Tang (四妙勇安湯)

THROMBOCYTOPENIC PURPURA (血小板減少性紫癜)
1. Deficiency of Qi and Spleen: (脾虛氣弱)
    Gui Pi Tang (歸脾湯)
2. Bleeding due to Heat in the Blood system: (血熱妄行)
    Xi Jiao Di Huang Tang (犀角地黃湯)
3. Deficiency of Yin with excess Fire: (陰虛火旺)
    Da Bu Yin Wan (大補陰丸)

THROMBOSIS (CEREBRAL) (腦血栓)
    Bu Yang Huan Wu Tang (補陽還五湯)

THROMBOTIC PHLEBITIS (血栓性靜脈炎)
    Si Miao Yong An Tang (四妙勇安湯)

THYROID ADENOMA (甲狀腺瘤)
1. Stagnation of Qi and Phlegm: (痰氣郁結)
    Hai Zao Yu Hu Tang (海藻玉壺湯)
    Xiao Luo Wan (消瘰丸)
2. Deficiency of Spleen and stagnation of Liver Qi: (脾虛肝郁)
    Xiao Yao San (逍遙散)

THYROIDITIS (甲狀腺炎)
    Xiao Luo Wan (消瘰丸)

TIDAL FEVER (潮熱)
　　Da Bu Yin Wan (大補陰丸)
　　Qing Gu San (清骨散)
　　Liu Wei Di Huang Wan (六味地黃丸)

TINEA PEDIS (足癬)
　　Er Miao San (二妙散)
　　Si Miao San (四妙散)
　　Gui Zhi Tang (桂枝湯)

TINNITIS (耳鳴)
　　Ci Zhu Wan (磁硃丸)
　　Er Long Zuo Ci Wan (耳聾左慈丸)

TONSILLITIS (扁桃體炎)
　　Liu Shen Wan (六神丸)
　　Qiang Lan Tang (羌籃湯)
　　Yin Qiao San (銀翹散)
　　Pu Ji Xiao Du Yin (普濟消毒飲)

TOOTHACHE (牙齒痛)
　　Yu Nu Jian (玉女煎)
　　Chai Ge Jie Ji Tang (柴葛解肌湯)

TRACHITIS (TRACHEITIS) (氣管炎)
　　Ma Xing Shi Gan Tang (麻杏石甘湯)
　　Bei Mu Gua Lou San (貝母瓜蔞散)
　　Qing Qi Hua Tan Wan (清氣化痰丸)
　　Dao Tan Tang (導痰湯)

TRACHOMA (沙眼)
　　Yin Qiao San (銀翹散)

TRICHOMONAS VAGINITIS (陰道炎)
　　She Chuang Zi Chong Xi Ji (蛇床子沖洗劑)

TREMATODIASIS (see FLUKE INFESTATION) (吸蟲病)

TRIGEMINAL NEURALGIA (三叉神經痛)
　　Qian Zheng San (牽正散)
　　Zhi Jing San (止痙散)
　　Tian Ma Gou Teng Yin (天麻鉤藤飲)

TUBERCULOSIS (see PULMONARY TUBERCULOSIS) (結核)

TUBERCULOSIS of BONE and JOINTS （骨關節結核病）
    Zhi Bai Di Huang Wan （知柏地黄丸）
    Ren Shen Yang Ying Tang （人參養營湯）

TYPHOID & PARATYPHOID FEVER （傷寒、副傷寒）（腸熱病、副腸熱病）
1. Stagnation of Heat and Dampness:（濕熱郁結）
    San Ren Tang （三仁湯）
2. Heat in the Ying (Nutrient) and Blood systems:（熱入營血）
    Qing Ying Tang （清營湯）& An Gong Niu Huang Wan （安宫牛黄丸）
3. Depletion of Qi and Yin, with remaining Heat:（氣陰兩傷，餘熱未清）
    Zhu Ye Shi Gao Tang （竹葉石膏湯）

ULCER (GASTRIC & DUODENAL) （胃與十二指腸潰瘍）
1. Stagnation of Liver Qi:（肝氣滯）
    Chai Hu Shu Gan Tang （柴胡舒肝湯）
2. Stagnation of Heat:（郁熱）
    Xiao Yao San （逍遙散）
3. Deficiency of Yin:（陰虚）
    Yi Guan Jian （一貫煎）
    Zuo Jin Wan （左金丸）
    Yi Wei Tang （益胃湯）
4. Asthenia with Cold:（虚寒）
    Li Zhong Wan （理中丸）& Huang Qi Jian Zhong Tang （黄芪建中湯）
5. Blood stasis:（血瘀）
    Ge Xia Zhu Yu Tang （膈下逐瘀湯）
    Xie Xin Tang （瀉心湯）
    Huang Tu Tang （黄土湯）

ULCERATIVE COLITIS (CHRONIC) （慢性非特异性潰瘍性結腸炎）
1. Heat and dampness in the lower part of body:（濕熱下注）
    Bai Tou Weng Tang （白頭翁湯）
2. Hyperactivity of Liver with Spleen asthenia:（肝旺脾虚）
    Tong Xie Yao Fang （痛瀉要方）
3. Asthenia of Spleen and Stomach:（脾胃虚弱）
    Shen Ling Bai Zhu San （參苓白术散）
    Zhen Ren Yang Zang Tang （真人養臟湯）
4. Deficiency of Spleen and Kidney:（脾腎陽虚）
    Si Shen Wan （四神丸）

UNDULANT FEVER (see BRUCELLOSIS) （布氏桿菌病、波浪熱）

UPPER RESPIRATORY TRACT INFECTION （上呼吸道感染）
1. Invasion of Wind and Cold:（風寒）
    Jing Fang Bai Du San （荆防敗毒散）
    Ma Xing Shi Gan Tang （麻杏石甘湯）

2. Invasion of Wind and Heat: (風熱)
   Yin Qiao San (銀翹散)
   Qiang Lan Tang (羌籃湯)
3. Invasion of Wind, Heat and Drought: (風、熱、燥)
   Qing Zao Jiu Fei Tang (清燥救肺湯)
   Sang Xing Tang (桑杏湯)
4. Invasion of Summer Heat with Dampness: (暑濕熱)
   Xiang Ru San (香薷散)

UREMIA (尿毒症)
1. Obstruction of Qi flow, with interior accumulation of Dampness and Turbidity:
      (氣滯，濕濁內阻)
   Shu Chi Yin Zi (疏齒飲子)
2. Deficiency of Spleen and Kidney Yang, with interior accumulation of Cold
   and Dampness: (脾腎陽虛，寒濕內蘊)
   Wu Zhu Yu Tang (吳茱萸湯) & Fu Zi Li Zhong Tang (附子理中湯)
3. Asthenia of Spleen and Kidney, with Heat and Dampness:
      (脾腎兩虛，濕熱互結)
   Huang Lian Wen Dan Tang (黃連溫膽湯) & Wen Pi Tang (溫脾湯)
4. Pathogenic factors lingering in the Pericardium, causing interior Heat in Blood
   and endogenous Wind: (邪陷心包，血熱風動)
   Xi Jiao Di Huang Tang (犀角地黃湯)
   Ling Yang Gou Teng Tang (羚羊鉤藤湯)

URETHRITIS (尿道炎)
   Ba Zheng San (八正散)
   Shi Wei San (石葦散)
   Long Dan Xie Gan Tang (龍膽瀉肝湯)

URINARY TRACT INFECTION (泌尿系感染)
1. Heat and Dampness in the Urinary Bladder: (膀胱濕熱)
   Ba Zheng San (八正散)
2. Stagnation of Heat in Heart, Liver, and Gallbladder: (心肝膽郁熱)
   Dao Chi San (導赤散)
   Long Dan Xie Gan Tang (龍膽瀉肝湯)
   Huang Lian Jie Du Tang (黃連解毒湯)
3. Deficiency of both Spleen and Kidney: (脾腎兩虛)
   Si Jun Zi Tang (四君子湯)
     & Liu Wei Di Huang Wan (六味地黃丸)
   Zhi Bai Di Huang Wan (知柏地黃丸)

URINATION DISORDERS (LIN ZHENG) (淋証)
1. Urolithiasis: (石淋、尿石症)
   Ba Zheng San (八正散)
   Shi Wei San (石葦散)

2. Related with Qi--with dysuria and pain in urethra after urination: （氣淋）
   a. Shi (excessive) syndrome: （實証）
      Chen Xiang San （沉香散）
   b. Xu (deficiency) syndrome: （虛証）
      Bu Zhong Yi Qi Tang （補中益氣湯）
3. Hematuria: （血淋、血尿）
   a. Shi (Excessive) syndrome: （實証）
      Xiao Ji Yin Zi （小薊飲子）
   b. Xu (Deficiency) syndrome: （虛証）
      Zhi Bai Di Huang Wan （知柏地黃丸）
4. Chyluria: （膏淋、乳糜尿）
   a. Shi (Excessive) syndrome: （實証）
      Bei Xie Fen Qing Yin （卑薢分清飲）
   b. Xu (Deficiency) syndrome: （虛証）
      Liu Wei Di Huang Wan （六味地黃丸）
5. Related with Stress--dull pain and drippling of urine: （勞淋）
      Bu Zhong Yi Qi Tang （補中益氣湯）
      Zhi Bai Di Huang Wan （知柏地黃丸）
6. Related with Heat--acute urinary tract infection: （熱淋）
      Ba Zheng San （八正散）
      Dao Chi San （導赤散）

UROLITHIASIS （尿石症）
      San Jin Tang （三金湯）
      Ba Zheng San （八正散）
      Shi Wei San （石葦散）

URTICARIA （蕁麻疹）
      Yu Ping Feng San （玉屏風散）& Dang Gui Yin Zi （當歸飲子）

UTERINE BLEEDING （子宮出血）
1. Heat in Blood: （血熱）
      Gu Jing Tang （固經湯）
      Dan Zhi Xiao Yao San （丹梔逍遙散）
2. Blood stasis: （血瘀）
      Tao Hong Si Wu Tang （桃紅四物湯）
       & Shi Xiao San （失笑散）
3. Deficiency of Kidney Yin: （腎陰虛）
      Zuo Gui Wan （左歸丸）
4. Deficiency of Kidney Yang: （腎陽虛）
      You Gui Wan （右歸丸）

VAGINAL BLEEDING （陰道出血）
      Jiao Ai Tang （膠艾湯）

VEGETATIVE NEUROSIS（植物性神經機能病，神經系官能病）
1. Deficiency of Heat and Gallbladder Qi, with insufficient Blood:
  （心膽氣虛，營血不足）
    Yang Xin Tang（養心湯）
2. Disharmony between Liver and Stomach:（肝胃不和）
    Si Ni San（四逆散）

VERTICAL HEADACHE（頭顱頂頭痛）
    Dang Gui Si Ni Jia Wu Zhu Yu Sheng Jiang Tang
    （當歸四逆加吳茱萸生薑湯）

VERTIGO（眩暈）
1. Hyperactivity of Liver Yang:（肝陽上亢）
    Tian Ma Gou Teng Yin（天麻鉤藤飲）
    Da Ding Feng Zhu（大定風珠）
    Dang Gui Lu Hui Wan（當歸蘆薈丸）
    Qi Ju Di Huang Wan（杞菊地黃丸）
2. Deficiency of Qi and Blood:（氣血虧虛）
    Gui Pi Tang（歸脾湯）
    Bu Zhong Yi Qi Tang（補中益氣湯）
3. Deficiency of Kidney essence:（腎精不足）
  a. Deficiency of Kidney Yin:（腎陰虛）
    Zuo Gui Wan（左歸丸）
  b. Deficiency of Kidney Yang:（腎陽虛）
    You Gui Wan（右歸丸）
4. Obstruction of turbid Phlegm:（痰濁中阻）
    Wen Dan Tang（溫胆湯）
    Ban Xia Bai Zhu Tian Ma Tang（半夏白术天麻湯）

VIRAL HEPATITIS（病毒性肝炎）
1. Acute hepatitis:（急性肝炎）
    Yin Chen Hao Tang（茵陳蒿湯）
    Yin Chen Wu Ling San（茵陳五苓散）
2. Hepatitis without jaundice:（無黃疸）
  a. Heat and Dampness in the Liver and Gallbladder:（肝膽濕熱）
    Yin Chen Hao Tang（茵陳蒿湯）
      & Long Dan Xie Gan Tang（龍膽瀉肝湯）
  b. Stagnation of Liver Qi with deficiency of Spleen:（肝郁脾虛）
    Xiao Yao San（逍遙散）
  c. Stagnation of Qi and Blood stasis:（氣滯血瘀）
    Tao Hong Si Wu Tang（桃紅四物湯）

VIRAL MYOCARDITIS（病毒性心肌炎）
1. Heat and Fire acting on the Heart:（火熱擾心）
    Zhu Sha An Shen Wan（硃砂安神丸）

2. Deficiency of Blood in Heart: (心血不足)
    Jia Jian Fu Mai Tang (加減復脈湯)
    Gui Pi Tang (歸脾湯)
    Sheng Mai San (生脈散)
3. Blood stasis in the cardiovascular system: (瘀血內阻)
    Xue Fu Zhu Yu Tang (血府逐瘀湯)

VOMITING (嘔吐)
1. Shi (excessive) syndrome: (實証)
    a. Exterior pathogenic factors affecting the Stomach: (外邪犯胃)
       Huo Xiang Zheng Qi San (藿香正氣散)
    b. Stagnation of Food: (飲食停滯)
       Bao He Wan (保和丸)
    c. Interior accumulation of Phlegm and Fluid: (痰飲內停)
       Wen Dan Tang (溫胆湯)
       Xiao Ban Xia Tang (小半夏湯) & Ling Gui Zhu Gan Tang (苓桂术甘湯)
    d. Liver Qi affecting the Stomach: (肝氣犯胃)
       Ban Xia Hou Po Tang (半夏厚朴湯) & Zuo Jin Wan (左金丸)
2. Xu (deficiency) syndrome: (虛証)
    a. Asthenia of Spleen and Stomach with Cold: (脾胃虛寒)
       Li Zhong Wan (理中丸)
    b. Deficiency of Stomach Yin fluid: (胃陰不足)
       Mai Men Dong Tang (麥門冬湯)

VOMITING (PERNICIOUS) (惡性嘔吐)
    Xiang Sha Liu Jun Zi Tang (香砂六君子湯)

WHEEZING (XIAO ZHENG) (哮証、喘息、哮鳴)
1. Acute stage: (發作期)
    a. Cold type: (寒哮)
       She Gan Ma Huang Tang (射干麻黄湯)
       Xiao Qing Long Tang (小青龍湯)
       Su Zi Jiang Qi Tang (蘇子降氣湯)
    b. Heat type: (熱哮)
       Yue Bi Jia Ban Xia Tang (越婢加半夏湯)
       Ding Chuan Tang (定喘湯)
2. Recovery stage: (緩解期)
    a. Asthenia of Lung: (肺虛)
       Yu Ping Feng San (玉屏風散)
    b. Asthenia of Spleen: (脾虛)
       Liu Jun Zi Tang (六君子湯)
    c. Asthenia of Kidney: (腎虛)
       Jing Kui Shen Qi Wan (金匱腎氣丸)
       Du Qi Wan (都氣丸)

WHOOPING COUGH（百日咳）
    Wei Jing Tang（葦莖湯）
    Zhi Sou San（止嗽散）

WILSON'S DISEASE（肝豆狀核變性）
    Da Ding Feng Zhu（大定風珠）

WOUNDS（創傷）
    Qi Li San（七釐散）

BIBLIOGRAPHY

Common Terms of Traditional Chinese Medicine in English
    by Beijing Medical College,
    China, 1981

Commonly used Chinese Herbal Formulas with Illustrations
    by Hong-yen Hsu, Ph.D. and Chau-shin Hsu, Ph.D.,
    Los Angeles, 1980

Encyclopedia of Chinese Material Medica
    by Jiang Su Medical College,
    China, 1975

Enumeration of Chinese Materia Medica, An
    by Shiu-ying Hu,
    Hong Kong, 1980

How to Treat Yourself with Chinese Herbs
    by Hong-yen Hsu, Ph.D.,
    Los Angeles, 1980

Illustrated Chinese Material Medica, Crude Drugs, The
    by Kung-ying Yen, Ph.D.,
    Taipei, 1980

Illustrated Chinese Materia Medica, Prepared Drugs, The
    by Kung-ying Yen, Ph.D.,
    Taipei, 1980

Pharmacology of Chinese Drugs
    by Scientific Technology Publishing Company of Shanghai,
    China, 1986

Textbook of Chinese Internal Medicine
    by Shanghai Medical College,
    China, 1983

Textbook of Chinese Prescriptions
    by Shanghai Medical College,
    China, 1977

Textbook of the Pharmacopeia
    by Cheng Du College of Traditional Chinese Medicine,
    China, 1978

CHINESE INDEX

ACCORDING TO DISEASES

CHINESE INDEX ACCORDING TO DISEASES

中文病名指引

二劃

十二指腸潰瘍	Ulcer (Duodenal)
儿童发育不良	Retarded growth of children

三劃

三叉神經痛	Trigeminal neuralgia
干呕	Retch
大腸病辯證	Differentiation according to Zang-fu (Large Intestine)
大葉肺炎	Pneumonia (Lobar)
下葉肺炎	Pneumonia (Lobular)
上呼吸道感染	Upper respiratory tract infection
小腸病辯證	Differentiation according to Zang-fu (Small Intestine)
小兒腹瀉	Infantile Diarrhea
小兒營養不良	Infantile Malnutrition
小兒麻痹症	Infantile Paralysis
小兒驚厥	Infantile Convulsion
口眼歪斜	Deviation of the eye & mouth (see Apoplexy or Apoplectiform)
口腔潰瘍	Oral ulceration
口炎（潰瘍性）	Stomatitis (ulcerative)
干嘔	Retch
子宮出血	Bleeding (Uterine)
子宮內膜移位	Endometriosis
子宮肌瘤	Hysteromyoma, uterine leiomyoma
子宮下垂	Hysteroptosis, Prolapse of the uterus
子癇、產驚	Puerperal eclampsia
卫气营血	Differentiation according to the 4 conditions in "Wen Bin Lung" (syndromes of Wei, Qi, Ying and Xue)

四劃

不寐	Insomnia
支氣管擴張	Bronchiectasis
支氣管哮喘	Bronchial asthma
支氣管癌	Bronchogenic carcinoma
支氣管炎	Bronchitis
不孕、不育症	Infertility

牙齦炎	Gingivitis
牙關緊閉	Lock-jaw
牙周炎	Periodontitis
牙齒痛	Toothache
太陽病辯證	Differentiation according to the Tai-Yang channel
太陰病辯證	Differentiation according to the Tai-Yin channel
中風	Apoplexy, stroke
中暑	Heat-stroke
中耳炎	Otitis media
反胃	Acid regurgitation
中毒	Poisoning
食物中毒	Food poisoning
蘑菇中毒	Mushroom Poisoning
气虚	Deficiency of Qi (vital energy); see Consumptive disease
气管炎	Trachitis, tracheitis
化膿性感染	Suppurative infection
少陽病辯證	Differentiation according to the Shao-Yang channel
少陰病辯證	Differentiation according to the Shao-Yin channel
丹毒	Erysipelas
手足徐動症	Athetosis
风湿热	Rheumatic fever
风湿病	Rheumatism
月經、行經	Menstruation
月經先期	Early menstruation
月經後期	Delayed menstruation
經期延長	Prolonged menstruation
月經失調	Irregular menstruation
血尿症	Hematuria
六經辯證	Differentiation according to the six channels
心絞痛	Angina pectoris
心率不齊	Arrhythmia
心力衰竭	Cardiac failure
充血性心力衰竭	Congestive Heart Failure
心病辯證	Differentiation according to Zang-fu (Heart)
心肌梗塞	Myocardial infarction
心肌炎	Myocarditis
心悸	Palpiration
心包炎	Pericarditis
心動過緩—持續性竇性	Persistent sinus bradycardia
心臟風濕病	Rhematic heart disease
心肌炎—病毒性	Viral myocarditis
水腫	Edema
水腫—心性	Cardiac edema
水痘	Chickenpox

五劃

布氏桿菌病	Brucellosis (undulant fever)
打嗝	Hiccough
甲狀腺機能亢進	Hyperthyroidism
甲狀腺機能減退	Hypothyroidism
甲狀腺瘤	Thyroid adenoma
甲狀腺炎	Thyroiditis
半身不遂	Hemiplegia, see Apoplectiform
头疼	Headache
头颅顶头痛	Vertical headache
出血	Bleeding
衄血	Epistaxis; see Bleeding
吐血	Spitting blood; see Bleeding
便血	Blood in the stools; see Bleeding
尿血	Blood in the urine; see Bleeding
痔瘡出血	Hemorrhoid bleeding; see Bleeding
子宮出血	Uterine bleeding; see Bleeding
手術後出血	Post-surgical bleeding; see Bleeding
產後出血	Post-partum bleeding; see Bleeding
出血性發熱	Hemorrhagic fever
白內障	Cataract
白喉病	Diphtheria
白血病—急性	Leukemia (acute)
白血病—慢性	Leukemia (chronic)
白細胞減少	Leukocytopenia
血小板減少性紫癜	Thrombocytopenic purpura
失音症	Aphonia
失語症	Aphasia
失眠	Insomnia
失嗅覺	Loss of smell
半身不遂	Hemiplegia
半月板損傷	Meniscus injury of the knee; see Knee Injury
皮膚炎—接觸性	Dermatitis (contact)
皮膚瘙痒症	Prutitus (cutaneous)
发烧、发热	Fever
丝虫病	Filariasis

六劃

耳聾	Deafness
耳性眩暈病	Meniere's disease
耳鳴	Tinnitis
巩膜炎	Scleritis
百日咳	Whooping cough

厌食	Anorexia
动脉粥样硬化	Atherosclerosis; see Coronary atherosclerosis
吐血	Spitting blood; see Bleeding
吸蟲蛭感染	Fluke infestation
先兆流产	Threatened abortion
舌炎	Glottitis
自汗	Spontaneous perspiration; see Perspiration
血証	Bood disorder; see Bleeding
血瘀	Blood stasis (Yu syndrome)
血栓闭塞性脉管炎	Buerger's disease (thromboangiitis obliterans)
血虚	Deficiency of blood; see Consumptive disease
血管球性腎炎	Glomercular nephritis
血吸虫病	Schistosomiasis
血小板减少性紫癜	Thrombocytopenic purpura
血栓性静脉炎	Thrombotic phlebitis
伤寒论辩证	Differentiation according to "Shang Han Lun" (Treatise on Febrile Disease)
伤寒、肠热病	Typhoid fever
行痹	Arthralgia (Migratory)
创伤	Wound
肋骨痛	Hypochondriac pain
肋間神經痛	Intercostal neuralgia
肌肉疼痛	Muscle-ache
肌肉萎缩	Muscular atrophy
孕嘔	Morning sickness
多神經根炎	Polyradiculitis
产后出血	Postpartum bleeding
产后调理	Postpartum care
产后发热	Postpartum fever
闭证	Syndrome of Tension; see Coma
关节痛	Arthralgia
关节炎—慢性	Arthritis (Chronic)
关节炎—化脓性	Suppurative arthritis
汗証	Perspiration disorders (Han Zheng)
自汗	Spontaneous perspiration
盗汗	Night perspiration
红眼症	Blood-shot eyes
阳虚	Deficiency of Yang; see Consumptive diseases
阳萎	Impotence
阳明病辩证	Differentiation according to the Yang-Ming channel
阴虚	Deficiency of Yin; see Consumptive diseases
阴囊湿疹	Scrotal eczema
阴囊水囊肿	Scrotal hydrocele
阴囊疝气	Scrotal hernia
阴道炎	Trichomonas vaginitis

| 阴道出血 | Vaginal bleeding |
| 寻常性痤疮 | Acne vulgaris |

七劃

更年期綜合症	Climacteric syndromes; Menopause
麦粒肿	Hordeolum
呕血	Hematemis
呕吐	Vomiting; see Nausea and Vomiting
足癣	Tinea pedia
吸蟲病	Trematodiasis; see Fluke infestation
低鈣血症	Hypocalcemia
坐骨神經痛	Sciatica
饮证	Fluid retention (Yin Zheng)
卵巢囊腫	Ovarian cyst
狂症	Mania, madness; see Psychosis
系統性紅斑狼瘡	Systemic lupus erythematosus
系統性膿性感染	Systemic pyogenic infection
肝病辩證	Differentiation according to Zang-fu (Liver)
肝昏迷	Hepatic coma
肝炎	Hepatitis
肝硬化	Hepato-cirrhosis; liver cirrhosis
肝豆狀核變性病	Hepatocuticular degeneration (Wilson's disease)
肝癌	Liver carcinoma
肝炎—病毒性	Viral hepatitis
肠炎	Enteritis
肠胃炎	Gastroenteritis
肠脓肿	Intestinal abscess
肠堵塞、肠梗阻	Intestinal obstruction
肠结核	Intestinal tuberculosis
行經	Menstruation
禿髮、斑禿	Alopecia areata; baldness
角膜潰瘍—匐行性	Corneal ulcer (serpiginous)
角膜炎	Keratitis
角後弓反張	Opisthotonos
坐立不安	Restlessness
疖	Boils, furuncle
美尼爾氏病	Meniere's disease
冻疮	Cold sores, frostbite
沙眼	Trachoma
尿血	Blood in the urine; see Bleeding
尿道結石	Urolithiasis, calculus in the urinary tract
尿崩病	Diabetes insipitus
尿頻	Frequent urination
尿失禁	Incontinence

尿毒症	Uremia
尿道炎	Urethritis
妊娠痛症	Eclampsia gravidarum
阿米巴病	Amebiasis
阿米巴痢疾	Amoebic dysentery
阿狄森病、慢性肾上腺皮質功能减退症	
	Addison's disease; hypoadrenalcorticism

八劃

郁証	Depressive syndrome (Yu Zheng)
青春豆	Acne vulgaris
青光眼	Glaucoma
肾病辩证	Differentiation according to Zang-fu (Kidney)
肾炎—血管球性	Glomerular nephritis
肾炎—急性	Nephritis (acute)
肾炎—慢性	Nephritis (chronic)
肾病综合症	Nephrotic syndrome
肾盂炎	Pyelitis
肾盂肾炎	Pyelonephritis
肾结核	Renal tuberculosis
败血病	Septicemia
兒童發育不良	Retarded growth of children
肥胖症	Obesity
肠胃炎	Gastroenteritis
便秘	Constipation
便血	Blood in the stools; see Bleeding
贫血—再生障碍性	Anemia (aplastic)
贫血—缺铁性	Anemia (iron deficiency)
贫血—营养不良性	Anemia (nutritional deficiency)
乳房漲痛	Breast distention
乳腺炎—急性	Mastadenitis
昏迷	Coma
肩關節周圍炎	Scapulo-humeral periarthritis
肩頸背僵硬	Stiff neck and shoulder
夜尿	Nocturia
卒中	Apoplexy
疟	Malaria
疝	Hernia
波動性發熱	Brucellosis (undulant fever)
泌尿系感染	Urinary tract infection
炎症	Inflammation
视力模糊	Blurriness of vision
视神经炎	Optic neuritis
视网膜炎	Retinitis

视网膜炎—色素性	Pigmentary degeneration of retina
驼背	Kyphosis
细菌性痢疾	Bacillary dysentery
细螺旋体病	Leptospirosis
经闭	Amenorrhea
经痛	Dysmenorrhea
经绝期	Menopause
经前期紧张症	Premenstrual tension syndrome

九劃

荨麻疹	Uriticaria
带状疱疹	Herpes zoster
带下病	Leukorrhea
面瘫	Bells's palsy (facial paralysis)
咳嗽	Cough
咳血	Cough with Blood; see Bleeding
咽炎	Pharyngitis
咽喉痛	Sore throat
咯血	Hemoptysis
哮証、哮鳴	Wheezping (Xiao Zheng)
胃潰瘍	Ulcer (gastric)
胃病辯證	Differentiation according to Zang-fu (Stomach)
胃脘痛	Epigastric pain
胃擴張	Gastrectasis
胃癌	Gastric carcinoma
胃神經官能症	Gastric neurosis
胃下垂	Gastroptosis
胃炎—慢性	Gastritis (chronic)
胃腸炎	Gastroenteritis
胃腸出血	Gastro-intestinal bleeding
胃腸感染	Gastro-intestinal flu
胃腸神經官能症	Gastro-intestinal neurosis
胃腸痙攣	Gastro-intestinal spasm
便血	Bloody stool; see Bleeding
衄血	Epistaxis; see Bleeding
食管癌	Esophageal carcinoma
食管痙攣	Esophagiospasm
重症肌無力	Myasthenia gravis
盆腔炎	Pelvic inflammation
肺病—消耗性	Consumptive pulmonary disease
肺氣腫—慢性	Cor pulmonale (chronic)
肺病辯證	Differentiation according to Zang-fu (Lung)
肺氣腫	Emphysema, pulmonary emphysema
肺膿腫	Lung abscess, pulmonary abscess

肺炎—小兒	Pneumonia (infantile)
肺炎—大葉	Pneumonia (lobar)
肺炎—下葉	Penumonia (lobular)
肺炎—支原菌	Pneumonia (mycoplasma)
肺矽炎	Pneumosilicosis
肺不張、肺膨脹不全	Pulmonary atelectasis
肺結核	Pulmonary tuberculosis
胆石病、胆結石	Cholelithiasis, biliary calculus
胆囊炎	Cholecystitis
胆囊病辩证	Differentiation according to Zang-fu (Gallbladder)
脉管炎—血栓闭塞性	Thromboangiitis obliterans
風濕熱	Rheumatic fever
風濕病	Rheumatism
風疹塊	Urticaria
恍惚	Absent-mindedness
類中風性的	Apoplectiform
前列腺增生	Prostate hyperplasia
前列腺炎	Prostatitis
前巩膜炎	Scleritis (anterior)
神經衰弱	Neurasthenia
神經官能症	Neurosis
神經機能病—植物性	Vegetative neurosis
扁桃體炎	Tonsillitis
语言困难	Difficulty of Speech; see Apoplectiform
結石	Calculus
结核病	Tuberculosis; see Pulmonary tuberculosis
结肠炎	Colitis
急性结肠炎	Acute colitis
慢性结肠炎	Chronic colitis
过敏性结肠炎	Allergenic colitis
结肠癌	Colon carcinoma
结肠过敏	Colon irritable
结肠结核	Colon tuberculosis
紅眼症	Blood-shot eyes

十劃

获得性免疫缺陷综合症	Aids (acquired immune deficiency syndrome)
恶心	Nausea
恶露	Lochia, retention of lochia
破傷風	Tetanus
损伤	Injury
热痹	Arthralgia (Heat)
热射病、中暑	Thermoplegia
哮喘	Asthma

蜂窩纖炎—急性	Phlegmon (acute)
骨骼肌肉鬆弛	Flaccidity of bones and muscles
骨髓炎—化膿性	Osteomyelitis (pyogenic)
骨關節結核病	Tuberculosis of articular joints
眩暈	Vertigo
氣虛	Deficiency of Qi; see Consumptive diseases
氣管炎	Trachitis; tracheitis
積聚	Mass
脊髓側索硬化	Sclerosis of funiculus lateralis
愛滋病	AIDS (Acquired Immune Deficiency Syndrome)
狼瘡	Lupus (see Systemic lupus erythematosus)
臟腑辩证	Differentiation according to Zang-fu (internal visceras)
脓肿	Abscess
脓疱病	Impetigo
脈管炎—血栓閉塞性	Thromboangiitis obliterans
脑震荡	Cerebral concussion
脑血栓	Cerebral thrombosis
脑血管意外	Cerebral vascular accident (CVA)
脑炎	Encephalitis
脑膜炎	Meningitis
胸痛	Chest pain
胸膜炎	Pleuritis (pleurisy)
胰腺炎	Pancreatitis
健忘症	Forgetfullness
脊柱後凸	Kyphosis
高脂蛋白血症	Hyper-lipoproteinemia
高血壓	Hypertension, high blood pressure
衰竭	Prostration
病態竇房結綜合征	Sick sinus syndrome (fibrosis of sinoatrial node)
疲勞	Fatigue
痈	Carbuncle
凍瘡	Cold sores, frostbite
酒齄鼻	Rosacea
流鼻涕	Running piggies
消化不良	Indigestion
消化性潰瘍	Peptic ulcer
粉刺	Acne vulgaris
幽門梗阻	Pyloric obstruction (incomplete)
冠心病	Coronary heart disease
陰虛	Deficiency of Yin; see Consumptive diseases
陰囊濕疹	Scrotal eczema
陰囊水囊腫	Scrotal hydrocele
陰囊疝氣	Scrotal hernia
陰道炎	Trichomonas vaginitis
陰道出血	Vaginal bleeding

十一劃

黃褐斑	Chloasma (yellow pigmentation)
黃疸	Jaundice, icteric
黃疸—新生兒	Jaundice (neonatal)
乾嘔	Retch
梅核氣	Globus hystericus
夢魘	Nightmare
麥粒腫	Hordeolum
掉牙	Loss of teeth
惡露	Lochia, retention of lochia
帶狀疱疹	Herpes zoster
副鼻竇炎	Acessory nasal sinusitis
副傷寒病	Paratyphoid fever
帶下病	Leukorrhea
虛勞	Consumptive diseases
虛脫	Prostration
晨吐	Morning sickness
酗酒	Crapulence
眼痛	Ophthalmalgia
敗血病	Septicemia
閉証	Syndrome of tension, see Coma
銀屑病	Psoriasis
停經	Menopause
斜視	Strabismus
貧血—再生障礙性	Anemia (aplastic)
貧血—缺鐵性	Anemia (iron deficiency)
貧血—營養不良性	Anemia (nutritional deficiency)
動脈粥樣硬化	Atherosclerosis; see Coronary atherosclerosis
腳氣	Beri-beri
脫髮	Loss of hair
脫肛	Prolapse of anus
脫証	Syndrome of Prostration; see Coma
麻痺	Paralysis (Wei Zheng)
痔瘡	Hemorrhoid
痔瘡出血	Hemorrhoid bleeding; see Bleeding
瘧	Malaria
產後出血	Postpartum bleeding
產後調理	Postpartum care
產後發熱	Postpartum fever
惊厥	Convulsion
惊厥病	Convulsive disease
寄生虫感染	Parasitic infestation
着痺	Arthralgia (Fixed)
視力模糊	Blurriness of vision

視神經炎	Optic neuritis
視網膜炎	Retinitis
視網膜炎—色素性	Pigmentary degeneration of retina
淋病	Gonorrhea
淋巴腺炎	Lymphadenitis
淋巴管炎	Lymphangitis
淋巴管回流梗阻	Obstructed backflow of lymph ducts
淋証	Urination disorders (Lin Zheng)
盜汗	Night perspiration
粒狀白血球過少症	Granulocytopenia; see Leukocytopenia
頸肩背僵硬	Stiff neck and shoulder
細菌性痢疾	Bacillary dysentery
絲蟲病	Filariasis
細螺旋體病	Leptospirosis
陽虛	Deficiency of Yang; see Consumptive diseases
陽萎	Impotence
陽明病辯證	Differentiation according to the Yang-Ming channel

十二劃

斑點	Macula
营养不良性貧血	Anemia (nutritional deficiency)
鼓脹	Distention
腎上腺皮質功能減退症	Addison's disease; hypoadrenocorticism
腎病辯證	Differentiaton according to Zang-fu (Kidney)
腎炎—血管球性	Glomerular nephritis (chronic)
腎炎—急性	Nephritis (acute)
腎炎—慢性	Nephritis (chronic)
腎病綜合症	Nephrotic syndrome
腎盂炎	Pyelitis
腎盂腎炎	Pyelonephritis
腎結核	Renal tuberculosis
駝背	Kyphosis
硬皮病	Scleroderma
硬皮病—初生兒	Scleroderma neonatorum
厥陰証辯證	Differentiation according to the Jue-Yin channel
厥証	Syncope
喉炎	Laryngitis
蛔蟲病	Ascariasis
蛔蟲病—膽囊性	Biliary ascariasis
遺尿	Bed-wetting, enuresis
紫癜—血小板減少性	Thrombocytopenic purpura
紫癜—過敏性	Purpura (allergic)
創傷	Wound
飲証	Fluid retention (Yin Zheng)

猩紅熱	Scarlet fever
脾病辯證	Differentiation according to Zang-fu (Spleen)
膽結石	Gallstone
腺炎	Adenitis
癆瘵	Phthiasis; see Pulmonary tuberculosis
痢疾	Dysentery
痢疾—細菌性	Bacillary dysentery
痛痺	Arthralgia (Pain)
痙症	Convulsive disease
寒熱交戰	Chills and fever
闌尾炎	Appendicitis
濕阻	Dampness obstruction
濕疹	Eczema
渴	Thirst
潰疡性结肠炎—慢性	Ulcerative colitis (chronic)
溫病論辯證	Differentiation according to "Wen Bin Lun" (Treastise on Epidemic Febrile Disease)
結石	Calculus
結腸炎	Colitis
結腸炎—過敏性	Allergenic colitis
結腸癌	Colon cardinoma
結腸過敏	Colon irritable
結腸結核	Colon tuberculosis
結核病	Tuberculosis; see Pulmonary tuberculosis
尋常性痤瘡	Acne vulgaris

十三劃

暈厥	Syncope
感冒	Flu, common Cold, influenza
損傷	Injury
睪丸下垂	Orchidiptosis
睪丸炎	Testitis
嗜鉻細胞瘤	Chromaffinoma
噯气	Belching
傷寒論辯證	Differention according to "Shang Han Lun" (Treatise on Febrile Disease)
傷寒、腸熱病	Typhoid fever
愛滋病	AIDS (Acquired Immune Deficiency Syndrome)
腰背痛、腰肌痛	Lumbago, low back pain
腰肌損傷	Sprain/strain of the lumbar muscles
腸炎	Enteritis
腸胃炎	Gastroenteritis
腸膿腫	Intestinal abscess
腸堵塞、腸梗阻	Intestinal obstruction

腸結核	Intestinal tuberculosis
膀胱炎	Cystitis
膀胱病辯證	Differentiation according to Zang-fu (Urinary-bladder)
腹痛	Abdominal Pain
腹上部疼痛	Epigastric pain
腹水	Ascites
腹鳴	Borborygmus
腹瀉	Diarrhea
腹股溝疝	Inguinal hernia
腹膜炎	Peritonitis
腮腺炎	Mumps, parotitis
腦震盪	Cerebral concussion
腦血栓	Cerebral thrombosis
腦血管意外	Cerebral Vascular Accident (CVA)
腦炎	Encephalitis
腦膜炎	Meningitis
痿証	Paralysis (Wei Zheng)
痲疹	Measles
痰証	Phlegm disorder (Tan Zheng)
瘀証	Blood stasis (Yu syndrome)
煩躁	Fidgetiness
經閉	Amenorrhea
經痛	Dysmenorrhea
經絕期	Menopause
經前期緊張症	Premenstrual tension syndrome
發燒、發熱	Fever
發熱—出血性	Hemorrhagic fever

十四劃

嘔血	Hematemesis
嘔吐	Vomiting; see Nausea and Vomiting
惡性嘔吐	Vomiting (pernicious)
厭食	Anorexia
鼻衄	Epistaxis
鼻竇炎	Nasal-sinusitis
鼻出血	Nose bleeding
鼻炎	Rhinitis
鼻塞	Stuffy nose
銀屑病	Psoriasis
膈痙攣	Phrenospasm
語言困難	Difficulty of speech; see Apoplectiform
痺証	Arthralia (Bi Syndrome)
精神病	Psychosis
精神分裂症	Schizophrenia

十五劃

蕁麻疹	Urticaria
熱痺	Arthralgia (Heat)
熱射病、中暑	Thermoplegia
鞏膜炎	Scleritis
遺尿	Bed-wetting, enuresis
遺精	Spermatorrhea
膝關節韌帶損傷	Ligamentous injury of the knee joint; see Knee injury
潮熱	Tidal fever
潰瘍性結腸炎—慢性	Ulcerative colitis (chronic)

十六劃

頭疼	Headache
頭顱頂頭痛	Vertical headache
靜脈炎—血栓性	Thrombotic phlebitis
霍亂	Cholera
醛甾酮過多症	Hyperaldersteronism (Conn's syndrome)
惡心	Nausea and vomiting
噪雜	Epigastric upset
噯氣	Belching
積聚	Mass
衛氣營血	Differentiation according to the 4 conditions in "Wen Bin Lung" (syndromes of Wei, Qi, Ying, Xue)
頸肩背僵硬	Stiff neck and shoulder
膝損傷	Knee injury
膽結石	Biliary calculus, cholelithiasis
膽囊炎	Cholecystitis
膽囊病辯證	Differentiation according to Zang-fu (Gallbladder)
癃閉	Dysuria

十七劃和十七劃以上

驚厥	Convulsion
驚厥病（痙症）	Convulsive disease
蘑菇中毒	Mushroom Poisoning
躁狂	Mania
闌尾炎	Appendicitis
關節痛	Arthralgia
關節炎—慢性	Arthritis (Chronic)
關節炎—化膿性	Suppurative arthritis
臟腑辯證	Differentiation according to Zang-fu (internal visceras)

膿腫	Abscess
膿皰病	Impetigo
獲得性免疫缺陷綜合症	AIDS (Acquired Immune Deficiency Syndrome)
癆瘵	Phthiasis; see Pulmonary tuberculosis
糖尿病	Diabetes mellitus
營養不良性貧血	Anemia (nutritional deficiency)
譫妄	Delirium
癲癇	Epilepsy
癤	Boils, furuncle
癰	Carbuncle
癲症	Depressive syndrome; see Psychosis
癔病	Hysteria
濕阻	Dampness obstruction
濕疹	Eczema
竇炎	Sinusitis

INDEX OF THE

CHINESE HERBAL FORMULAS

(CHINESE)

INDEX of the CHINESE HERBAL FORMULAS (Chinese)

中文方劑索引

一劃

一貫煎   Yi Guan Jian

二劃

二陳湯   Er Chen Tang
二妙散   Er Miao San
二仙湯   Er Xian Tang
十補丸   Shi Bu Wan
十灰散   Shi Hui San
十全大補湯   Shi Quan Da Bu Tang
十棗湯   Shi Zao Tang
丁香柿蒂湯   Ding Xiang Shi Di Tang
七里散   Qi Li San
七味白术散   Qi Wei Bai Zhu San
人參湯   Ren Shen Tang
人參敗毒散   Ren Shen Bai Du San
人參胡桃湯   Ren Shen Hu Tou Tang
人參養營湯   Ren Shen Yang Rong Tang
八味地黃丸   Ba Wei Di Huang Wan
八仙長壽丸   Ba Xian Chang Shou Wan
八珍湯   Ba Zhen Tang
八珍益母丸   Ba Zhen Yi Mu Wan
八正散   Ba Zheng San
九味羌活湯   Jiu Wei Qiang Huo Tang

三劃

三仁湯   San Ren Tang
三妙散   San Miao San
三拗湯   San Niu Tang
三金湯   San Jin Tang
三子養親湯   San Zi Yang Qing Tang
三甲復脈湯   San Jia Fu Mai Tang
三黃四物湯   San Huang Si Wu Tang
大補丸   Da Bu Wan

大補陰丸	Da Bu Yin Wan
大柴胡湯	Da Chai Hu Tang
大承氣湯	Da Cheng Qi Tang
大定風珠	Da Ding Feng Zhu
大黃附子湯	Da Huang Fu Zi Tang
大黃牡丹皮湯	Da Huang Mu Dan Pi Tang
大建中湯	Da Jian Zhong Tang
大青龍湯	Da Qing Long Tang
大陷胸湯	Da Xian Xiong Tang
小半夏湯	Xiao Ban Xia Tang
小承氣湯	Xiao Cheng Qi Tang
小柴胡湯	Xiao Chai Hu Tang
小活絡丹	Xiao Huo Luo Dan
小薊飲子	Xiao Ji Yin Zi
小建中湯	Xiao Jian Zhong Tang
小青龍湯	Xiao Qing Long Tang
小青龍加石膏湯	Xiao Qing Long Jia Shi Gao Tang
小陷胸湯	Xiao Xian Xiong Tang
川芎茶調散	Chuan Xiong Cha Tiao San
己椒藶黃丸	Ji Jiao Li Huang Wan

四劃

天麻鉤藤飲	Tian Ma Gou Teng Yin
天台烏药散	Tian Tai Wu Yao San
天王補心丹	Tian Wang Bu Xin Dan
不換金正氣散	Bu Huan Jin Zheng Qi San
木香檳榔丸	Mu Xiang Bin Lang Wan
五苓散	Wu Ling San
五磨飲子	Wu Mo Yin Zi
五皮飲	Wu Pi Yin
五皮散	Wu Pi San
五味消毒飲	Wu Wei Xiao Du Yin
止痙散	Zhi Jing San
止嗽散	Zhi Sou San
貝母瓜蔞散	Bei Mu Gua Lou San
丹參飲	Dan Shen Yin
丹梔逍遙散	Dan Zhi Xiao Yao San
少腹逐瘀湯	Shao Fu Zhu Yu Tang
升麻葛根湯	Sheng Ma Ge Gen Tang
牛黃解毒片	Niu Huang Jie Du Pian
乌梅丸	Wu Mei Wan
乌头湯	Wu Tou Tang
六一散	Liu Yi San

六君子湯	Liu Jun Zi Tang
六神丸	Liu Shen Wan
六味地黄丸	Liu Wei Di Huang Wan

五劃

玉女煎	Yu Nu Jian
玉真散	Yu Zhen San
玉屏風散	Yu Ping Feng San
甘草瀉心湯	Gan Cao Xie Xin Tang
甘露消毒丹	Gan Lu Xiao Du Dan
甘麥大棗湯	Gan Mai Da Zao Tang
甘遂通結湯	Gan Sui Tong Jie Tang
平胃散	Ping Wei San
左歸丸	Zuo Gui Wan
左歸飲	Zuo Gui Yin
右歸丸	You Gui Wan
右歸飲	You Gui Yin
龙胆泻肝汤	Long Dan Xie Gan Tang
布袋丸	Bu Dai Wan
石葦散	Shi Wei San
四生丸	Si Sheng Wan
四妙散	Si Miao San
四物湯	Si Wu Tang
四苓散	Si Ling San
四神丸	Si Shen Wan
四逆湯	Si Ni Tang
四逆散	Si Ni San
四磨飲	Si Mo Yin
四君子湯	Si Jun Zi Tang
四妙勇安湯	Si Miao Yong An Tang
四逆加人參湯	Si Ni Jia Ren Shen Tang
归脾汤	Gui Pi Tang
白术散	Bai Zhu San
白虎湯	Bai Hu Tang
白頭翁湯	Bai Tou Weng Tang
白术芍藥散	Bai Zhu Shao Yao San
白虎加人參湯	Bai Hu Jia Ren Shen Tang
白虎加桂枝湯	Bai Hu Jia Gui Zhi Tang
生化湯	Sheng Hua Tang
生脈散	Sheng Mai San
生薑瀉心湯	Sheng Jiang Xie Xin Tang
失笑散	Shi Xiao San
失笑丸	Shi Xiao Wan

瓜蒂散	Gua Di San
瓜蔞薤白半夏湯	Gua Lou Xie Bai Ban Xia Tang
瓜蔞薤白白酒湯	Gua Lou Xie Bai Bai Jiu Tang
半夏瀉心湯	Ban Xia Xie Xin Tang
半夏厚朴湯	Ban Xia Hou Po Tang
半夏白术天麻湯	Ban Xia Bai Zhu Tian Ma Tang
加減復脈湯	Jia Jian Fu Mai Tang
加減葳蕤湯	Jia Jian Wei Rui Tang
加味二妙散	Jia Wei Er Miao San

六劃

耳聾左慈丸	Er Long Zuo Ci Wan
百合固金湯	Bai He Gu Jin Tang
地黄飲子	Di Huang Yin Zi
至寶丹	Zhi Bao Dan
达原饮	Da Yuan Yin
朱砂安神丸	Zhu Sha An Shen Wan
异功散	Yi Gong San
曲麥枳术丸	Qu Mai Zhi Zhu Wan
当归补血汤	Dang Gui Bu Xue Tang
当归健中汤	Dang Gui Jian Zhong Tang
当归六黄汤	Dang Gui Liu Huang Tang
当归龙荟丸	Dang Gui Long Hui Wan
当归芍药散	Dang Gui Shao Yao San
当归四逆汤	Dang Gui Si Ni Tang
当归四逆加吴茱萸生姜汤	Dang Gui Si Ni Jia Wu Zhu Yu Sheng Jiang Tang
竹葉石膏湯	Zhu Ye Shi Gao Tang
舟車丸	Zhou Che Wan
血府逐瘀湯	Xue Fu Zhu Yu Tang
安宫牛黄丸	An Gong Niu Huang Wan
导赤散	Dao Chi San
导气汤	Dao Qi Tang
导痰汤	Dao Tan Tang
红花桃仁煎	Hong Hua Tao Ren Jian
防風通聖散	Fang Feng Tong Sheng San
防己茯苓湯	Fang Ji Fu Ling Tang
防己黄芪湯	Fang Ji Huang Qi Tang

七劃

杏蘇散	Xing Su San
苏合香丸	Su He Xiang Wan
苏子降气汤	Su Zi Jiang Qi Tang
苇茎汤	Wei Jing Tang
苍耳散	Cang Er San
麦门冬汤	Mai Men Dong Tang
麦味地黄丸	Mai Wei Di Huang Wan
杞菊地黄丸	Qi Ju Di Huang Wan
吴茱萸湯	Wu Zhu Yu Tang
牡蠣散	Mu Li San
龟鹿二仙胶	Gui Lu Er Xian Jiao
身痛逐瘀湯	Shen Tong Zhu Yu Tang
完帶湯	Wan Dai Tang
良附丸	Liang Fu Wan
补肺汤	Bu Fei Tang
补肝汤	Bu Gan Tang
补阳还五汤	Bu Yang Huan Wu Tang
补中益气汤	Bu Zhong Yi Qi Tang
辛夷散	Xin Yin San
沙參麥門冬湯	Sha Shen Mai Men Dong Tang
鸡鸣散	Ji Ming San
附子湯	Fu Zi Tang
附子理中湯	Fu Zi Li Zhong Tang
附桂理中湯	Fu Gui Li Zhong Tang
附子瀉心湯	Fu Zi Xie Xin Tang

八劃

青娥丸	Qing E Wan
青蒿鱉甲湯	Qing Hao Bie Jia Tang
苓甘五味薑辛湯	Ling Gan Wu Wei Jiang Xin Tang
苓桂术甘湯	Ling Gui Zhu Gan Tang
固冲湯	Gu Chong Tang
固經丸	Gu Jing Wan
吴茱萸湯	Wu Zhu Yu Tang
虎潛丸	Hu Qian Wan
明目地黄丸	Ming Mu Di Huang Wan
金匱腎氣丸	Jin Kui Shen Qi Wan
金水六君煎	Jin Shui Liu Jun Jian
金鎖固經丸	Jin Suo Gu Jing Wan
知柏地黄丸	Zhi Bai Di Huang Wan
炙甘草湯	Zhi Gan Cao Tang

实脾散	Shi Pi San
定喘湯	Ding Chuan Tang
羌籃湯	Qiang Lan Tang
羌活勝濕湯	Qiang Huo Sheng Shi Tang
河車大造丸	He Che Da Zao Wan
泻心汤	He Che Da Zao Wan
泻白散	Xie Bai San
泻肺散	Xie Fei San
参附汤	Shen Fu Tang
参蚧散	Shen Jie San
参苓白术散	Shen Ling Bai Zhu San
参苏饮	Shen Su Yin

九劃

枳實消痞丸	Zhi Shi Xiao Pi Wan
枳术丸	Zhi Zhu Wan
柿蒂湯	Shi Di Tang
柿錢散	Shi Qian San
厚朴溫中湯	Hou Po Wen Zhong Tang
牽正散	Qian Zheng San
胃苓湯	Wei Ling Tang
香薷散	Xiang Ru San
香砂二陳湯	Xiang Sha Er Chen Tang
香砂六君子湯	Xiang Sha Liu Jun Zi Tang
香砂枳术丸	Xiang Sha Zhi Zhu Wan
香蘇散	Xiang Su San
复脉汤	Fu Mai Tang
复元活血汤	Fu Yuan Huo Xue Tang
保和丸	Bao He Wan
胆道排石汤	Dan Dao Pai Shi Tang
养阴清肺汤	Yang Yin Qing Fei Tang
济川煎	Ji Chuan Jian
紅花桃仁煎	Hong Hua Tao Ren Jian
独活寄生汤	Du Huo Ji Sheng Tang

十劃

真人養臟湯	Zhen Ren Yang Zang Tang
真武湯	Zhen Wu Tang
泰山磐石散	Tai Shan Pan Shi San
桂附地黄丸	Gui Fu Di Huang Wan
桂枝茯苓丸	Gui Zhi Fu Ling Wan

桂枝加葛根湯	Gui Zhi Jia Ge Gen Tang
桂枝加厚朴杏仁湯	Gui Zhi Jia Hou Po Xing Ren Tang
桂枝加龍骨牡蠣湯	Gui Zhi Jia Long Gu Mu Li Tang
桂枝芍藥知母湯	Gui Zhi Shao Yao Zhi Mu Tang
桂枝湯	Gui Zhi Tang
桃核承氣湯	Tao He Cheng Qi Tang
桃花湯	Tao Hua Tang
都氣丸	Du Qi Wan
柴葛解肌湯	Chai Ge Jie Ji Tang
柴胡舒肝散	Chai Hu Shu Gan San
健脾丸	Jian Pi Wan
胶艾汤	Jiao Ai Tang
消風散	Xiao Feng San
涼膈散	Liang Ge San
消瘰丸	Xiao Luo Wan
逍遙散	Xiao Yao San
调肝汤	Tiao Gan Tang
调味承气汤	Tiao Wei Cheng Qi Tang
益元散	Yi Yuan San
射干麻黄湯	She Gan Ma Huang Tang
通脈四逆湯	Tong Mai Si Ni Tang
通竅活血湯	Tong Qiao Huo Xue Tang
桑菊飲	Sang Ju Yin
桑螵蛸散	Sang Piao Xiao San
桑杏湯	Sang Xing Tang

十一劃

黄連阿膠湯	Huang Lian E Jiao Tang
黄連解毒湯	Huang Lian Jie Du Tang
黄連湯	Huang Lian Tang
黄龍湯	Huang Long Tang
黄芪建中湯	Huang Qi Jian Zhong Tang
黄芪桂枝五物湯	Huang Qi Gui Zhi Wu Wu Tang
黄土湯	Huang Tu Tang
菊花茶調散	Ju Hua Cha Tiao San
草薢分清飲	Bi Xie Fen Qing Yin
理中湯	Li Zhong Tang
硃砂安神丸	Zhu Sha An Shen Wan
麥門冬湯	Mai Men Dong Tang
異功散	Yi Gong San
蛇床子沖洗劑	She Chuang Zi Chong Xi Ji
銀翹敗毒散	Yin Qiao Bai Du San
銀翹散	Yin Qiao San

羚羊鈎藤湯	Ling Yang Gou Teng Tang
牽正散	Qian Zheng San
麻子仁丸	Ma Zi Ren Wan
麻黃附子細辛湯	Ma Huang Fu Zi Xi Xin Tang
麻黃加术湯	Ma Huang Jia Zhu Tang
麻黃連翹赤小豆湯	Ma Huang Lian Qiao Chi Xiao Dou Tang
麻黃湯	Ma Huang Tang
麻杏石甘湯	Ma Xing Shi Gan Tang
旋覆代赭湯	Xuan Fu Dai Zhe Tang
清骨散	Qing Gu San
清氣化痰丸	Qing Qi Hua Tan Wan
清暑益氣湯 I	Qing Shu Yi Qi Tang (I)
清暑益氣湯II	Qing Shu Yi Qi Tang (II)
清胰湯	Qing Yi Tang
清營湯	Qing Ying Tang
清瘟敗毒飲	Qing Wen Bai Du Yin
清燥救肺湯	Qing Zao Jiu Fei Tang
透膿散	Tou Nong San
參附湯	Shen Fu Tang
參蚧散	Shen Jie San
參苓白术散	Shen Ling Bai Zhu San
疏齒飲子	Shu Chi Yin Zi
陽和湯	Yang He Tang

十二劃

葶藶子大棗瀉肺湯	Ting Li Da Zao Xie Fei Tang
葱豉湯	Cong Chi Tang
葛根黃芩黃連湯	Ge Gen Huang Qin Huang Lian Tang
葛根湯	Ge Gen Tang
越婢加术湯	Yue Bi Jia Zhu Tang
越婢湯	Yue Bi Tang.
越麴丸	Yue Qu Wan
達原飲	Da Yuan Yin
紫雪丹	Zi Xue Dan
當歸補血湯	Dang Gui Bu Xue Tang
當歸健中湯	Dang Gui Jian Zhong Tang
當歸六黃湯	Dang Gui Liu Huang Tang
當歸龍薈丸	Dang Gui Long Hui Wan
當歸芍藥散	Dang Gui Shao Yao San
當歸四逆湯	Dang Gui Si Ni Tang
當歸四逆加吳茱萸生薑湯	Dang Gui Si Ni Jia Wu Zhu Yu Sheng Jiang Tang
復脈活血湯	Fu Mai Huo Xue Tang
復脈湯	Fu Mai Tang

舒肝丸	Shu Gan Wan
補肺湯	Bu Fei Tang
補肝湯	Bu Gan Tang
補陽還五湯	Bu Yang Huan Wu Tang
補中益氣湯	Bu Zhong Yi Qi Tang
普劑消毒飲	Pu Ji Xiao Du Yin
痛瀉要方	Tong Xie Yao Fang
溫胆湯	Wen Dan Tang
溫經湯	Wen Jing Tang
溫脾湯	Wen Pi Tang
犀角地黃湯	Xi Jiao Di Huang Tang

十三劃

蒿芩清膽湯	Hao Qin Qing Dan Tang
葦莖湯	Wei Jing Tang
槐花散	Huai Hua San
槐角丸	Huai Jiao Wan
暖肝煎	Nuan Gan Jian
愈帶丸	Yu Dai Wan
新加黃龍湯	Xin Jia Huang Long Tang
新加香薷飲	Xin Jia Xian Ru Yin

十四劃

蒼耳散	Cang Er San
碧玉散	Bi Yu San
酸棗仁湯	Suan Zao Ren Tang
磁硃丸	Ci Zhu Wan
膈下逐瘀湯	Ge Xia Zhu Yu Tang
實脾散	Shi Pi San
縮泉丸	Suo Quan Wan

十五劃

增液承氣湯	Zeng Ye Cheng Qi Tang
增液湯	Zeng Ye Tang
震靈丹	Zhen Ling Dan
膠艾湯	Jiao Ai Tang
鎮肝熄風湯	Zhen Gan Xi Feng Tang
導赤散	Dao Chi San
導氣湯	Dao Qi Tang

導痰湯	Dao Tan Tang
養心湯	Yang Xin Tang
養陰清肺湯	Yang Yin Qing Fei Tang
濟川煎	Ji Chuan Jian

十六劃以上

蘇合香丸	Su He Xiang Wan
蘇子降氣湯	Su Zi Jiang Qi Tang
藿香正氣散	Huo Xiang Zheng Qi San
橘半枳朮丸	Ju Ban Zhi Zhu Wan
橘核丸	Ju He Wan
橘皮竹茹湯	Ju Pi Zhu Ru Tang
銀翹敗毒散	Yin Qiao Bai Du San
銀翹散	Yin Qiao San
膽道排石湯	Dan Dao Pai Shi Tang
歸脾湯	Gui Pi Tang
龜鹿二仙膠	Gui Lu Er Xian Jiao
雞鳴散	Ji Ming San
龍膽瀉肝湯	Long Dan Xie Gan Tang
瀉白散	Xie Bai San
瀉肺散	Xie Fei San
瀉心湯	Xie Xin Tang
蠲痺湯I	Juan Bi Tang (I)
蠲痺湯II	Juan Bi Tang (II)
獨活寄生湯	Du Huo Ji Sheng Tang

INDEX OF THE

CHINESE HERBAL FORMULAS

(ENGLISH)

INDEX of the CHINESE HERBAL FORMULAS (English)

Anemarrhena, Phellodendron and Pills of Six Herbs with Rehmannia
(Zhi Bai Di Huang Wan) (知柏地黄丸)
Anti-bruises Powder (Qi Li San) (七釐散)
Anticonvulsant Powder (Zhi Jing San) (止痙散)
Antiphlogistic Decoction for Epidemic Diseases
(Qing Wen Bai Du Yin) (清瘟敗毒飲)
Antiphlogistic Decoction of Coptis
(Huang Lian Jie Du Tang) (黄連解毒湯)
Antiphlogistic Pills with Ox Calculus
(Niu Huang Jie Du Pian) (牛黄解毒片)
Antiphlogistic Pills of Dew (Gan Lu Xiao Du Dan) (甘露消毒丹)
Antiphlogistic Powder of Ginseng
(Ren Shen Bai Du San) (人參敗毒散)
Antiphlogistic Powder of Lonicera Flower and Forsythia
(Yin Qiao Bai Du San) (銀翹敗毒散)
Antiphlogistic Powder of Schizonepeta and Ledebouriella
(Jing Fang Bai Du San) (荊防敗毒散)
Aromatic Formula with Five Herbs (Wu Mo Yin Zi) (五磨飲子)

Baked Licorice Decoction (Zhi Gan Cao Tang) (炙甘草湯)
Bezoar Resurrection Pills (An Gong Niu Huang Wan) (安宮牛黄丸)
Biliary Lithagogue Decoction (Dan Dao Pai Shi Tang) (膽道排石湯)
Blood Tonifying Decoction with Chinese Angelica
(Dang Gui Bu Xue Tang) (當歸補血湯)

Cinnabar Sedative Pills (Zhu Sha An Shen Wan) (硃砂安神丸)
Cock-a-doodle-doo Powder (Ji Ming San) (雞鳴散)
Conducting the Vital Energy Decoction (Dao Qi Tang) (導氣湯)
Cough Relieving Powder (Zhi Sou San) (止嗽散)

Decoction Acting on the Half-exterior & Half-interior Portion
of the Body (Da Yuan Yin) (達原飲)
Decoction for Acute Pancreatitis (Qing Yi Tang) (清胰湯)
Decoction for Arthralgia I (Juan Bi Tang I) (蠲痺湯I)
Decoction for Arthralgia II (Juan Bi Tang II) (蠲痺湯II)
Decoction for Asthma (Ding Chuan Tang) (定喘湯)
Decoction for Blood Stasis (Tong Yu Jian) (通瘀煎)
Decoction for Edema (Yue Bi Tang) (越婢湯)
Decoction for Invigorating Blood Circulation for Recovery
(Fu Yuan Huo Xue Tang) (復元活血湯)
Decoction for Morbid Leukorrhea (Wan Dai Tang) (完帶湯)

Decoction for Reinforcing the Middle Burner and Replenishing the Vital Energy
(Bu Zhong Yi Qi Tang) (補中益氣湯)

Decoction for Reinforcing the Vital Function and Restoring Normal Function
of the Five Visceras (Bu Yang Huan Wu Tang) (補陽還五湯)

Decoction for Removing Blood Stasis in Chest
(Xue Fu Zhu Yu Tang) (血府逐瘀湯)

Decoction for Removing Blood Stasis in the Lateral Abdomen
(Shao Fu Zhu Yu Tang) (少腹逐瘀湯)

Decoction for Removing Stagnant Blood and Promoting Hemogenesis
(Sheng Hua Tang) (生化湯)

Decoction for Restoring the Normal Function of the Middle Burner
with Astragalus (Huang Qi Jian Zhong Tang) (黃芪建中湯)

Decoction for Restoring the Normal Function of the Middle Burner
with Chinese Angelica (Dang Gui Jian Zhong Tang) (當歸健中湯)

Decoction for Thromboangiitis with Four Effective Ingredients
(Si Miao Yong An Tang) (四妙勇安湯))

Decoction for Treating Vital Prostration with Cold Limbs
(Si Ni Tang) (四逆湯)

Decoction for Treating Vital Prostration with Cold Limbs by
Invigorating the Vascular System
(Tong Mai Si Ni Tang) (通脈四逆湯)

Decoction for Warming the Liver Channel (Nuan Gan Jian) (暖肝煎)

Decoction of Allium Bulb and Soya (Cong Chi Tang) (葱豉湯)

Decoction of Antelope Horn and Uncaria
(Ling Yang Gou Teng Tang) (羚羊鉤藤湯)

Decoction of Artemisia and Donkey-hide Gelatin
(Jiao Ai Tang) (膠艾湯)

Decoction of Bamboo Leaf and Gypsum
(Zhu Ye Shi Gao Tang) (竹葉石膏湯)

Decocotion of Belamcanda and Ephedra
(She Gan Ma Huang Tang) (射干麻黃湯)

Decoction of Bupleurum and Pueraria
(Chai Ge Jie Ji Tang) (柴葛解肌湯)

Decoction of Magnolia to warm the Spleen and Stomach
(Hou Po Wen Zhong Tang) (厚朴溫中湯)

Decoction of Peach Flower (Tao Hua Tang) (桃花湯)

Decoction of Pueraria (Ge Gen Tang) (葛根湯)

Decoction of Capillaris (Yin Chen Hao Tang) (茵陳蒿湯)

Decoction of Carthamus and Persica Seed
(Hong Hua Tao Ren Jian) (紅花桃仁煎)

Decoction of Chinese Angelica and Six Yellow Ingredients)
(Dang Gui Liu Huang Tang) (當歸六黃湯)

Decoction of Cimicifuga and Pueraria
(Sheng Ma Ge Gen Tang) (升麻葛根湯)

Decoction of Cinnamon Twig (Gui Zhi Tang) (桂枝湯)

Decoction of Dinnamon Twig, Paeonia and Anemarrhena
(Gui Zhi Shao Yao Zhi Mu Tang)（桂枝芍藥知母湯）

Decoction of Citrus Peel and Bamboo Shavings
(Zu Pi Zhu Ru Tang)（橘皮竹茹湯）

Decoction of Cloves and Kaki Calyx
(Ding Xiang Shi Di Tang)（丁香柿蒂湯）

Decoction of Cnidium Fruit for Vaginitis
(She Chuang Zi Chong Xi Ji)（蛇床子沖洗劑）

Decoction of Coptis and Gelatin
(Huang Lian E Jiao Tang)（黃連阿膠湯）

Decoction of Curculigo and Epimedium
(Er Xian Tang)（二仙湯）

Decoction of Cyperus and Perilla Leaf
(Xiang Su San)（香蘇散）

Decoction of Elsholtzia (Xiang Ru San)（香薷散）

Decoction of Ephedra (Ma Huang Tang)（麻黃湯）

Decoction of Ephedra, Aconite and Asarum
(Ma Huang Fu Zi Xi Xin Tang)（麻黃附子細辛湯）

Decoction of Ephedra, Apricot Seed, Gypsum and Licorice
(Ma Xing Shi Gan Tang)（麻杏石甘湯）

Decoction of Evodia (Wu Zhu Yu Tang)（吳茱萸湯）

Decoction of Gastrodia and Uncaria
(Tian Ma Gou Teng Yin)（天麻鉤藤飲）

Decoction of Ginseng (Ren Shen Tang)（人參湯）

Decoction of Ginseng and Aconite (Shen Fu Tang)（參附湯）

Decoction of Ginseng and Perilla Leaf (Shen Su Yin)（參蘇飲）

Decoction of Ginseng and Walnut
(Ren Shen Hu Tao Tang)（人參胡桃湯）

Decoction of Glehnia/Adenophora and Ophiopogon
(Sha Shen Mai Men Dong Tang)（沙參麥門冬湯）

Decoction of Hypoglauca Yam
(Bi Xie Fen Qing Yin)（萆薢分清飲）

Decoction of Ignited Yellow Earth (Huang Tu Tang)（黃土湯）

Decoction of Inula Flower and Hematite
(Xuan Fu Dai Zhe Tang)（旋覆代赭湯）

Decoction of Kansui for Intestinal Obstruction
(Gan Sui Tong Jie Tang)（甘遂通結湯）

Decoction of Licorice, Light Wheat and Jujube
(Gan Mai Da Zao Tang)（甘麥大棗湯）

Decoction of Lily Bulb to Consolidate the Lung
(Bai He Gu Jin Tang)（百合固金湯）

Decoction of Morus and Apricot Seed (Sang Xing Tang)（桑杏湯）

Decoction of Morus Leaf and Chrysanthemum
(Sang Ju Yin)（桑菊飲）

Decoction of Nine Ingredients with Notopterygium
(Jiu Wei Qiang Huo Tang) （九味羌活湯）

Decoction of Notopterygium and Isatis Root
(Qiang Lan Tang) （羌藍湯）

Decoction of Notopterygium to Dispel Dampness
(Qiang Huo Sheng Shi Tang) （羌活勝濕湯）

Decoction of Ophiopogon Root (Mai Men Dong Tang) （麥門冬湯）

Decoction of Perilla Seed to Descend the Flow of Qi
(Su Zi Jiang Qi Tang) （蘇子降氣湯）

Decoction of Phragmites Stem (Wei Jing Tang) （葦莖湯）

Decoction of Pinellia and Magnolia Bark
(Ban Xia Hou Po Tang) （半夏厚朴湯）

Decoction of Pinellia, White Atractylodes and Gastrodia
(Ban Xia Bai Zhu Tian Ma Tang) （半夏白朮天麻湯）

Decoction of Polygonatum Rhizome
(Jia Jian Wei Rui Tang) （加減葳蕤湯）

Decoction of Poria, Licorice, Schisandra, Ginger and Asarum
(Ling Gan Wu Wei Jiang Xin Tang) （苓甘五味薑辛湯）

Decoction of Poria, Cinnamon, Atractylodes and Licorice
(Ling Gui Zhu Gan Tang) （苓桂朮甘湯）

Decoction of Prepared Aconite (Fu Zi Tang) （附子湯）

Decoction of Pubescent Angelica and Loranthus
(Du Huo Ji Sheng Tang) （獨活寄生湯）

Decoction of Pueraria, Scutellaria and Coptis
(Ge Gen Huang Qin Huang Lian Tang) （葛根黃芩黃連湯）

Decoction of Pulsatilla (Bai Tou Weng Tang) （白頭翁湯）

Decoction of Rhinoceros Horn and Rehmannia
(Xi Jiao Di Huang Tang) （犀角地黃湯）

Decoction of Rhubarb and Aconite
(Da Huang Fu Zi Tang) （大黃附子湯）

Decoction of Rhubarb and Moutan Bark
(Da Huang Mu Dan Pi Tang) （大黃牡丹皮湯）

Decoction of Salvia Root (Dan Shen Yin) （丹參飲）

Decoction of Sichuan Aconite (Wu Tou Tang) （烏頭湯）

Decoction of Small Thistle (Xiao Ji Yin Zi) （小薊飲子）

Decoction of Stephania and Astragalus
(Fang Ji Huang Qi Tang) （防己黃芪湯）

Decoction of Stephania and Poria
(Fang Ji Fu Ling Tang) （黃芪茯苓湯）

Decoction of Sweet Wormwood and Turtoise Shell
(Qing Hao Bie Jia Tang) （青蒿鱉甲湯）

Decoction of Ten Jujubes (Shi Zao Tang) （十棗湯）

Decoction of the Four Ingredients and Three Yellow Colored
Herbs (San Huang Si Wu Tang) （三黃四物湯）

Decoction of Three Golds (San Jin Tang) （三金湯）

Decoction of Three Kinds of Seeds (San Ren Tang)（三仁湯）
Decoction of Three Seeds/Sons Nursing the parents
    (San Zi Yang Qing Tang)（三子養親湯）
Decoction of Three Shells to Recover the Pulse
    (San Jia Fu Mai Tang)（三甲復脈湯）
Decoction of Trichosanthes, Macostem Onion and White Wine
    (Gua lou Xie Bai Bai Jiu Tang)（瓜蔞薤白白酒湯）
Deoction of Two Old Herbs -- Citrus Peel and Pinellia
    (Er Chen Tang)（二陳湯）
Decoction of Wild Jujube Seed (Suan Zao Ren Tang)（酸棗仁湯）
Decoction of Zhen-wu, the God Who Controls Water
    (Zhen Wu Tang)（真武湯）
Decoction or Powder with Five Kinds of Peels
    (Wu Pi Yin)（五皮飲）
    (Wu Pi San)（五皮散）
Decoction or Tea with Ligustricum
    (Chua Xiong Cha Tiao San)（川芎茶調散）
Decoction to Clear Summer-heat and Replenish Qi (I)
    (Qing Shu Yi Qi Tang (I)（清暑益氣湯 (I)
Decoction to Clear Summer-heat and Replenish Qi (II)
    (Qing Shu Yi Qi Tang (II)（清暑益氣湯 (II)
Decoction to Conduct the Heart Fire Downward
    (Dao Chi San)（導赤散）
Decoction to Dispel Dampness in the Spleen and Stomach
    (Wei Ling Tang)（胃苓湯）
Decoction to Dispel Pathogenic Heat from the Ying System
    (Qing Ying Tang)（清營湯）
Decoction to Disperse the Vital Energy in Liver
    (Chai Hu Shu Gan San)（柴胡舒肝散）
Decoction to Eliminate the Dryness in the Lung
    (Qing Zao Jiu Fei Tang)（清燥救肺湯）
Decoction to Increase Body Fuilds (Zeng Ye Tang)（增液湯）
Decoction to Inigorate Blood Circulation and Open the Orifices
    (Tong Qio Huo Xue Tang)（通竅活血湯）
Decoction to Nourish the Heart (Yang Xin Tang)（養心湯）
Decoction to Nourish the Yin and Cleanse the Lung
    (Yang Yin Qing Fei Tang)（養陰清肺湯）
Decoction to Purge the Heat from the Heart and Stomach
    (Xie Xin Tang)（瀉心湯）
    (San Huang Xie Xin Tang)（三黄瀉心湯）
Decoction to Purge the Liver Fire with Gentiana
    (Long Dan Xie Gan Tang)（龍膽瀉肝湯）
Decoction to Purge the Lung Heat
    (Xie Bai San)（瀉白散）
    (Xie Fei San)（瀉肺散）

Decoction to Purge the Lung with Lepidium and Jujube
      (Ting Li Da Zao Xie Fei Tang)（葶藶大棗瀉肺湯）
Decoction to Reinforce the Chong Channel (Gu Chong Tang)（固冲湯）
Decoction to Regulate the Spleen and Stomach
      (Li Zhong Wan)（理中丸）
      (Ren Shen Tang)（人參湯）
Decoction to Regulate the Spleen and Stomach with Aconite
      (Fu Zi Li Zhong Wan)（附子理中丸）
Decoction to Regulate the Spleen and Stomach with Aconite and
      Cinnamon Bark (Fu Gui Li Zhong Wan)（附桂理中丸）
Decoction to Relieve Muscle-ache
      (Shen Tong Zhu Yu Tang)（身痛逐瘀湯）
Decoction to Remove Blood Stasis Below the Diaphragm
      (Ge Xia Zhu Yu Tang)（膈下逐瘀湯）
Decoction to Strengthen the Heart and the Spleen
      (Gui Pi Tang)（歸脾湯）
Decoction to Subdue the Endogenous Wind in the Liver
      (Zhen Gan Xie Feng Tang)（鎮肝熄風湯）
Decoction with Chinese Angelica for Treating Vital Prostration
      with Cold Limbs (Dang Gui Si Ni Tang)（當歸四逆湯）
Decoction with Chinese Angelica, Evodia and Fresh Ginger for
      Vital Prostration with Cold Limbs
      (Dang Gui Si Ni Jia Wu Zhu Yu Sheng Jiang Tang)
      （當歸四逆加吳茱萸生薑湯）
Decoction with Rehmannia for Aphasia and Paralysis
      (Di Huang Yin Zi)（地黃飲子）
Drastic Purgative Decoction (Da Cheng Qi Tang)（大承氣湯）

Febrifugal Decoction with Sweet Wormwood and Scutellaria
      (Hao Qin Qing Dan Tang)（蒿芩清膽湯）
Five Ingredients Decoction with Astragalus and Cinnamon
      (Huang Qi Gui Zhi Wu Wu Tang)（黃芪桂枝五物湯）
Formula for Dispersing Pathogenic Wind (Xiao Feng San)（消風散）
Formula for Edema by Irrigation (Shu Chi Yin Zi)（疏齒飲子）
Formula for Hemoptysis (Ke Xue Fang)（咳血方）

Improving Eyesight Formula with Pills of Six Herbs with Rehmannia
      (Ming Mu Di Huang Wan)（明目地黃丸）

Less Drastic Purgative Decoction
      (Xiao Cheng Qi Tang)（小承氣湯）
Liver Soothing Pills (Shu Gan Wan)（舒肝丸）
Losing the Smile Pills (Shi Xiao Wan)（失笑丸）
Losing the Smile Powder (Shi Xiao San)（失笑散）

Lycium Fruit, Chrysanthemum and Pills of Six Herbs with Rehmannia
(Qi Ju Di Huang Wan) (杞菊地黃丸)

Magic Glue of Tortoise Plastron and Antler Horn
(Gui Lu Er Xian Jiao) (龜鹿二仙膠)
Major Bupleurum Decoction (Da Chai Hu Tang) (大柴胡湯)
Major Decoction for Restoring the Normal Function of the Middle
Burner (Da Jian Zhong Tang) (大建中湯)
Major Decoction of Blue Dragon (Da Qing Long Tang) (大青龍湯)
Major Decoction Sinking into the Chest
(Da Xian Xiong Tang) (大陷胸湯)
Manthis Egg-case Powder (Sang Piao Xiao San) (桑螵蛸散)
Minor Bupleurum Decoction (Xiao Chai Hu Tang) (小柴胡湯)
Minor Decoction for Restoring the Normal Function of the Middle
Burner (Xiao Jian Zhong Tang) (小建中湯)
Minor Decoction of Blue Dragon (Xiao Qing Long Tang) (小青龍湯)
Minor Decoction Sinking into the Chest
(Xiao Xian Xiong Tang) (小陷胸湯)
Modified Baked Locorice Decoction
(Jia Jian Fu Mai Tang) (加減復脈湯)
Modified Decoction of Two Effective Ingredients
(Jia Wei Er Miao San) (加味二妙散)

Nutrient System Nourishing Decoction with Ginseng
(Ren Shen Yang Ying Tang) (人參養營湯)

Ophiopogon, Schisandra and Pills of Six Herbs with Rehmannia
(Mai Wei Di Huang Wan) (麥味地黃丸)
(Ba Xian Chang Shou Wan) (八仙長壽丸)
Oyster Shell Powder (Mu Li San) (牡蠣散)

Pills for Activating Circulation in Collateral Channels--Minor
(Xiao Huo Luo Dan) (小活絡丹)
Pills for Enuresis (Suo Quan Wan) (縮泉丸)
Pills for Goitre (Xiao Luo Wan) (消瘰丸)
Pills for Indigestion (Bao He Wan) (保和丸)
Pills for Leukorrhea (Yu Dai Wan) (癒帶丸)
Pills for Menorrhagia (Gu Jing Wan) (固經丸)
Pills for Replenishing the Yin (Da Bu Yin Wan) (大補陰丸)
Pills for Restoring the Vital Energy and Function of the Kidney
(Jin Kui Shen Qi Wan) (金匱腎氣丸)
(Ba Wei Di Huang Wan) (八味地黃丸)
Pills for Shocking the Spirits (Zhen Ling Dan) (震靈丹)
Pills for Spermatorrhea (Jin Suo Gu Jing Wan) (金鎖固經丸)
Pills for the Deaf (Er Long Zuo Ci Wan) (耳聾左慈丸)

Pills of All Qi (Du Qi Wan)（都氣丸）

Pills of Chinese Angelica, Gentiana and Aloe
　　　　(Dang Gui Lu Hui Wan)（當歸蘆薈丸）

Pills of Cinnamon and Poria (Gui Zhi Fu Ling Wan)（桂枝茯苓丸）

Pills of Eight Ingredients with Rehmannia
　　　　(Ba Wei Di Huang Wan)（八味地黃丸）
　　　　(Jin Kui Shen Qi Wan)（金匱腎氣丸）

Pills of Four Fresh Ingredients (Si Sheng Wan)（四生丸）

Pills of Four Miraculous Drugs (Si Shen Wan)（四神丸）

Pills of Galanga and Cyperus (Liang Fu Wan)（良附丸）

Pills of Human Placenta (He Che Da Zao Wan)（河車大造丸）

Pills of Immature Bitter Orange and White Atractylodes
　　　　(Zhi Zhu Wan)（枳术丸）

Pills of Ledebouriella with Magical Therapeutic Effects
　　　　(Fang Feng Tong Sheng San)（防風通聖散）

Pills of Mume/Black Plums (Wu Mei Wan)（烏梅丸）

Pills of Saussurea and Areca Seed
　　　　(Mu Xiang Bing Lang Wan)（木香檳榔丸）

Pills of Six Miraculous Drugs (Liu Shen Wan)（六神丸）

Pills of Six Ingredients with Rehmannia
　　　　(Liu Wei Di Huang Wan)（六味地黃丸）

Pills of Sophora Fruit (Huai Jiao Wan)（槐角丸）

Pills of Stephania, Zanthoxylum, Lepidium Seed and Rhubarb
　　　　(Ji Jiao Li Huang Wan)（己椒藶黃丸）

Pills of Tangerine Seed (Ju He Wan)（橘核丸）

Pills to Relieve Stagnancy of All Kinds
　　　　(Yue Qu Wan)（越麴丸）

Pills with Immature Bitter Orange for Abdominal Distention
　　　　(Zhi Shi Xiao Pi Wan)（枳實消痞丸）
　　　　(Shi Xiao Wan)（失笑丸）

Powder for Dispelling Turbidity with Agastache
　　　　(Huo Xiang Zheng Qi Wan)（藿香正氣丸）

Powder for Tetanus (Yu Zhen San)（玉真散）

Powder for Relieving Depression with Cold Limbs
　　　　(Si Ni San)（四逆散）

Powder for Threatened Abortion
　　　　(Tai Shan Pan Shi San)（泰山盤石散）

Powder of Apricot Seed and Perilla (xing Su San)（杏蘇散）

Powder of Chinese Angelica and White Peony
　　　　(Dang Gui Shao Yao San)（當歸芍藥散）

Powder of Eight Ingredients to Correct Urinary Disturbances
　　　　(Ba Zheng San)（八正散）

Powder of Five Drugs with Poria (Wu Ling San)（五苓散）

Powder of Fritillary and Trichosanthes Fruit
　　　　(Bei Mu Gua Lou San)（貝母瓜蔞散）

Powder of Ginseng and Gecko (Shen Jie San)（參蚧散）

Powder of Ginseng, Poria and White Atractylodes
　　　　(Shen Ling Bai Zhu San)（參苓白术散）

Powder of Ingredients Six to One in Ratio
　　　　(Liu Yi San)（六一散）

Powder of Lonicera Flower and Forsythia
　　　　(Yin Qiao San)（銀翹散）

Powder of Magnolia Flower (Xin Yi San)（辛夷散）

Powder of Melon Pedicle (Gua Di San)（瓜蒂散）

Powder of Pyrrosia Leaf (Shi Wei San)（石葦散）

Powder of Sophora Flower (Huai Hua San)（槐花散）

Powder of Ten Ingredients in Ash
　　　　(Shi Hui San)（十灰散）

Powder of Two Effective Ingredients
　　　　(Er Miao San)（二妙散）

Powder of Xanthium Fruit (Cang Er San)（蒼耳散）

Powder of White Atractylodes and White Peony for Diarrhea
　　　　with Abdominal Pain
　　　　(Bai Zhu Shao Yao San)（白术芍藥散）
　　　　(Tong Xie Yao Fang)（痛瀉要方）

Powder to Activate the Vascular System (Sheng Mai San)（生脈散）

Powder to Clear the Heat in the Bone
　　　　(Qing Gu San)（清骨散）

Powder to Conduct the Heart Fire Downward
　　　　(Dao Chi San)（導赤散）

Powder to Disperse Vital Energy in Liver
　　　　(Chai Hu Shu Gan San)（柴胡舒肝散）

Powder to Purge the Lung Heat
　　　　(Xie Bai San)（瀉白散）
　　　　(Xie Fei San)（瀉肺散）

Purgative Decoction of Persica Seed
　　　　(Tao He Cheng Qi Tang)（桃核承氣湯）

Purple Snowy Powder (Zi Xue Dan)（紫雪丹）

Regulating the Liver Decoction (Tiao Gan Tang)（調肝湯）

Replenishing the Yang (Right) Decoction
　　　　(You Gui Yin)（右歸飲）

Replenishing the Yang (Right) Pills
　　　　(You Gui Wan)（右歸丸）

Replenishing the Yin (Left) Decoction
　　　　(Zuo Gui Yin)（左歸飲）

Replenishing the Yin (Left) Pills
　　　　(Zuo Gui Wan)（左歸丸）

Restoring to the Normal Position Powder
　　　　(Qian Zheng San)（牽正散）

Sedative Pills with Magnetite and Cinnabar
    (Ci Zhu Wan) (磁硃丸)
    (Shen Qu Wan) (神曲丸)
Saussurea, Cardamon and the Six Noble Ingredients Decoction
    (Xiang Sha Liu Jun Zi Tang) (香砂六君子湯)
Spleen and Stomach Tonic Pill (Jian Pi Wan) (健脾丸)
Spleen Tonic for Edema (Shi Pi San) (寶脾散)
Styrax Pills (Su He Xiang Wan) (蘇合香丸)

The Antiseptic Decoction with Five Ingredients
    (Wu Wu Xiao Du Yin) (五物消毒飲)
The Big Pearl for Endogenous Wind
    (Da Ding Feng Zhu) (大定風珠)
The Blood Replenishing Decoction (Ji Chuan Jian) (濟川煎)
The Blue Fairy Lady Pills for Lumbago
    (Qing E Wan) (青娥丸)
The Boat and Carriage Pills (Zhou Che Wan) (舟車丸)
The Cannabis Seed Pills (Ma Zi Ren Wan) (麻子仁丸)
The Collateral Warming Decoction (Wen Jing Tang) (溫經湯)
The Coptis Decoction (Huang Lian Tang) (黃連湯)
The Diaphragm Colling Powder (Liang Ge San) (涼膈散)
The Ease Powder (Xiao Yao San) (逍遙散)
The Ease Powder plus Moutan Bark and Gardenia
    (Dan Zhi Xiao Yao San) (丹梔逍遙散)
The Eight Precious Ingredients Decoction
    (Ba Zhen Tang) (八珍湯)
The Expectorant Pills (Qing Qi Hua Tan Wan) (清氣化痰丸)
The Fair Maiden Decoction (Yu Nü Jian) (玉女煎)
The Four Ingredients Decoction (Si Wu Tang) (四物湯)
The Four Noble Ingredients Decoction
    (Si Jun Zi Tang) (四君子湯)
The Gallbladder Warming Decoction (Wen Dan Tang) (溫胆湯)
The Jade Screen Powder (Yu Ping Feng San) (玉屏風散)
The King's Mind-easing Tonic Pills
    (Tian Wang Bu Xin Dan) (天王補心丹)
The Lindera Root Powder (Tian Tai Wu Yao San) (天台烏药散)
The Liver Reinforcing Decoction (Yi Guan Jian) (一貫煎)
The Longevity Pills (Ba Xian Chang Shou Wan) (八仙長壽丸)
The Most Precious Pellets (Zhi Bao Dan) (至寶丹)
The Phlegm Resolving Decoction (Dao Tan Tang) (導痰湯)
The Pills in a Bag (Bu Dai Wan) (布袋丸)
The Pustulant Powder (Tou Nong San) (透膿散)
The Six Noble Ingredients Decoction
    (Liu Jun Zi Tang) (六君子湯)

The Spleen Warming Decoction (Wen Pi Tang)（溫脾湯）
The Stomach Neutralizing Powder (Ping Wei San)（平胃散）
The Stomach Purging Decoction with Aconite
    (Fu Zi Xie Xin Tang)（附子瀉心湯）
The Stomach Purging Decoction with Fresh Ginger
    (Sheng Jiang Xie Xin Tang)（生薑瀉心湯）
The Stomach Purging Decoction with Licorice
    (Gan Cao Xie Xin Tang)（甘草瀉心湯）
The Stomach Purging Decoction with Pinellia
    (Ban Xia Xie Xin Tang)（半夏瀉心湯）
The Stomach Regulating Purgative Decoction
    (Tiao Wei Cheng Qi Tang)（調胃承氣湯）
The Stubborn Decoction with Three Ingredients
    (San Niu Tang)（三拗湯）
The Tiger Pills (Hu Qian Wan)（虎潛丸）
The Tonification Decoction with Ten Ingredients
    (Shi Quan Da Bu Tang)（十全大補湯）
The White Atractylodes Powder
    (Bai Zhu San)（白术散）
    (Qi Wei Bai Zhu San)（七味白术散）
The Yellow Dragon Decoction (Huang Long Tang)（黃龍湯）
Tonifying the Liver Formula (Bu Gan Tang)（補肝湯）
Tonifying the Lung Decoction (Bu Fei Tang)（補肺湯）

Universal Antiphlogistic Decoction
    (Pu Ji Xiao Du Yin)（普濟消毒飲）

Visceras Nourishing Decoction with Ginseng
    (Zhen Ren Yang Zang Tang)（真人養臟湯）

White Tiger Decoction (Bai Hu Tang)（白虎湯）
White Tiger Decoction plus Cinnamon
    (Bai Hu Jia Gui Zhi Tang)（白虎加桂枝湯）
White Tiger Decoction plus Ginseng
    (Bai Hu Jia Ren Shen Tang)（白虎加人參湯）

Yang Activating Decoction (Yang He Tang)（陽和湯）